PEDIATRIC
NEUROLOGIC
PHYSICAL THERAPY

CLINICS IN PHYSICAL THERAPY
VOLUME 5

Already Published

Vol. 1   Cardiac Rehabilitation
Louis R. Amundsen, Ph.D., guest editor

Vol. 2   Electrotherapy
Steven L. Wolf, Ph.D., guest editor

Vol. 3   Physical Therapy of the Geriatric Patient
Osa Jackson, Ph.D., guest editor

Vol. 4   Rehabilitation of the Burn Patient
Vincent R. DiGregorio, M.D., guest editor

Forthcoming Volumes in the Series

Vol. 6   Spinal Cord Injury
Hazel V. Adkins, R.P.T., guest editor

Vol. 7   Measurement in Physical Therapy
Jules M. Rothstein, Ph.D., guest editor

This book is to be returned on or before
the last date stamped below.

CAMPBELL

PEDIATRIC NEUROLOGIC PHYSICAL THERAPY

Edited by

Suzann K. Campbell, Ph.D., L.P.T.

Professor
Division of Physical Therapy
Department of Medical Allied Health Professions
School of Medicine
University of North Carolina at Chapel Hill
Chapel Hill, North Carolina

CHURCHILL LIVINGSTONE
NEW YORK, EDINBURGH, LONDON, AND MELBOURNE
1984

IML
R

Acquisitions editor: William R. Schmitt
Copy editor: Kim Loretucci
Production editor: Karen Goldsmith Montanez
Production supervisor: Joe Sita
Composition: Maryland Composition Company, Inc.
Printer/Binder: The Maple-Vail Book Manufacturing Group

© Churchill Livingstone Inc. 1984

Distributed in the United Kingdom by Churchill Livingstone, Robert
Stevenson House, 1–3 Baxter's Place, Leith Walk, Edinburgh EH1
3AF and by associated companies, branches and representatives
throughout the world.

First published 1984
Printed in U.S.A.

ISBN 0-443-08241-3
7 6 5 4 3 2 1

Library of Congress Cataloging in Publication Data
Main entry under title:

Pediatric neurologic physical therapy.

(Clinics in physical therapy; v. 5)
Includes bibliographies and index.
1. Pediatric neurology.   2. Physical therapy
for children.   I. Campbell, Suzann K.   II. Series.
[DNLM: 1. Nervous System Diseases—in infancy &
childhood.   2. Nervous System Diseases—therapy.
3. Physical Therapy—in infancy & childhood.
W1 CL831CN v.5 / WS 340 P3685]
RJ486.P32   1984   618.92′8   84-12038
ISBN 0-443-08241-3

Manufactured in United States of America

To Dick,
my mentor and friend

Contributors

Susan M. Attermeier, L.P.T., M.A.C.T.
Section Head, Physical Therapy, Division for Disorders of Development and Learning, Biological Sciences Research Center; Assistant Professor, Division of Physical Therapy, Department of Medical Allied Health Professions, School of Medicine, University of North Carolina at Chapel Hill, Chapel Hill, North Carolina

Jocelyn Blaskey, R.P.T., M.S.
Physical Therapy Instructor, Physical Therapy Department, County of Los Angeles, Downey, California

Lois Bly, P.T.
Private Practitioner, Piermont, New York

June E. Bridgford, P.T., M.A.C.T.
Associate Faculty Member, Division of Physical Therapy, Emory University School of Medicine, Atlanta, Georgia

Suzann K. Campbell, Ph.D., L.P.T.
Professor, Division of Physical Therapy, Department of Medical Allied Health Professions, School of Medicine, University of North Carolina at Chapel Hill, Chapel Hill, North Carolina

Barbara H. Connolly, Ed.D.
Associate Professor, Department of Rehabilitation Sciences, Program in Physical Therapy, University of Tennessee Center for the Health Sciences, Memphis, Tennessee

Susan R. Harris, Ph.D., P.T.
Physical Therapy Consultant, Seattle, Washington

Carolyn B. Heriza, P.T., M.A.
Associate Professor, Department of Physical Therapy, School of Allied Health Professions, St. Louis University Medical Center, St. Louis, Missouri

Karen Yundt Lunnen, L.P.T., M.S.
Physical Therapy Consultant, Developmental Evaluation Center, School of Education and Psychology, Western Carolina University, Cullowhee, North Carolina

Roberta B. Shepherd, Dip.Phty., F.A.C.P.
Senior Lecturer, School of Physiotherapy, Cumberland College of Health Sciences, Sydney, New South Wales, Australia

Thomas J. Stengel, L.P.T., M.S.
Executive Director, Intervention with PACT, Inc., Baltimore, Maryland

Darcy Umphred, Ph.D., P.T.
Private Practitioner, Rio Oso, California

Irma J. Wilhelm, L.P.T., M.S.
Research Assistant Professor, Division of Physical Therapy, Department of Medical Allied Health Professions, University of North Carolina at Chapel Hill, Chapel Hill, North Carolina

Janet M. Wilson, L.P.T., M.A.C.T.
Adjunct Associate Professor, Division of Physical Therapy, Department of Medical Allied Health Professions, School of Medicine, University of North Carolina at Chapel Hill, Chapel Hill, North Carolina

Foreword

Our knowledge and understanding of the developing nervous system have rapidly progressed during the past decade. Part of this progress has been the realization that the pathologic brain of the adult no longer serves as an adequate model for the nervous system of the infant. This point has been emphasized by recent ultrasound studies of fetal behavior. These studies have identified spontaneously generated fetal motility as a prenatal precursor of postnatal motor behavior and responses. Such findings have provided new insights into the developmental processes of neural functions and have replaced the reductionistic concepts of reflexology. This replacement is most strongly represented in the discipline of developmental neurology, with its emphasis on the age-specific properties of the neurologic and behavioral repertoires of the infant and child.

The introduction of new concepts in developmental mechanisms of neural functions has affected the design of new assessment techniques and the critical evaluations of existing ones. We are now in a better position to know the "why" and "what" of neurologic diagnostic procedures. Seeing the nervous system of the newborn and young infant as consisting of complex patterns of behavior (most of which are spontaneously generated) rather than as a bundle of primitive reflexes has obvious consequences in early therapy.

The chapters in this book note the new concepts and discuss the many problems of assessment and therapy in light of these new concepts. I hope the book serves as an important guide and source of reference for those who are directly confronted with the interrelated problems of developmental diagnosis and therapy in their daily work.

Prof. Dr. Heinz F. R. Prechtl
Groningen, The Netherlands

Preface

Physical therapy involvement in pediatric neurology is as old as the field itself. From the earliest days of "physical therapeutics," management of the child with central nervous system (CNS) dysfunction has appeared as a topic of discussion in the professional journals and conferences. Cerebral palsy has undoubtedly been the most commonly treated disorder, but medical and historical trends reflecting increasing concern for the health and development of *all* children eventually led to expansion of physical therapy services into the areas of mental retardation and other developmental disabilities, including minimal brain dysfunction and the learning problems of children in educational environments. Most recently, we are engaged in the exciting study of whether early intervention can reduce or prevent CNS dysfunction in high-risk infants. Whatever the problem, our purpose has always been to facilitate the maximum attainment of each child's potential and to be ever mindful that our patients are *children*, with special needs for fun, play, and love, and that parents and other professionals are our partners in this enterprise.

The primary purpose of this book is to bring to the practicing pediatric specialist in physical therapy the most current information on management of typical problems in pediatric neurology. The material included emphasizes current research in evaluation and management of nervous system dysfunction in children, as well as the theory and treatment approaches of prominent physical therapists working in the specialty of pediatric neurology. As editor, I have questioned, probed, and suggested ideas; each author, however, is an experienced clinician with a unique point of view, and no attempt has been made to forge a unified approach.

The first three chapters of this book provide a survey of neurologic dysfunction in children; a review of advanced methods of evaluation, including standardized tests of child development and sensorimotor dysfunction, quality of movement or coordination, and developmental reflexes; and an integrated approach to management of patients with neurologic dysfunction. The chapters that follow are devoted to the management of a typical neurologic problem treated by pediatric physical therapists.

Taken as a whole, the chapters reveal that our challenges for the future are (1) to develop improved theory and new measurement tools for use in evaluation and outcome assessment, (2) to produce a large volume of clinical studies on which to base theory building and research, and (3) to conduct large-scale research on the efficacy of physical therapy in pediatric neurologic disorders, based on past research and new information on the pathokinesiology of CNS dysfunction. Our challenges are great, not least of all because we are dealing with damage to a developing nervous system. I hope that these chapters will facilitate the work of pediatric specialists in physical therapy and stimulate the production of greatly needed research on the outcome of our therapeutic efforts.

While I worked on this project, I was supported by a training grant from the Division of Maternal and Child Health, Bureau of Health Care Delivery and Assistance of the U.S. Public Health Service, DHHS, and by a research grant from the American Academy for Cerebral Palsy and Developmental Medicine. I am also grateful to the following for assistance to the editor and several authors: Gregg Kemp, illustrations; Patsy Tickle, typing and editorial assistance; Linda King-Thomas, Irma J. Wilhelm, and Debbie and Dianne Campbell, editorial assistance. Although she is in no way responsible for any misinterpretations I may have made, I would like to express my appreciation to Shirley Sahrmann for the extended series of conversations we had over the past several years. She has stimulated my thinking, questioned my ideas, and caused me to reconsider many "truths." Few people have done this in such a way since I was guided in my development as a neurophysiologist by Wally Welker, in my clinical skills by Leila Green and Georgia Shambes, and in my research by Dick Campbell. Finally, I owe special thanks to Irma J. Wilhelm, Margaret L. Moore, Charles P. Schuch, Ernest N. Kraybill, and Earl Siegel for their support in past and present projects.

Suzann K. Campbell, Ph.D., L.P.T.

Contents

1 | Central Nervous System Dysfunction in Children

Suzann K. Campbell

The treatment of pediatric patients with neurologic dysfunction is both an exciting challenge and a frustrating dilemma for the physical therapist. The problems are so complex, so enigmatic, we barely understand the simplest facts about the neuromuscular dysfunction we treat. Still, helping a child to function better so that he or she can participate more fully in life is a joyous undertaking.

The first purpose of this introductory chapter is to review selected information from the literature on brain dysfunction in children (primarily spastic cerebral palsy because this is the most frequently encountered subject of research), including the effects of lesions at various ages, the neuropathology and pathokinesiology of central nervous system (CNS) dysfunction, and recovery following injury to the developing nervous system. The second purpose is to propose a model for studying the effects of physical therapy on children with central nervous system dysfunction.

THE VARYING PICTURE OF SENSORIMOTOR DYSFUNCTION WITH AGE

The clinical literature provides evidence that the effects on sensorimotor function of a brain lesion in the exceptionally premature infant differ from those in the full-term infant,[1,2] and that the 5-year-old trauma victim presents yet another picture.[3] Differing etiologies and sites of injury may be factors accounting for significant variance, but the clinical outcome varies primarily because the insult is inflicted upon brains that are tremendously different in structure and physiology. Indeed, the brain of the very premature infant may resemble that of the full-term infant less than the full-term infant's brain resembles the adult brain.[2] Even similar lesions may produce strikingly different results at different chronologic ages.

It is not accidental that the incidence of spastic diplegia is greater among survivors of extreme prematurity than in full-term babies who experience asphyxia.[2] Cerebral convolutions first appear in the fetal human brain during the fifth month of gestation and continue to develop into the first postnatal year.[4] During the sixth and seventh months of gestation, the cerebral cortex remains largely underdeveloped with smooth surfaces quite uncharacteristic of the full-term brain with its many cerebral cortical convolutions.[2] The blood supply of the fetal brain is directed toward the most metabolically active parts; thus, the area of germinal matrix near the caudate nucleus and the periventricular area are especially vulnerable in the preterm infant.[1,2] Asphyxia or intracranial hemorrhage in the newborn of less than 32 weeks gestation is likely to cause damage to tracts in the periventricular area of the internal capsule, including those axons projecting to motoneurons to the lower extremities and trunk, and resulting in the typical outcome of spastic diplegia. Relative sparing of intellect is typical, although perceptual problems are not uncommon.

This type of cerebral palsy is rarely seen in the full-term child who has been asphyxiated.[1,2] Here the more likely area of vulnerability is the now highly developed cerebral cortex with resultant spastic quadriplegia or, if more localized, hemiplegia. The basal ganglia and brainstem nuclei are also highly metabolically active; if the basal ganglia are damaged by lack of blood supply or oxygen, athetosis results.

In research on monkeys, Goldman-Rakic[5] demonstrated that prenatal injury to a localized area of cerebral cortex results in widespread changes in the configuration of brain convolutions, corresponding to those areas of cerebral cortex that normally receive inputs from the damaged areas during the final weeks of gestation. On the other hand, the subcortical areas normally projecting to the now damaged cortex were more normal in neuronal structure than expected, presumably because their projections were directed to new sites. These results were not seen in postnatally damaged infant animals whose brains showed little signs of reorganization of connections. If the same is true in humans, early central nervous system damage may create abnormal function in areas far removed from the initial insult; on the other hand, the ability of circuits to reorganize may provide a basis for ameliorating the effects of brain damage in the preterm infant, which would not be possible in those with later injury.

In the preschool-age child, the cerebral hemispheres have become increasingly specialized, individualized, and committed in function,[6,7] with resulting effects on muscle tone, cognition, and language that differ from those in children experiencing prenatal or perinatal insults.[3] Chapters 4, 8, and 11 on the high-risk infant, head trauma, and cerebral palsy further clarify some of the ways in which these patients differ from each other.

Musculoskeletal Changes with Age and Sensorimotor Dysfunction

Clearly movement coordination is affected by the disruption in neural circuits produced by a brain lesion; however, little attention has been paid to the fact that the musculoskeletal system is undergoing developmental changes in the early months and years of life as well. A perinatal brain injury results in an abnormal nervous system attempting to direct the growth and development of muscles that are largely composed of slowly contracting fibers[8-10] but are genetically programmed to gradually differentiate into at least three types of fibers specialized in their endurance and force production properties.[11] These properties of individual muscle fibers can be varied, within certain limits, in accordance with the task demands of exercise.[12] Because brain injury affects the coordination, force, speed, and duration of movement and therefore the quality of exercise engaged in by the individual, it is possible, though unproven, that abnormalities in muscle fiber development are produced secondarily by brain dysfunction.

In the older child, brain damage will also create movement problems, but these difficulties will be imposed on a muscular system unlike that of the newborn who has only begun to move against the force of gravity. Nevertheless, muscular dysfunction is likely to occur in the older child as well. In addition to the possible pathologic effects of abnormal patterns of posture and movement on individual muscle fibers, such as abnormal hypertrophy in some and atrophy in others,[13] developing contracture in a muscle increases its stiffness (unit change in force per unit change in length) and may contribute to increasing spasticity.[14] Thus spasticity may be more than just a primary problem in the nervous system, for muscle stiffness is determined not only by the neural components of the neuromuscular system, but also by the passive viscoelastic properties of muscle and connective tissue.

Further effects on the muscular system derive from general poverty of movement. Muscular atrophy and disuse weakness are inevitable results of lack of exercise, and stretch weakness is likely to develop in muscles that are excessively elongated for prolonged periods by overactive antagonists.[15]

Inactivity and abnormal muscle physiology undoubtedly can have a negative effect on the development of the skeletal system, although the effects may once again vary with the age and plasticity of the bones. The deforming forces of contractured muscle are well known to physical therapists, and prevention of bony deformities is a major goal of physical therapy for the client with central nervous system dysfunction. Indeed, the work we do with our hands in aiding the muscles to work in normal ranges and with more normal force, and the repetition afforded by active exercise in the overload range, may be our most important contributions to the health and habilitation or rehabilitation of children with sensorimotor dysfunction.

Pathokinesiology

The complexity of the outcome of brain lesions in childhood is also revealed by new studies of patterns of muscular activity recorded by electromyography (EMG). These studies demonstrate the inadequacy of many of our clinical methods, including supposedly differential tests for individual muscle function and observational analysis of muscle dysfunction underlying individual patterns of movement coordination. They also bring into question the maxim that abnormal tone is the *major* problem that must be treated to improve movement in the child with cerebral palsy.

Electromyographic studies of children with cerebral palsy have revealed that clinically similar patterns of movement can be produced by several different patterns of muscular activity.[16-19] Chong and colleagues,[16] for example, identified three types of abnormal patterns of muscle activity during gait characterized by abnormal medial rotation at the hip. These patterns included: (1) activation of hip adductor and medial rotator muscles at the normal time during the gait cycle but phasically prolonged medial hamstring activity so that muscular force creating medial rotation was applied at an inappropriate point in the cycle; (2) on–off patterning of phasic muscle activity but with no relationship to gait cycle; and (3) mass turning on and off at the same time of all muscles used in gait leading to a stumplike progression pattern. Knutsson[20] reported that the latter pattern was the most common in patients with cerebral palsy; however, Chong and associates[16] reported the first pattern to be most frequent in children with abnormal medial rotation.

Orthopedists have made a major point of the finding that clinically similar patterns, such as the presence of medial rotation of the hip during gait, can be produced by different patterns of muscle activation that are not identifiable with visual observation. This finding has made electromyography a powerful tool for making decisions regarding orthopedic surgery. Offending muscles are identified by electromyographic recordings during locomotion.[16-19] If the suspect muscle is overactive during its normal place in the gait cycle, it can be lengthened. If a muscle acts at the wrong point in the gait cycle, it might be considered for transplantation. In the situation where numerous muscles work together to produce a dysfunctional pattern, surgery is unlikely to be successful. One can only guess that the future holds similar promise for physical therapists that electromyographic analysis might lead to differential treatments depending on the pattern of muscle dysfunction present. A challenge for the future must be the introduction of more sophisticated quantitative assessment into the typical clinical environment.

Two types of restraint of movement are found in patients with spasticity.[20] One is the result of activation of tonic stretch reflexes by muscle stretch. The forces produced by stretch reflex activation are weak relative to normal forces of muscle used to restrain movement; however, they occur at the wrong point in a cycle of movement. Restraint of movement by stretch reflex activation may, *or may not*, appear in the patient with strong stretch reflex activity upon passive motion; therefore, assessment of tone during passive manipulation is not highly predictive of ability to control voluntary movement. More common, indeed almost diagnostic, of cerebral palsy of either the spastic or hypertonic athetoid type is pathologic coactivation of muscles when reciprocal inhibition should occur during voluntary movement.[20–22] Abnormal restraint of movement occurs because muscles outbalance the action of each other. Abnormal reciprocal innervation through spinal circuits, rather than spasticity, is then a cause of disrupted voluntary control, contributing to delayed initiation of movement.[21,22]

These findings suggest that most patients would have difficulty coordinating movement even if muscle tone and reflexes were normal.[21] Spasticity is only one of the symptoms of a central nervous system lesion. It is one of the positive symptoms, along with clonus, disinhibition of primitive reflexes, and increased size of reflexogenic zones.[21,23,24] Spasticity is defined as "a motor disorder characterized by a velocity-dependent increase in tonic stretch reflexes ('muscle tone') with exaggerated tendon jerks, resulting from hyperexcitability of the stretch reflex, as one component of the upper motoneuron syndrome."[25] Negative symptoms, such as paresis, inadequate force production, delayed initiation of movement, and inappropriate cocontraction of antagonists to prime movers may be far more significant in producing dysfunction and difficult to improve with therapy. Indeed, this has been the case with some patients in controlled studies of the effect of baclofen on cerebral or spinal spasticity and voluntary movement in which tone was decreased by the drug without notable improvement in function.[26] Results such as these should be taken into account when attempting to develop a theory for treatment of central nervous system dysfunction.

RECOVERY OF FUNCTION FOLLOWING BRAIN INJURY

As Blaskey suggests (Chapter 8) the therapist probably does not produce recovery in a patient with neurologic damage, but rather takes advantage of the recovery and maturation that are occurring, directing energy into the most functional paths to encourage maximal use of returning and developing functions. Recovery of function following nervous system injury is not well understood. Animal studies are the primary source of information, because very few natural history studies of the recovery of function in humans are available in the literature, and almost no studies of quantitative changes across time in neurologic functions following lesions have been done. Although species differences must be kept firmly in mind, the animal studies suggest that several variables are important in determining extent of recovery, including site and extent of lesion, whether lesions were staged, age at time of lesion, and pre- and postlesion experience and training.[27,28]

The effects of each of these variables in recovery are complex and poorly understood. For example, young age is no longer considered to be the significant advantage suggested by early studies.[28,29] Careful reanalysis of some of the data suggests that delayed deficits appeared in animals lesioned at young ages and that few differences between immature- and adult-lesioned animals were evident when tests were made several years postlesion rather than only immediately after damage. Indeed, the period of shock that follows any nervous system lesion may have an effect on maturation of the nervous system that irreversibly compounds the damage caused by the lesion. Such an effect is suggested by the work of Myklebust and colleagues[30] who reported that stretch of the soleus muscle produces a reciprocal *excitation*, rather than the expected inhibition, in the antagonist tibialis anterior muscle only in patients who suffered perinatal injury and not in adult-injured subjects. This finding suggests that either abnormal circuits were formed in the immature spinal cord as a result of cerebral injury, or that primitive spinal cord circuits that should have regressed or been altered during early development failed to do so. One of the prime areas of dysfunction affecting movement in children with central nervous system dysfunction is the aberrant spread of excitation to many muscles from afferent stimulation of sensory receptors,[23] making the production of isolated, or disassociated, movements difficult or impossible. The interaction, therefore, between the course of maturation and the attempts of the nervous system to compensate for damage may alter the usual regressions and transformations of neural circuitry,[31] the normal decrease with maturation of dependence on sensory cues,[32] and the ability to use flexible combinations of sensory modalities in coping with postural and environmental demands.[31,33] The stimulus-bound nature of movement in central nervous system dysfunction results.

Numerous theories, not necessarily mutually exclusive, exist regarding recovery of function after brain damage.[34] They are summarized in the following sections.

Diaschisis.   Diaschisis suggests that return of function following brain damage occurs as the nervous system recovers from a period of shock, having widespread effects on areas of the brain not directly damaged by the lesion. As diaschisis resolves, some previously lost functions reappear.

Equipotentiality/Vicariation.   Equipotentiality and vicariation refer to the idea that undamaged parts of the nervous system have the potential to take over functions previously subserved by damaged areas. Equipotentiality specifically refers to assumption of control by undamaged parts of the same neural system; here, size of the lesion would be important in determining whether sparing or recovery of function would occur. Vicariation refers to takeover by other parts of the nervous system. Age is an important variable in this theory because the degree to which vicariation can occur appears to depend to a great extent on how committed to other functions a potential substitute area is at the time of damage. During early development, an uncommitted area may easily substitute for the damaged one; however, the substitute area's commitment may mean a consequent impairment in performance of its own intended function at the appointed time, resulting in the delayed appearance of deficits.[35]

Takeover of language functions by the right hemisphere in early left hemisphere-damaged children, for example, is postulated to decrease overall intellectual functioning as a cost of vicariation.[3]

Reorganization of Circuits.   Regrowth of damaged axons or sprouting of undamaged axons to assume vacated synaptic sites have been demonstrated to occur under some conditions in the central nervous system of experimental animals.[36] Goldman-Rakic[5] has also demonstrated significant redirection of fiber projections in the cerebral cortical development of prenatally brain-damaged primates. Although theories involving establishment of new circuits are under investigation and are frequently suggested as underlying the effects of treatment of central nervous system dysfunction, actual analysis of the effects on behavior of such nervous system remodeling are rare. The effects may more often be harmful and responsible for aberrant behavior rather than necessarily beneficial and responsible for recovery. Great caution is warranted in using these types of theories as possible rationale for treatment effects when no firm evidence is available to support this supposition.

Supersensitivity.   Target neurons of the damaged system develop supersensitivity to remaining neurotransmitter molecules, thus enhancing their ability to function in a deprived state and producing a degree of recovery. This response to damage could obviously provide a molecular basis for vicariation or equipotentiality.

Compensation.   The theory of compensation suggests that, rather than true recovery occurring, the functions damaged by the nervous system lesion are taken over by other circuits that accomplish the same goal but by different means, such as using a different sensory system to guide performance. This means that the function is not really recovered, though defects may be extremely subtle, but rather compensated for with varying degrees of abnormality in achieving the performance goal. LeVere and LeVere[37] believe that compensation is the critical process: as soon as damage occurs, compensations begin to develop as the organism struggles to function with an inadequate system. If these compensations are relatively effective in helping the individual to meet its goals, recovery of the original function may actually be retarded or prevented. They suggest that the aim of early intervention after brain damage must be to prevent the establishment of compensatory mechanisms and to force the organism to use the function that may be present but temporarily suppressed. In support of this argument, LeVere and LeVere cite studies of monkeys with deafferented limbs whose normal limbs were restrained, demonstrating that this intervention could produce significant recovery of function in the deafferented limb which did not occur if the animal was allowed to compensate for the useless limb by use of undamaged parts. Although the theory of LeVere and LeVere does not take into account the maturational forces directing change in the developing nervous system, their ideas are commensurate with several of the major approaches to early management of central nervous system dysfunction in children. Preventing the development of compensatory patterns of movement by early treatment may in turn prevent or limit the development of spasticity, which may itself be a compensation engaged in by the nervous system for the inadequate force production generated by a defective central nervous system. This is a generally accepted goal of neuro-developmental treatment.

A THEORETICAL MODEL FOR THE EFFECTS OF CENTRAL NERVOUS SYSTEM DYSFUNCTION IN CHILDHOOD

I believe that it is time to develop a model for the effects of CNS dysfunction based on *clinical* observations and *human* experimentation with subjects with neurologic dysfunction and to abandon our perseveration on constructing neurophysiologic theories of a stimulus-response nature to rationalize what we do. These theories neglect many important factors involved in the response of the nervous system to injury and exercise, some of which I have tried to describe in this chapter. I would like to present here a model for the effects of central nervous system dysfunction in the immature organism that can be used to develop a set of testable hypotheses regarding the effectiveness of treatment of neurologic dysfunction in children. Lest this model be used to provide yet another rationale for the effects of treatment, I hasten to emphasize that it is a theoretical model with a set of resulting hypotheses, one or more of which are likely to be proved wrong by research. We must avoid perpetuating what are mere hypotheses by accepting them as truth and not subjecting them to experimental test. I encourage and challenge clinicians to test, support, or refute the hypotheses presented.

The model I propose suggests that a central nervous system lesion in childhood of the type that typically produces cerebral palsy results in three primary problems: abnormal movement, sensory deprivation, and disturbed patterns of social interaction. Each of these major areas of deficit results in typical outcomes if no intervention is undertaken. The outcomes vary with age because the neuromusculoskeletal system response to damage varies with age and previous experience.

In general, however, abnormal movement is characterized by increased latency of movement onset, poor force production, and decreased speed of movement, all at least partially related to the presence of abnormal amounts of cocontraction in antagonists opposing prime movers. These problems eventually result in increasingly abnormal muscle tone, stretch weakness in muscles antagonistic to hypertonic muscles, poor endurance and motivation for movement, lack of adequate exercise, compensatory postures, and contractures and skeletal deformities.

Deprivation is experienced because of lack of opportunity to move as well as because of possible damage to sensory circuits and abnormal feedback from poorly coordinated movement. These problems result in impaired sensory processing, perceptual motor dysfunction, and deviant cognitive development. Finally, abnormal social interaction is engendered by poor ability to signal emotions and intent, difficulty expressing body and vocal language, and perhaps autonomic instability, resulting in frustration, lowered motivation, and impaired cognitive development.

If this model is an accurate reflection of the problems created by CNS dysfunction in children, the following hypotheses regarding the effects of physical therapy might be tested by research:

1. Important effects of therapy are related to the well-documented (in animals and human adults) general effects of exercise, including prevention of disuse atrophy, promotion of normal posture preventing the development of stretch weakness and deformities, and improvement of strength and endurance for physical activity which are also thought to contribute to a subjective sense of well-being and self-esteem.

2. More normal patterns of muscular coordination result from improving force production, decreasing latency of movement initiation, increasing speed of movement, improving postural set for movement, and decreasing the amount of abnormal cocontraction in groups of muscles including prime movers.

3. Abnormal compensatory patterns, including development of abnormal tone and assumption of abnormal postures, can be prevented if the above effects occur.

4. Primary and secondary deprivation and lack of social interaction can be decreased by providing the opportunity for more normal movement and endurance for physical activity.

5. The opportunity to be successful in movement performance leads to increased motivation to move and decreased frustration when doing so, with resulting improvement in self-confidence and self-esteem, and improved ability to learn.

Research designed to test these hypotheses would require quite different measurement tools in addition to the typical assessments of motor milestones, reflexes, and presence of contractures and deformities. Research outcome measures might then be extended to include electromyographic analysis of patterns of muscular coordination during gait and other activities, posture, endurance, muscle biopsies, quality and extent of social interaction, self-esteem, and perceptual and cognitive abilities. Because exercise and other intervention effects are typically specific to the type of experience provided,[12,27] we must direct our efforts, as Shepherd and Harris suggest (Chapters 5 and 6), toward finding successful means for treating the specific problems that children with neurologic dysfunction have, e.g., genu recurvatum during stance phase of gait, lack of scapular muscle cocontraction during reaching into space, head posture characterized by excessive upper cervical and capital extension. This problem-solving approach to documenting treatment effectiveness focuses on the specific abnormalities of the child with central nervous system dysfunction. It may free us to consider new treatment adjuncts such as functional electrical stimulation.[20] Lest critics suggest that this would mean a return to technique-oriented approaches to management of children's problems, I hasten to add that this type of treatment planning and clinical research need not preclude consideration of the whole child in the overall plan of management. Indeed, the effects of treatment are likely to be related to numerous factors, such as age at time of injury, site of lesion, severity and type of involvement, intellectual potential, home environment, age at initiation of treatment, and other variables which should be considered in the analysis of outcome, as well as in the planning of a management program.

The challenge for the future of physical therapy is to develop our potential as a scientific, as well as compassionate, clinical field. To do this we need testable theories, quantitative analysis of movement dysfunction, common terminology, creative scholars and clinicians with well-educated minds, and motivation to demonstrate accountability for our methods to clients and the public. I hope that the chapters that follow will be a source of knowledge and a prod to further investigation for all who read them.

REFERENCES

1. Hill A, Volpe JJ: Seizures, hypoxic-ischemic brain injury, and intraventricular hemorrhage in the newborn. Ann Neurol 10:109, 1981.
2. Pape K, Wigglesworth JS: Haemorrhage, Ischaemia and the Perinatal Brain. Clinics in Developmental Medicine, No 69/70. Lippincott, Philadelphia, 1979.
3. Woods BT, Teuber H-L: Early onset of complementary specialization of cerebral hemispheres in man. Trans Am Neurol Assoc 98:113, 1973.
4. Richman DP, Stewart RM, Hutchinson JW, et al: Mechanical model of brain convolutional development. Science 189:18, 1975.
5. Goldman-Rakic PS: Morphological consequences of prenatal injury to the primate brain. Prog Brain Res 53:3, 1980.
6. Buser P: Higher functions of the nervous system. Annu Rev Physiol 38:217, 1976.
7. Galaburda AM, LeMay M, Kemper TL, et al: Right-left asymmetries in the brain. Science 199:852, 1978.
8. Spielholz NI: Skeletal muscle: A review of its development in vivo and in vitro. Phys Ther 62:1757, 1982.
9. Slaton D: Muscle fiber types and their development in the human fetus. Phys Occup Ther Pediatr 1:47, 1981.
10. Kelly AM, Rubinstein NA: Why are fetal muscles slow? Nature 288:266, 1980.
11. English AWM, Wolf SL: The motor unit: Anatomy and physiology. Phys Ther 62:1763, 1982.
12. Rose SJ, Rothstein JM: Muscle mutability: Part I. General concepts and adaptations to altered patterns of use. Phys Ther 62:1773, 1982.
13. Castle ME, Reyman TA, Schneider M: Pathology of spastic muscle in cerebral palsy. Clin Orthop 142:223, 1979.
14. Perry J: Rehabilitation of spasticity. In: Feldman RG, Young RR, Koella WP (eds): Spasticity: Disordered Motor Control. Year Book Medical Publishers, Chicago, 1980.
15. Gossman MR, Sahrmann SA, Rose SJ: Review of length-associated changes in muscle: Experimental evidence and clinical implications. Phys Ther 62:1799, 1982.
16. Chong KC, Vojnic CD, Quanbury AO, et al: The assessment of the internal rotation gait in cerebral palsy—An electromyographic gait analysis. Clin Orthop 132:145, 1978.

17. Perry J, Hoffer MM: Preoperative and postoperative dynamic electromyography as an aid in planning tendon transfers in children with cerebral palsy. J Bone Jt Surg 59A:531, 1977.
18. Perry J, Hoffer MM, Antonelli D, et al: Electromyography before and after surgery for hip deformity in children with cerebral palsy: A comparison of clinical and electromyographic findings. J Bone Jt Surg 58A:201, 1976.
19. Perry J, Hoffer MM, Giovan P, et al: Gait analysis of the triceps surae in cerebral palsy. A preoperative and postoperative clinical and electromyographic study. J Bone Jt Surg 56A:511, 1974.
20. Knutsson E: Restraint of spastic muscles in different types of movement. In Feldman RG, Young RR, Koella WP (eds): Spasticity: Disordered Motor Control. Year Book Medical Publishers, Chicago, 1980.
21. Milner-Brown HS, Penn RD: Pathophysiological mechanisms in cerebral palsy. J Neurol Neurosurg Psychiatr 42:606, 1979.
22. Neilson PD: Voluntary control of arm movement in athetotic patients. J Neurol Neurosurg Psychiatr 37:162, 1974.
23. Barolat-Romana G, David R: Neurophysiological mechanisms in abnormal reflex activities in cerebral palsy and spinal spasticity. J Neurol Neurosurg Psychiatr 42:333, 1980.
24. Lance JW: The control of muscle tone, reflexes and movement: Robert Wartenberg lecture. Neurology 30:1303, 1980.
25. Lance JW: Symposium synopsis. In Feldman RG, Young RR, Koella WP (eds): Spasticity: Disordered Motor Control. Year Book Medical Publishers, Chicago, 1980.
26. Hattab JR: Review of European clinical trials with baclofen. In Feldman RG, Young RR, Koella WP (eds): Spasticity: Disordered Motor Control. Year Book Medical Publishers, Chicago, 1980.
27. Herdman SJ: Effect of experience on recovery following CNS lesions. Phys Ther 63:51, 1983.
28. Johnson D, Almli CR: Age, brain damage, and performance. In Finger S (ed): Recovery from Brain Damage: Research and Theory. Plenum Press, New York, 1978.
29. St. James-Roberts I: Neurological plasticity, recovery from brain insult, and child development. Adv Child Dev Behav 14:253, 1979.
30. Myklebust BM, Gottlieb GL, Penn RD, et al: Reciprocal excitation of antagonistic muscles as a differentiating feature in spasticity. Ann Neurol 12:367, 1982.
31. Prechtl HFR: Regressions and transformations during neurological development. In Bever TG (ed): Regressions in Mental Development: Basic Phenomena and Theories. Lawrence Erlbaum Associates, Hillsdale, NJ, 1982.
32. Broom DM: Behavioural plasticity in developing animals. In Garrod DR, Feldman JD (eds): Development in the Nervous System. Cambridge University Press, New York, 1981.
33. Nashner LM: Analysis of stance posture in humans. In Towe AL, Luschei ES (eds): Handbook of Behavioral Neurobiology. Vol 5: Motor Coordination. Plenum Press, New York, 1981.
34. Laurence S, Stein DG: Recovery after brain damage and the concept of localization of function. In Finger S (ed): Recovery from Brain Damage: Research and Theory. Plenum Press, New York, 1978.
35. Goldman PS: An alternative to developmental plasticity: Heterology of CNS structures in infants and adults. In Stein DG, Rosen JJ, Butters N (eds): Plasticity and

Recovery of Function in the Central Nervous System. Academic Press, New York, 1974.

36. Marx JL: Regeneration in the central nervous system (Research News). Science 209:378, 1980.

37. LeVere ND, LeVere TE: Recovery of function after brain damage: Support for the compensation theory of the behavioral deficit. Physiol Psychol 10:165, 1982.

2 | Evaluation of Sensorimotor Dysfunction

Thomas J. Stengel   Susan M. Attermeier
Lois Bly   Carolyn B. Heriza

The evaluation of a child with a neurologic disorder is a multidimensional process involving assessment of various aspects of development. Motor, communication, social, cognitive, and sensory-perceptual development may be assessed individually and in relationship to each other, in an attempt to obtain a comprehensive and yet understandable profile of a child's strengths and weaknesses.

Subareas of the five aspects of development mentioned above may vary in organization and content according to the experience, interest, and educational background of an individual tester or the developmental orientation of an individual service agency. Subareas of motor development include gross and fine motor performance, reflexes, range of motion, muscle tone, coordination or quality of movement, muscle strength, and posture. Subareas of communication include expressive language, receptive language, and nonverbal communication. Social subareas are feeding (including the oral motor area), dressing, caregiver-child interaction and attachment, and behavior. Cognitive subareas are attention, problem-solving, and responses to eliciting situations described initially by Piaget[1] involving assessment of concepts such as imitation, operational causality, object permanence, and object relations. Sensory perceptual subareas are the processing and organization of sensory information and the concepts described by Ayres,[2] including form and space perception, and postural and bilateral integration.

It is essential to mention other areas that require assessment for comprehensive program planning for the child with neurologic dysfunction, for example, cardiopulmonary status, medical and developmental history, family structure, home environment, and adaptive equipment.

This chapter is limited to two general topics. The first topic is a discussion of formalized developmental assessment tools used for the evaluation of motor, cognitive, social, communication, and sensory-perceptual development. The second is the less formalized, but comprehensive, assessment of motor development, including specific topics such as quality of movement, role of central state, components of movement, and postural reactions and reflexes, based primarily on the principles of Bobath[3] and Rood.[4]

Implicit in the decision to emphasize these areas is the following framework for evaluation of the child with neurologic dysfunction: overall evaluation of the child's general developmental level should be completed, first, to obtain an assessment of the child's performance in relation to age peers and, second, to develop hypotheses regarding specific areas of dysfunction. Typically, problems of coordination of movement that require further detailed observation of posture and movement will be revealed during developmental assessment. During these observations, the physical therapist may develop further hypotheses, suggesting that abnormal reflexes are interfering with the production of coordinated movement. Formal reflex testing may then be used to document such problems in more detail.

In this chapter Stengel discusses the utilization of formalized developmental tests, Attermeier discusses motor assessment from a Rood perspective, Bly contributes a neurodevelopmental therapy perspective, and finally, Heriza discusses the assessment of reflexes and reactions.

FORMALIZED DEVELOPMENTAL TESTING

The purpose of this section is to provide the physical therapist with a format for evaluating developmental tests, to review the structure and uses of various formal testing instruments, to critically review selected instruments, and to propose a clinical application for some of the tests. The tests that are reviewed measure social, motor, behavioral, cognitive, language, and functional development, and are divided into three categories: (1) newborn assessments, (2) comprehensive developmental tests, and (3) intervention tools. Screening tests will not be reviewed.

Specific developmental tests were chosen for discussion for several reasons. Some of the tests have been used by the author for clinical and research purposes and are considered useful and reliable measurement tools. Some of the tests are viewed to be potentially useful for physical therapists as intervention tools. The more popular tests are discussed, excluding those that have a similar conceptual and structural framework. Finally, some tests were included because they seemed to be appropriate for a specific clinical setting. Primary sources of information other than the specific test manuals are the

Mental Measurements Yearbook,[5] *Psychological Abstracts,* periodicals such as *Physical and Occupational Therapy in Pediatrics,* and books such as *Screening Growth and Development of Preschool Children: A Guide for Test Selection,*[6] *Handbook of Infant Development,*[7] and *Linking Developmental Assessment and Curricula.*[8]

The need for physical therapists to become more informed about formal developmental testing was highlighted by Lewko[9] in a survey assessing current practices in evaluating motor behavior in a sample of 207 facilities providing services to children in the United States and Canada. The 207 respondents, of whom 59 were physical therspists, identified 256 different motor evaluations being used[9]; 91 of these tests were published and 165 were not published. Furthermore, the data indicated that the motor functioning of a great number of children was not being evaluated, particularly in larger facilities. Only 4 of the 91 published tests were used with any consistenty: the Denver Developmental Screening Test,[10] the Gesell Developmental Schedules,[11] the Lincoln-Oseretsky Motor Development Scale,[12] and the Purdue Perceptual-Motor Survey.[13] The respondents generally indicated they misused the tests in some fashion, particularly in terms of the ages and populations for whom they were developed and on whom they were standardized. Finally, 61 percent of the total number of respondents reported they knew of normative data regarding a particular test but only 44 percent of this group could specify the source of this information. Based on these findings, Lewko recommended that a single reference source including a large number of published tests of motor development should be made available to guide practitioners in the selection of appropriate tests.

Stangler and colleagues[6] have partially fulfilled Lewko's recommendation in a book on selection of screening tools. The authors proposed six criteria for evaluating a screening tool: (1) acceptability, (2) simplicity, (3) cost, (4) appropriateness, (5) reliability, and (6) validity.

Acceptability is defined as acceptance by all who will be affected by screening, including the children and families screened, the professionals who receive resulting referrals, and the community as a whole. Screening test simplicity is determined by the ease of teaching, learning, and administering the tool. The cost of a screening test includes the cost of equipment, training and paying personnel, and inaccurate test results. Also included are the costs to the individual being screened, for example, charges and transportation, and the total screening test cost in relation to the benefits of early detection. Test appropriateness is based on the prevalence of developmental delay in the population to be screened and on the application of the test to the population under consideration.

Reliability is the ability of a test to yield consistent results when the same test is given to the same individual more than once.[14] The two types of reliability are stability over time (test-retest reliability) and observer consistency (interobserver reliability).[15] Acceptable reliability is usually indicated by a correlation coefficient above 0.80 or a percentage of agreement above 90 percent.[16]

Test-retest reliability is measured when the same test is given to the same child twice with some interval of time between the two administrations.[6] When this measure, expressed as a correlation coefficient or as a percent of agreement, is high, it is likely that a test is reflecting the actual abilities of a child. Distractions in the environment that may cause children to perform differently at each test administration are inconsistent methods of test administration, the child's state of health, and the time of day when the tests are administered.

Observer consistency or interobserver reliability is defined as the amount of agreement between two persons interpreting the same test performance.[15] This reliability coefficient is obtained by having two people independently observe and score the behavior of the same individual or by having two people read and interpret the same set of test results.[6] When interobserver reliability is high, the behavior under consideration is relatively easily observed and scored in the same way by more than one person.

The final criterion, the validity of a developmental test, is defined as its ability to separate persons with a developmental problem from those without a problem.[14] Validity is concerned with what a test measures and how well it measures it.[16] Validity is determined by comparing performance on one instrument with other independent observations of the same characteristic.[15]

Important validity aspects for screening tests are percent of agreement with a diagnostic measure, sensitivity, specificity, over- and underreferral rates, and predictive validity of positive and negative findings.[6] These aspects of test validity pertain to how well a screening test in question relates to a diagnostic measure. Screening test validity may be expressed as a correlation coefficient between screening test results and the results of corresponding diagnostic tests. The higher the validity, the more efficient is the screening test. Sensitivity of an instrument is defined as how well the instrument identifies abnormal cases as being abnormal.[17] Instrument specificity is defined as how well an instrument identifies normal cases.

In nonscreening tests, four types of validity should be considered.[17] They are predictive validity, concurrent validity, content validity, and construct validity. Predictive validity, expressed as a validity coefficient, indicates the extent to which an individual's future level of functioning or performance on a criterion variable, for example, intellect at age 15 can be predicted from the results of a developmental test administered to a preschool child. Concurrent validity, also expressed as a validity coefficient, represents the relationship between a test, for example, the Neurological Examination of the Full Term Newborn Infant,[18,19] and a concurrent criterion variable, for example, a clinical diagnosis of brain damage. Content validity is applicable when it is necessary to measure the extent to which a test, for example, a school test, covers some field of study.[17] It is not expressed as a validity coefficient. "The test items can be regarded as a sample from a population representing the content and the aims of the course. Content validity is determined by the extent to which the sample of items in a test is representative of the total population."[17] When examining a developmental test of "motor" function, one might assess how well the items cover both gross and fine motor performance, as well as motor planning.

The construct validity concept is useful when tests measure traits for which external criteria are not readily available.[17] Construct validity is not a single measure of correlation between test scores and criterion scores; it is determined by showing that consequences are predicted by a theory developed on the basis of test results. These consequences can be confirmed by a series of testings or experiments.

Newborn Tests

In this section, several newborn tests will be reviewed, including the Neurological Examination of the Full Term Newborn Infant by Prechtl and Beintema,[18,19] the Neonatal Behavioral Assessment Scale by Brazelton,[20] and the Neurological Assessment of the Preterm and Full-Term Newborn Infant by Dubowitz and Dubowitz.[21] These tests represent three types of newborn assessments: (1) neurologic, (2) behavioral, and (3) behavioral-neurologic.

Parmelee and Michaelis[22] proposed that a newborn neurologic examination has three purposes:

1. The immediate diagnosis of an evident neurological problem, such as extreme hypotonia, convulsions, coma or localized paralysis, to determine what therapy to institute.
2. The evaluation of the day to day changes of a known neurological problem to determine the evolution of a pathological process, such as an hypoxic episode, or to follow the evolution of the neurological signs of a systematic disease such as respiratory distress.
3. The long term prognosis of a newborn who is recovering from some neonatal neurological problem or is considered at risk due to abnormalities of the pregnancy, or delivery.

The neurologic examination should contain a properly balanced selection of items to represent the important subsystems of the neural repertory.[23] It is essential to consider that the occurrence and/or intensity of many newborn responses are determined by the behavioral state in which they are examined. The Prechtl and Beintema scale[18,19] is an example of a neurologic examination and is discussed in detail later in this section.

The purpose of a behavioral test is to determine the behavioral makeup of an individual newborn.[23] Behavioral tests should cover a wide selection of behavior patterns which are important in the infant's daily life. The process of selecting test items should be based empirically on an extensive ethogram of the mother-infant dyad and not on preconceptions about what newborns should do. Finally, the obtained behavioral test results should correspond with the actual behavior of the individual baby in the natural mother-infant interaction. The Brazelton scale[20] is an example of a behavioral test.

The third test discussed in this section, the Dubowitz and Dubowitz scale,[21] is an example of a behavioral-neurologic newborn examination, combining elements of both the neurologic and the behavioral assessments.

Neurologic Examination of the Full-Term Newborn Infant. Prechtl and Beintema[18] published a standardized neurologic test for the full-term newborn infant, which was revised slightly in 1977.[19] The manual states that the test is valid for full-term infants between the gestational ages of 38 and 42 weeks and for preterm infants once they have reached the same postconceptional age. The test was developed to diagnose neurologic abnormalities and to predict future neurologic problems. In addition, a screening test is available to determine the need for low-risk neonates to undergo more detailed testing.[19]

The test[18] was standardized on a large sample of infants whose mothers had a history of obstetric complications. The aspects of the test that were standardized are the external conditions, for example, the testing environment, the behavioral state of the infant, and the handling of the infant, for example, position and stimulation. Prechtl[24] reported that interobserver reliability on the test was high (0.80–0.96). Beintema[25] tested 49 infants with the neurologic examination starting at 1 day of age and ending at 9 days of age. He found that the infants changed considerably over that time. Beintema concluded that neurological examinations administered to infants during the first 3 days of postnatal life were less valid than those administered later in the neonatal period. He also pointed out that an infant's behavioral state during testing significantly influenced test results.

The items of the test are scored on variable scales.[18] No total score is obtained, but Prechtl and Beintema have noted that abnormal neurologic findings in full-term newborn infants frequently appear in particular combinations. They have identified four syndromes: (1) the apathy syndrome, characterized by generally depressed responses; (2) the hyperexcitability syndrome, characterized by a low-frequency, high-amplitude tremor and easily elicited Moro reflex; (3) the hemisyndrome, consisting of at least three asymmetries of motility, posture, or response; and (4) the comatose syndrome, characterized by depressed respiration and absent or weak arousal to various stimuli. In a study of 150 newborns with one of more of the abnormal syndromes, Prechtl[26] found that 73 had neurologic abnormalities at 2 to 4 years of age. Certain patterns of movement identified in the neonatal testing were also found to be predictive of later CNS dysfunction.[27] These were (1) consistent lateral asymmetry of reflex responses; (2) hypertonic or hypotonic muscular responses, (3) athetoid movements, (4) obligatory tonic neck responses, (5) constant strabismus and poor suck, and (6) Moro reflexes.

Some major strengths of the Prechtl and Beintema assessment are its well-standardized instructions for administration of each item, the fact that reflexes and responses are quantified as to intensity, reflex or response asymmetry is noted, and the state of the infant is recorded before each major section of the assessment. A disadvantage is that it is a long and complex test to administer, but the authors caution against abbreviating it because in the course of the examination sequence, findings are consistently verified by repeating certain items. The authors believe this adds to test validity.

Brazelton Neonatal Behavioral Assessment Scale. The Brazelton Neonatal Behavioral Assessment Scale (BNBAS)[20] is an infant behavior analysis instrument developed to distinguish individual differences among normal infants, especially with respect to social interactive behaviors.[28] The test is appropriate for infants from birth to the approximate postterm age of 1 month. The BNBAS was developed on the view that full-term healthy newborns are essentially social beings structured in such a way that they reliably elicit from the caretaker that organization which they themselves still lack.[29] The test includes 26 behavioral items that assess the neonate's capacity (1) to organize states of consciousness, (2) to habituate reactions to disturbing events, (3) to attend to and process simple and complex environmental events, (4) to control motor activity and postural tone while attending to these events, and (5) to perform integrated motor acts.[20,30] The test also includes 20 reflex items[20] purported to assess the neonate's neurologic intactness.[28] Contrary to this viewpoint, Prechtl[23] maintains that the BNBAS reflex items are inadequate to assess neural intactness or impairment. Prechtl points out that even though the BNBAS reflex items are based on the descriptions of neurologic assessment he and Beintema outlined in 1964,[18] they are not tested in the same way as was originally described.[23] In addition, the BNBAS reflex scale does not include the most sensitive items for detection of neurologic deviancy.

The reflex items and the biobehavioral items of the BNBAS are scored individually, reflecting the infant's best performance. No total score is obtained; however, the items can be clustered into four categories—interactive processes, motoric processes, state control, and physiologic response to stress.[29] Each of these clusters are then graded as exceptional, average, or worrisome. Als[29] recommends that specific clusters should be developed for the population of infants being tested, and to fit the purposes for testing in any given setting.

No formal standardization sample has been used in the development of the BNBAS nor have norms been derived for any large sample. Instead, researchers using the scale have provided their own normative data with the population they were testing.[29] In addition, Brazelton reported that the mean score for each item is based on the expected behavior of an infant who is an average 7 pounds, full-term, normal, white infant; whose mother did not have more than 100 mg of barbiturates for pain or 50 mg of other sedative drugs as premedication in the 4 hours prior to delivery; and whose Apgar ratings were no lower than 7,8,8 at 1, 5, and 15 minutes after delivery, respectively.[20] Tester-observer reliability and test-retest reliability are reported to be high (≥ 0.85 and ≥ 0.80, respectively).

The predictive validity of the BNBAS was investigated by Tronick and Brazelton[30] in a study involving 53 children examined during the neonatal period and at 7 years of age. They found that a standard but crude neurologic examination and the BNBAS were similar in their capacity for detecting abnormal infants, but that the BNBAS was far superior to the neurologic examination in detecting suspect-abnormal infants. The latter conclusion is rejected by Prechtl[23] because of the small number of subjects and because neurologic conditions during early life may be transient. The low number of

BNBAS false positives, therefore, may indicate an insensitivity on the part of the BNBAS to detect the presence of abnormal neurologic conditions.

Divitto and Goldberg[31,32] found that sick and healthy premature infants had significantly more worrisome scores on the interactive and motoric clusters of the BNBAS than did the full-term infants they tested. When the infants were retested, the same pattern was found, but the differences were not significant. Goldberg and Divitto[31] also tested the same infants on the Bayley Scales of Infant Development during the first year and found that the premature infants lagged behind the full-term infants and were less responsive to testing materials and tasks, more difficult to test, and less attentive. Finally, Bakow and colleagues[33] reported that the BNBAS items of alertness, motor maturity, tremulousness, habituation, and self-quieting were correlated with infant temperament at 4 months.

The following clinical uses of the BNBAS have been proposed[34]: (1) screen infants for behavioral or motor problems, (2) educate parents about their infant's development and behavior, (3) assess, in part, what impact an infant's behavior will have on the process of parent-infant bonding, (4) help plan a behavioral and/or motor intervention program, (5) provide a developmental and behavioral baseline on infants who will receive future developmental assessments, and (6) help objectively monitor the medical status of an insulted infant, for example, one with a central nervous system bleed.

Horowitz and Dunn[35] and Lancioni and colleagues[36] revised the Brazelton Neonatal Behavioral Assessment Scale with the Kansas Supplements (BNBAS-K). The BNBAS-K provides for scoring both best and most typical behavior on several items in order to better reflect the range and variability of infant behavior observed during an assessment.

Field and associates[37] also modified the BNBAS so it could be used by mothers. The instrument was named The Mother's Assessment of the Behavior of Her Infant (MABI). To determine the validity of this instrument, Field and associates trained testers to administer the BNBAS to 32 normal infants and to 32 postterm postmature infants; the mothers in this group administered the MABI to the same infant groups. No differences were found between mothers' and testers' assessments, except that the testers assigned more optimal interactive process scores. Normal-term infants received more optimal scores than postmature infants from both mothers and testers. The mothers' motoric process scores and the testers' motoric process scores correlated with 8-month Bayley motor scores at the 0.34–0.42 level. Widmayer and Field[38] found that teenage mothers who observed the BNBAS administered to their preterm infants and who also administered the MABI to their infants during the first month and another group of mothers who only administered the MABI to their infants demonstrated more optimal interactions during feeding and play with their babies than the mothers who did not administer the MABI or observe the BNBAS.

The BNBAS is not intended for use with infants of a gestational age of less than 37 weeks; its use is inappropriate for premature or stressed newborns whose normative performance is not known.[39] Als and Brazelton[40,41] are currently developing a scale for use with premature infants. They propose a method to document systematically a premature infant's behavioral organization along five dimensions: physiologic, motor, state, interactional and attentional, and self-regulatory. This scale is not yet available for general use; because of its length it may not be feasible for routine clinical use.

3. Neurological Assessment of the Preterm and Full-Term Infant. The Neurological Assessment of the Preterm and Full-Term Infant by Dubowitz and Dubowitz[21] was devised in response to the authors' need for a single instrument that would meet a number of basic requirements: (1) to be suitable for use by staff without expertise in neonatal neurology; (2) to be usable with preterm and full-term neonates; (3) to be reliable very soon after birth; (4) to require no more than 10 to 15 minutes to administer and score to encourage routine clinical use; and (5) to be suitable for sequential assessment of infants after birth.[21] The opportunity to test sequentially permits the clinician (1) to compare preterm infants after birth with newborn infants of corresponding postmenstrual age, (2) to document the normal evolution of neurologic behavior in the preterm infant after birth, and (3) to detect deviations in neurologic signs and their subsequent resolution.

The test incorporates items from the systems of Saint-Anne Dargassies,[42] Prechtl,[19] Parmelee,[22] and Brazelton,[20] and a recording method similar to the gestational age assessment of Dubowitz and associates.[43] Items are scored on a five-point ordinal scale, and it is not essential that all items be administered.[21] No single total score is recorded; rather, the patterns of responses may reflect variations in neurologic function. Some patterns typical of particular groups of infants have begun to be identified and are described in the manual in a series of case histories.

No reliability information on the final version of the scale is presented in the manual. Concurrent validity was investigated by Dubowitz and associates.[44] The investigation consisted of a comparative study of neurologic assessment and ultrasound examination of 100 infants consecutively admitted to a neonatal unit over a 9-month period. All infants received at least three neurologic assessments consisting of six items from the Dubowitz and Dubowitz scale. These items were selected because they could be elicited in even the most severely ill infants. The infants also received a variable number of ultrasound scans, depending on their gestational age and medical condition. The results revealed that 24 of the 31 infants born at less than 36 weeks gestation with ultrasound evidence of an intraventricular bleed had three or more abnormal clinical signs, compared with only 2 of 37 infants without intraventricular hemorrhage who were also born at less than 36 weeks gestation. Of the 37 infants without intraventricular hemorrhage, 21 had no abnormal signs. In comparison, only 1 of 31 infants with an intraventricular bleed had no abnormal signs. The researchers suggested that repeated, careful examination of the infants in the sample and the recognition of abnormal signs provide an objective means of alerting the clinician to the probable presence of an intraventricular hemorrhage, which can be verified by ultrasound. Unfortunately, long-term studies of predictive validity for later outcome are not yet available.

Graziani and Korberly[45] address the issue of predictive limitations of neurologic and behavioral assessments in the newborn period. They suggest that several factors may influence the predictability of these instruments. One of these is the ability of the infant who is severely depressed in the newborn period, because of perinatal hypoxia or trauma, to recover completely, provided that brain structures are not damaged. The severity and acuteness of the insult and the maturation and capacities of the infant's subcortical neuroanatomic structures may influence this ability to recover. Other factors are the effects of the environment, human maturation, and psychosocial influences on developmental outcome.

Another factor influencing the predictability of neonatal measures is test-retest reliability. Despite standardization procedures, for example, testing an infant on the Brazelton Neonatal Behavioral Assessment Scale midway between feedings, test-retest reliability may be affected by changes in an infant's chronological age, behavioral state, and internal physiologic state. The standardization procedures themselves may alter test performance. Casear and Akiyama[46] found that an infant's postural position during assessment may affect the heart rate, respirations, and motor activity. Reliability is also affected by the training, experience, and bias of the examiner.

Prechtl[23] suggests that the prognostic value of a neonatal instrument may be increased by repeated testings; however, he also suggests that there is overconcern when neonatal behavioral tests have low test-retest reliability. This overconcern stems from insufficient appreciation of discontinuities in developmental processes. The ability to detect developmental change during the neonatal period should therefore be considered a positive characteristic for any of the instruments discussed in this section. This characteristic has been demonstrated by the Brazelton Neonatal Behavioral Assessment Scale in a study involving 10 Zambian and 10 American infants.[47] The Zambian infants demonstrated significant behavioral changes when tested the third time at 10 days of age. The first test was administered on day 1 and the second on day 5.

Graziani and Korberly[45] point out that abnormal neurobehavior in the neonate does not imply abnormal or different brain structure. In addition, an absent or abnormal infant response or reflex is frequently of uncertain significance because local dysfunction within the immature brain is not manifested by a *specific* change in behavior or reflexes.

Although there appears to be no completely satisfactory and valid clinical method for the behavioral or neurologic assessment of the neonate, valuable information may be obtained from any of the instruments discussed in this section. Prechtl[23] has suggested that a standardized neurologic assessment be administered along with the Brazelton Scale. The Dubowitz and Dubowitz scale designed to assess premature and term infants and the behavioral and neurologic areas may prove to be the most practical and useful clinical instrument for physical therapists.

Comprehensive Developmental and Sensorimotor Tests

The following tests are discussed in this section: the Bayley Scales of Infant Development,[48] the Gesell Developmental Scales,[11,49] the Preschool Attainment Record,[50] the Bruininks-Oseretsky Test of Motor Proficiency,[51] the Southern California Sensory Integration Test,[2] and the Miller Assessment for Preschoolers.[52]

These instruments are used as diagnostic tools by clinicians because they are more comprehensive than screening tests. They are also familiar to clinicians from a variety of disciplines involved in the management of the child with neurologic dysfunction. Common knowledge of these instruments facilitates communication between disciplines, thereby aiding multidisciplinary management. Finally, these comprehensive developmental tests are statistically designed primarily for diagnostic purposes.

Bayley Scales of Infant Development. The California First-Year Mental Scale by Bayley,[53] the California Preschool Mental Test by Jaffa,[54] and the California Infant Scale of Motor Development by Bayley[55] contributed heavily to the unpublished 1958 version of the Bayley Scales of Infant Development (BSID) and most of the specific test items for these early Bayley Scales[53,55] were drawn from the Gesell Scales. The 1958 version of the BSID was revised and a 1958–1960 version was published for use in assessing children from 1 to 15 months of age. The BSID was again revised, renormed, and expanded to its current form in 1969.

The current BSID[48] edition allows assessment of children from 2 to 30 months of age and consists of three parts—a Mental Scale, a Motor Scale, and an Infant Behavior record. The Mental Scale is designed to assess sensory-perceptual acuities, discriminations, and the ability to respond to these; the early acquisition of "object constancy" and memory, learning, and problem-solving ability; vocalizations and the beginning of verbal communication; and early evidence of the ability to form generalizations and classifications, which is the basis of abstract thinking. The Motor Scale is designed to provide a measure of the degree of control of the body, of coordination of the large muscles, and of finer manipulatory skills of the hands and fingers. The Infant Behavior Record helps the clinician assess the nature of the child's social and objective orientations toward his or her environment as expressed in attitudes, interests, emotions, energy, activity, and tendencies to approach or withdraw from stimulation.

Each test item of the Mental and Motor Scales is scored passed, failed, or not testable.[48] All scoring is based on tester observations. By adding the number of passes, a raw score is obtained for each of the scales. These scores are then converted to standard scores (MDI-mental, PDI-motor). Basal and ceiling levels and an age equivalency can also be obtained. For the Infant Behavior Record, no total score is obtained. The items are scored individually and may be compared to the range of scores and the modal scores obtained from the 14 age groups of the normative sample.

The 1958–1960 version of the BSID was normed on a national sample of 1400 normal children.[48] The current 1969 version was normed on a national

Table 2-1. Coefficients of Correlation Between MDI's on the Bayley Scales of Infant Development (BSID) and IQ's on the Stanford-Binet (Form L-M) for Children 24, 27, and 30 Months of Age

Age in Months	N	r	BSID MDI		Stanford-Binet IQ	
			Mean	SD	Mean	SD
24	22	.53	117.7	14.2	112.0	9.5
27	41	.64	108.6	14.1	109.0	13.1
30	57	.47	104.1	11.3	106.7	10.0
Total	120	.57	108.1	13.8	108.5	11.2

sample of 1262 normal children ranging in age from 2 to 30 months. The original sample design called for testing 100 children at 14 different ages. The sample was controlled for sex, race, residence (urban-rural), and education of the head of the household. This sample reflected the proportions of children from 2 months through 30 months of age in selected strata of the United States population, as described in the 1960 U.S. Census of Population. Using the 1958–1960 version of the scale, Bayley[56] demonstrated that in a nationwide sample of 1400 children, there were no differences in test scores due to sex, birth order, geographical location, or parents' education; however, a consistent tendency for black children to obtain significantly higher scores on the Motor Scale at all ages from 3 through 14 months was found.

Four different methods were used to measure reliability for the BSID.[48] Split-half reliability coefficients were obtained from each of the 14 age groups of the standardization sample. The reliability coefficient for the Mental Scale ranged from 0.81 to 0.93 with a median value of 0.88. The reliability coefficients for the Motor Scale ranged from 0.68 to 0.92 with a median value of 0.84. The second statistic calculated was the standard error of measurement (SEM). The SEM for the Mental Scale ranged from 4.2 to 6.9 standard score points; the SEM for the Motor Scale ranged from 4.6 to 9.0. Finally, high tester-observer reliability (>89 percent agreement) and test-retest reliability (>75 percent agreement) were demonstrated by Werner and Bayley[57] using the 1958–1960 version of the Mental and Motor Scales. No reliability information was reported for the Infant Behavior Record.

The validity of the BSID was investigated by several researchers. Bayley studied the degree of correspondence between the 1969 version of the BSID (Mental Scale) and the IQ scores obtained from the Stanford-Binet Intelligence Scale.[48] The sample for this study consisted of 120 California children aged 24, 27, and 30 months. Table 2-1 indicates a substantial degree of agreement between results of both tests given at the same age. Correlation between an earlier version of the BSID and the Stanford-Binet Form L was investigated by Bayley[58] and by Honzik and colleagues.[59] Neither of those studies demonstrated prediction of 8-year IQ scores from Bayley Mental Test scores, but both show increasing power of prediction during the age period of 1 to 3 years. An additional study by Ramey and associates[60] suggested that, in situations where natural environmental variation is reduced, there is a high correlation between the scores of the Bayley Mental and Motor Scales and Stanford-Binet scores. Their sample consisted of 24 subjects who attended day-care facilities and were tested on the Bayley Scales at 6 to 8 months, at 9 to 12 months, and at 13 to 16 months, and on the Standford-Binet at 36 months. Mental Scale–Stanford-Binet correlations were 0.49, 0.71, and 0.90, respectively, while Motor Scale–Stanford-Binet correlations were 0.77, 0.56, and 0.43, respectively. Additional validity studies can be found in the chapters by Self and Horowitz and by Yang in the *Handbook of Infant Development.*[7]

The next topic of discussion is the usefulness of the BSID in diagnosing handicapping conditions. Honzik and associates[61] compared the 8-month Bayley Mental Test scores of a group of infants suspected of having neurologic handicaps with the scores of a matched normal control group from the same hospital. The total numer of infants tested was 197. The testers were blind to the grouping of the infants they tested. The Bayley Mental Test scores differentiated the suspect from the control group at a probability of less than 0.05.

Berk[62] conducted a study to determine the discriminative efficiency of the BSID for identifying infants with possible neurologic impairments. The sample consisted of 194 subjects, including 105 randomly selected normal subjects and 89 neurologically suspicious subjects selected incidentally. The Bayley Mental and Motor Scales were administered at 8 months of age. Neurologic examinations were administered to all subjects at ages 1 and 7 years for classification of the children as neurologically normal or suspicious. Berk concluded that the Bayley Motor Scale provides modest discriminating power and that the information contributed by the Mental Scale in linear combination with the Motor Scale is not substantial and meaningful enough to warrant its administration when attempting to discriminate infants with neurologic impairment; however, the findings should be considered tentative until cross-validation studies are completed.

The Infant Behavior Record was standardized on 886 infants between the ages of 2 and 30 months.[48] In regard to validity, Bayley found that certain Infant Behavior Record items correlated positively with contemporary current Bayley Mental Scale standard scores. Mental Scale scores correlated positively and moderately with ratings of goal-directed behavior, reactivity to stimuli, interest in vocalizing, smooth manual coordination, and attention span. Honzik and colleagues[61] reported that the "infants for whom there was the most concern at birth about positive neurological involvement were, at the age of 8 months, most likely to be poorly coordinated, have a short span of attention, to be markedly more distractible, hypo- or hyperactive, and to perform less well on tests involving eye-hand coordination and problem solving."

Clinically, the BSID provides the physical therapist with a comprehensive evaluation of an infant's level of development.[48] The standard scores (MDI, PDI) provide the basis for establishing a child's current status, in comparison to children in the normative sample, and the extent of any deviation from normal expectancy. The mean standard score for each age range of the standardization sample is 100. A standard deviation (SD) is 16 standard score points; 68 percent of the children in the standardization sample for a particular age range scored between 1 SD below the mean of 100 and 1 SD above the mean of 100. Based on the author's experience with the BSID, a standard score above the 16th percentile indicates normal development; a score between 1 and 2 SD below the mean of 100 indicates a possible developmental problem or environmental deprivation, and a score 2 or more SD below the mean indicates retarded development relative to age peers.

The Mental Scale is not intended to measure an infant's IQ,[48] yet it is a common clinical practice in some areas to obtain an "IQ" by dividing the infant's mental age equivalency on the Bayley by the chronologic age, and then multiplying this figure by 100. In North Carolina, for example, state funding guidelines allow use of this score to help determine whether a child qualifies for continued participation in an early intervention program after 18 months of age or whether a child qualifies as a student at a developmental day-care facility.

The extensive research use of the BSID has shown that it is not a particularly good predictor of adult IQ. Reasons for this are immaturity of the infant, the infant's rapidly changing behaviors, or the overriding significance of other infant behavior, such as relative activity.[63] Prediction of later intelligence does not improve to an acceptable level until after an infant's second birthday.[58]

In regard to program planning, the instrument's (BSID) developmental sequencing of skills provides a useful starting point for goal planning.[8] The value of the instrument for program planning, however, is diminished for several reasons. The number of developmental items contained in the BSID is insufficient to allow the program planner to pinpoint targets precisely for interaction in any particular developmental domain. The time increments between sequenced developmental items are too broad for precision programming with handicapped children. However, an infant's performance on selected BSID items within the developmental sequences can provide the planner with an idea of the upper and lower intervention limits. The clustering of BSID items may be useful when planning intervention programs.[64]

Because of the motor requirements of many of the Mental Scale items, developmentally delayed children with motor deficits may be unfairly scored on certain items. The ability of the tester to recognize motor deficits and to accurately judge when these deficits interfere with the completion of a specific task is important. Another factor is the ability of the tester to adapt to the motor problem by changing the position of the child, by providing proximal stability through handling, or by changing some aspect of a test item; however, the tester must be cautious about deviating from standardized test procedures because of the possibility of invalidating a particular test item. Therefore, a thorough knowledge of each test item is imperative when adapting the BSID. The adaptations made should be documented and an adaptive and nonadaptive standard score and age equivalency should be recorded. Hoffman[65] proposes certain clinical procedures for substituting tasks, reconstructing objects, and altering the administration of activities for handicapped children.

Gesell Developmental Schedules. The Gesell Developmental Schedules (GDS)[11,49] is the patriarch of traditional developmental measures on which all other scales have been directly or indirectly modeled. It is a functional and clinical assessment of the infant's and preschooler's (1 to 72 months of age) broad range of developmental skills not contained in many developmental tests.[8] The scales are not an intellectual measure but a vivid sampling of interrelated behaviors across maturity-age levels and developmental areas. Scoring does not provide a global index. Instead, five areas, including language, fine motor, gross motor, adaptive (problem-solving), and personal-social skills are assessed. The purpose of the GDS is to estimate intellectual potential based upon an analysis of developmental maturity.[49] In addition, the test includes a developmental history and a neurologic survey.[11] Information is obtained from observation and parental reports.

The original standardization procedure involved three normative samples. The first normative sample was composed of 90 normal and abnormal infants who were tested from the time they were less than 3 months of age until they were more than 48 months of age.[66] The second was composed of 107 normal children of the middle socioeconomic class.[67] The third was composed of 107 normal children of the middle socioeconomic class who were examined at 15 months, 18 months, and at 2, 3, 4, 5, and 6 years of age.[68]

The normative basis and organizational format of the GDS for age levels 2.5 to 6 years was minimally revised in 1974.[11] The sample for this revision was composed of 640 normal children who were socioeconomically stratified according to the United States census figures for 1960. All the children lived in Connecticut and were mostly Caucasian. Ten items, primarily from the adaptive behavior scale, were moved to adjacent later points in the scale. Thirty-two items, primarily involving the personal-social and language scales, were moved to earlier age points. Finally, the original motor behavior category was divided into gross and fine motor behavior categories.

The most recent revision of the Gesell schedules was published in 1980.[49] It involved the birth-to-36-months age range and included alterations in item placement and sequence. The revision was based on tests conducted on 927 children in the Albany, New York, area. Here 24 children were tested at 4 weeks of age, 28 at 8 weeks and also at 12 weeks, 52 at 28 weeks, 47 at 36 months, and 50 at 15 other age levels. Race distribution for this sample reflected the United States distribution. The mean education in years for white mothers was similar to that of the United States population; for the black mothers it was slightly higher than the United States average.

The following GDS revisions were made. In the adaptive area, the test items were achieved 10 percent earlier by the children in the sample. The sequencing of the adaptive area items was almost entirely unaltered.[49] In the gross motor area, the items were achieved 17 percent earlier and the sequencing of the items was altered significantly. There was no change in the sequencing of fine motor items; however, these items were achieved 5 percent earlier only in the children in the age range of 56 weeks to 36 months. In the language area, the items were achieved 12 percent earlier, several new items were added, and a greater differentiation was made between expressive and receptive language. No sequencing changes were mentioned. In personal-social behavior, items were achieved 16 percent earlier with no mention of sequencing changes.

Performance is assessed by deriving separate developmental ages, instead of a global score, for each of the five developmental domains.[8] Thus, individual developmental differences are revealed. A flexible scoring system, although somewhat confusing, allows the rating of emerging capabilities and qualitative performance features. Developmental skills are rated as absent, fully acquired, advanced for age, or emerging. Developmental performance in a specific developmental area is described as an age range. A rating of 21 months in the language area represents a skill range of 18 to 24 months. This means that the child typically performs at the 21-month level, but shows scattered and emerging skills spanning the 18- to 24-month range. This scoring system is flexible, thereby facilitating the assessment of individual developmental variations, a useful asset when assessing handicapped children. A handicapped child may perform relatively well in the gross motor area but poorly in the fine motor and language areas. Such a developmental profile could be documented by the GDS scoring system. One drawback is that a specific age level cannot be derived if there is a wide scatter of items passed and failed in a particular area.

A developmental quotient (DQ) can be derived for each developmental area by using the formula[49]

$$DQ = \frac{\text{maturity age}}{\text{chronologic age}} \times 100$$

A child's intellectual potential is related to the adaptive area DQ, but is not rigidly defined by the DQ's numerical value. A diagnosis is not derived from an adaptive scale DQ. Instead, the determination of a DQ is aimed at providing a clinical estimate of intellectual potential. The theoretical rationale supporting this is that adaptive behavior is the forerunner of later intelligent behavior. An adaptive scale DQ below 85 indicates probable organic impairment in the cognitive area. Serious retardation in the cognitive area can be suspected when a DQ falls decisively below the 65–75 range.

Gesell never investigated the problem of examiner-observer reliability; however, Knobloch and Pasamanick[11] reported the reliability of DQ assignment to be 0.98 among 18 pediatric residents. Test-retest reliability was investigated by Gesell in 1928.[66] The sample for this investigation was composed of 90 infants tested 492 times. Reliability was found to be high. An 80 percent agreement was obtained when the scores were within the normal range; a 96 percent agreement was obtained when the scores were subnormal. In 1974 Knobeloch and Pasamanick[11] reported test-retest reliability for 65 infants over a two to three-day time span to be 0.82. An interobserver reliability study was also done using the 1980 version of the scale and a sample of 48 children ranging in age from 16 weeks to 21 months.[49] The overall percentage of agreement for 305 behavior patterns was 93.7 percent; however, agreement varied from 88 percent in fine motor behavior to 97 percent in language. Interrater reliability was also found to be high.

The concurrent validity coefficient obtained from a study of 195 children, 3 years of age, who were administered the GDS and the Stanford-Binet, was 0.87.[8] The predictive validity coefficient obtained from a study of 195 children who were administered the GDS at 40 weeks and the Stanford-Binet at 3 years was 0.48.[8] In another validity study, the GDS performances of 26 normal male children at 7, 9, and 15 months correlated significantly and consistently with performance on the Merrill-Palmer Scale[69] at 27 months, and the visual motor channel of the Illinois Test of Psycholinguistic Abilities[70] at 5 years.[71] It is important to point out that Gesell never intended the GDS to measure "intelligence," and, therefore, did not expect it to predict later IQ.[72]

A predictive validity study involving neurologically or intellectually abnormal infants was done by Knobloch and Pasamanick[73] in 1960. The sample consisted of 195 premature children tested on the GDS at the adjusted age of 40 weeks and on the Stanford-Binet at 3 years of age. The correlation coefficient for the GDS and Stanford-Binet scores was 0.43 for 147 children who were considered normal and 0.74 for those neurologically or intellectually abnormal. These results indicate that test results are more stable for low-scoring babies. Additional validity information for the GDS can be obtained from the Yang chapter and the Self and Horowitz chapter in *The Handbook of Infant Development.*[7]

In regard to program planning, the five domains tested by the GDS are congruent with the skills focused on in many early intervention curricula.[8] The results of research in programs for both handicapped and nonhandicapped preschoolers indicate that the GDS is highly correlated with developmental curriculums. The schedules also have utility as a diagnostic device for educational programming.

Preschool Attainment Record.   The Preschool Attainment Record (PAR)[50] is a downward extension of the Vineland Social Maturity Scale.[74] The PAR surveys the birth to 7-year age range by focusing upon three major developmental domains and eight subareas.[8] The major domains are physical, social, and intellectual. The subareas are ambulation, manipulation, rapport, communication, responsibility, information, ideation, and creativity. The scale is frequently used to assess "untestable" multihandicapped preschoolers because it is administered by interviewing parents or other significant caregivers. A child may also be "untestable" because of his or her behavior during a testing session. The interview can be supplemented by direct observation.

Caregivers are asked to reveal the "typical" behavior of the child.[8] The items are scored (+) if the child's behavior fits the task completely, (±) if the behavior is marginal or inconsistent, and (−) if the behavior is undeveloped. Attainment age scores and attainment quotients can be obtained but must be used with great care.

The PAR has no established technical and normative base.[8] No validity or reliability studies are reported in the manual. The scale's content validity comes from a literature review on child development plus expert opinion as to the placement and applicability of the items.

Clinically, the PAR should not be used to formally test a handicapped child but to obtain descriptions of the child's habitual behavior.[8] This can be beneficial when formulating intervention programs for handicapped children.

The scale has several drawbacks. The PAR manual fails to explain the relevance or use of an attainment age or quotient. Because several of the categories overlap, subjectivity during an interview may occur. A final drawback is lack of standardization.

Bruninks-Oseretsky Test of Motor Proficiency. The Bruninks-Oseretsky Test of Motor Proficiency (BOTMP)[51] assesses the gross and fine motor functioning of children from 4½ to 14½ years of age. The specific motor areas evaluated by subtests are running speed and agility, balance, bilateral coordination, strength, upper limb coordination, response speed, visual motor control, and upper limb speed and dexterity. The test was developed to provide educators, clinicians, and researchers useful information to assist them in assessing the motor skills of individual students, in developing and evaluating motor training programs, and in assessing serious motor dysfunctions and developmental handicaps in children. A shortened version of the BOTMP has also been developed.

The BOTMP provides global and differentiated information about a child.[51] The test yields a Gross Motor Composite Score, a Fine Motor Composite Score, and a Battery Composite Score; these are standard scores. Age equivalencies and standard scores are also obtained for each subtest.

The BOTMP[51] consists of 30 items previously contained in the Oseretsky Tests of Motor Proficiency.[75] The BOTMP was standardized on 765 subjects representative of the 1970 United States census according to sex, race, community size, and geographic distribution.[51]

The validity of the BOTMP is based on how well it assesses the construct of motor development or proficiency.[51] Several researchers proposed that motor development consists of a number of constructs.[76–81] The BOTMP measures (1) 6 of 7 constructs identified by Guilford,[76] (2) 4 of 6 constructs postulated by Cratty,[77,78] (3) 12 of 20 constructs described by Fleishman,[79] (4) 10 constructs identified by Harrow,[80] and (5) 6 of 8 constructs identified by Rarick and Dobbins.[81]

Construct validity of the BOTMP is also demonstrated by the statistical characteristics of the test.[51] One study reveals that the scores of each subtest correlated significantly with the chronologic age of the children in the standardization sample. For the total sample, the correlations ranged from 0.57 to 0.86 with a median of 0.78. For each subtest, the mean point scores showed the expected increase from one age group to the next.

The final method whereby validity is measured is by comparing contrast groups.[51] The manual reports that normal subjects perform significantly better than mildly retarded subjects, moderately to severely retarded subjects, and learning disabled subjects of the same chronologic age. Part of the difference may be due to difficulty encountered when testing retarded or learning disabled children, specifically giving instructions that are often complex.

Reliability for the BOTMP was measured by three methods.[51] A test-retest reliability study was conducted with a sample of 63 second graders and 63 sixth graders. The BOTMP was administered to each group twice within a 7- to 12-day period. The test-retest reliability coefficients for the Gross and Fine Motor Composites were 0.77 and 0.88, respectively, for the sixth graders. The reliability coefficient for the Battery Composite was 0.89 for the second graders and 0.86 for the sixth graders. Test-retest coefficients for the separate subtests ranged from 0.58 to 0.89 for the second graders and from 0.29 to 0.89 for the sixth graders. The second method to measure reliability was the determination of the standard error of measurement (SEM) for the composites and for the subtests. Generally, the SEM for the subtests was found to be 2 or 3 standard score points while the SEM for the composites was found to be 4 or 5 standard score points. The final method was the determination of interrater reliability on the eight items of the visual motor control subtest, chosen because the items in this subtest require more tester judgment than the items of the other subtests. The interrater reliability coefficient for one group of raters was 0.98; it was 0.90 for a second group.

Southern California Sensory Integration Tests. The Southern California Sensory Integration Tests (SCSIT)[2] are designed to explain the dysfunction in underlying neural systems that is believed to accompany the perceptual and learning problems presented by children of late preschool and school age (age 4 to 10 years).[82] The SCSIT aids diagnosis of dysfunction in form and space perception, postural and bilateral integration, tactile perception, and motor skills. The SCSIT consists of a battery of 17 tests: space visualization, figure-ground perception, kinesthesia, manual form perception, finger identification, graphesthesia, localization of tactile stimuli, double tactile stimuli perception, motor accuracy, imitation of postures, crossing midline of body, bilateral motor coordination, right-left discrimination, standing balance with eyes open, standing balance with eyes closed, design copying, and position in space.

The SCSIT was normed on 1004 children in the metropolitan Los Angeles area.[83] No blacks and few Hispanics were in the sample.[2] The number of children per normative age group was 30. Norms for ages 9 and 10 are available only for the areas of space visualization, figure-ground perception, position in space, and design copying.[83]

Except for one subtest, reliability was measured by the test-retest method.[83] The period between tests is unknown. Results are extremely variable with correlation coefficients ranging from 0.01 to 0.89. Reliability for motor accuracy was measured by internal consistency methods and the correlation coefficient values ranged from 0.67 to 0.94. Ayres[2] believes that the reliability coefficients vary because the nervous system of a child varies from day to day.

The only SCSIT validity data available were obtained from a study done by Kimball[84] who assessed 26 children between the ages of 5 and 9 years with the SCSIT and the Bender Gestalt.[85] He found that the motor accuracy and the design copy subtests were highly correlated between the two tests. The

Bender Gestalt was also found to be a predictor of scores on the form and space perception and the praxis tactile portions of the SCSIT. However, the Bender Gestalt was not found to tap either postural mechanisms or integration of the two sides as does the SCSIT.

The SCSIT has several weaknesses. The normative sample was small for specific age groups, and the background of the normative sample was not socioeconomically representative of the metropolitan Los Angeles area. Only one geographic area, Los Angeles, was represented. The normative data are incomplete for the 9- to 10-year age group. Finally, validity data are minimal. A strength is that the instrument is, nonetheless, a useful clinical tool.[86]

Miller Assessment for Preschoolers. The Miller Assessment for Preschoolers (MAP) assesses such developmental areas as ocular ability, quality of movement, and sensory integration.[52] It was developed for two reasons: (1) to provide a statistically sound, short developmental screening tool that could be used by educational and clinical personnel to identify those children in need of further evaluation, and (2) to provide a comprehensive, clinical framework that would be helpful in defining a child's developmental strengths and weaknesses, and indicate possible avenues of remediation.

A MAP research edition consisting of 530 items was administered nationwide to a randomly selected stratified sample of 600 normal preschool children and to a selected sample of 60 children with preacademic problems.[52] Based on the resulting data, 27 items and a series of structured observations were selected for the current version of the MAP. This version was standardized in all nine U.S. Census Bureau regions on a randomly selected sample of 1200 preschoolers, stratified to represent the United States population in regards to sex, age, race, size of residential community, and socioeconomic factors.

Several reliability studies were completed during the standardization project.[52] An interrater reliability coefficient of 0.98 was obtained in a study involving 40 children. A test-retest study involving 90 children resulted in scores remaining stable over time in 81 percent of the children. In terms of validity, the MAP identified as "at risk" 80 percent of a sample of 80 children identified by teachers, parents, or doctors as having preacademic problems.

Intervention Tools

In this section two selected instruments will be reviewed: the Vulpe Assessment Battery (VAB)[87] and the Ordinal Scales of Psychological Development (OSPD).[88] In the author's opinion, the primary usefulness of these instruments is in the formulation of developmental intervention programs because they have not been statistically designed for diagnostic purposes. These instruments were chosen for discussion because the author has found them to be helpful in the clinic. The Marshalltown Behavioral Development Profile[89] and the Haeussermann Educational Evaluation-Inventory of Development Levels[90] are additional intervention tools, which will not be discussed here but are reviewed, along with others, in the book *Linking Developmental Assessment and Curricula*.[8]

Vulpe Assessment Battery. The Vulpe Assessment Battery (VAB)[87] is comprised of assessment items that attempt to cover comprehensively essential areas of child development from birth through 6 years of age. The battery provides a method for obtaining and organizing the information necessary to plan an individualized learning program for an atypical child. The battery utilizes the child's strengths and compensates for areas of weakness using a teaching method approach with which the child learns most effectively. The VAB assesses basic senses and functions, gross motor behaviors, fine motor behaviors, the child's environment, language behaviors, activities of daily living, the organization of behavior, and cognitive processes and specific concepts, including cause-effect and means-ends relationships and object constancy. Also included in the VAB are tests of reflexes, motor planning, muscle strength, and balance.

Conceptually, the VAB views the child to be actively constructing an understanding of the world on the basis of perceptual organization and adaptation.[87] "The child interacts with the world in a manner which adds new content to learning and which progressively alters the structure of thinking so that the child can interact with the world in a developmentally more mature fashion."[87]

The VAB is not standardized in a formal sense; however, it is not designed to compare children with their age peers.[87] The battery is a product of the author's 15 years of experience working with children with a wide range of developmental disabilities. No reliability or validity information is provided in the manual.

The advantages of the VAB are numerous. First, it is applicable to normal, as well as handicapped, children. Second, it is comprehensive in nature. Third, the battery can be individualized to each child's learning and developmental pattern. Fourth, it is competency-oriented so that the child can succeed. Fifth, scoring of the child's performance considers the teaching technique utilized and the child's learning style; therefore, the VAB can be used simultaneously for assessment and programming. Sixth, an accountability schema is built into the assessment process which facilitates reported assessments and the evaluation of developmental programs. Seventh, references for the original inclusion of each item in the test are provided.

Ordinal Scales of Psychologic Development. The conception of the organization and the development of intelligence, which provided the theoretical basis for the construction of the Ordinal Scales of Psychological Development (OSPD), appears to differ substantially from the conceptions that underlie other existing tests of infant development, such as the Bayley.[88] The most marked difference pertains to the view of the nature of intellectual developmental change. Traditional test design assumes incremental developmental progress, without much consideration of the interrelationships between achievements at one level and those at the next. In contrast, the design of the OSPD implies a hierarchial relationship between intellectual achievements at different levels. Therefore, the achievements of the higher developmental level do not incidently follow, but are intrinsically derived from those at the preceding level and encompass them within the higher level.

Another difference between traditional test design and the design of the OSPD is the conception of the organization of intellectual achievement at any one level.[88] In traditional tests, achievements are grouped together on the basis of their cooccurrence at a particular chronologic age for the normative population. Also, there are no assumed inherent relationships between achievements. In contrast, the OSPD, by separating the issue of sequence from association with chronologic age, provides more inherent grounds for the cooccurrence of achievements. The developers of traditional tests such as the Bayley assumed that psychologic development in infancy reflects essentially a unitary process, for example, the MDI of the Bayley Scales subsumes all of cognitive development, and that individual differences in intelligence may be measured in terms of differential rates of achievement.[88] From these assumptions, the developmental quotient (DQ) was conceived for measuring differential rates of infant development, and the expectation arose that intellectual development in infancy, measured by a DQ, would be continuous in nature and, therefore, predictive of later intellectual achievement, measured by IQ. Traditional test designers assumed that rates of development are predetermined and that there is a linear relationship between increments in DQ scores or developmental age (DA) and increments in chronologic age (CA).

As discussed previously, Bayley DQ scores are not generally predictive of adult IQ scores. Therefore, longitudinal validity for traditional tests such as the Bayley has not been significantly demonstrated which discredits the assumptions that rates of development are predetermined and that there is a linear relationship between increments in DQ or DA scores and increments in CA. Furthermore, DA and DQ scores yield little information about the nature of development within individual infants as well as minimal information about the kinds of circumstances that will foster infant development.[88]

The OSPD have been designed in order to have better tools with which to investigate the effects of infants' encounters with various kinds of circumstances on the rate of their development.[88] The designers of the OSPD have presumed that competence is based not on a unitary ability but on a hierarchial organization of a number of abilities and motive systems with several relatively independent branches (six scales). They have also presumed that this hierarchial organization of abilities and motives consists of coordinations and differentiations among the several sensorimotor organizations already present at birth, and that progress toward the symbolic representations and regulations comprising competence and intelligence undergoes an epigenetic developmental change.

The epigenetic developmental point of view proposes that at each higher level of developmental complexity there emerges a new characteristic, one that simply was not present at a lower organizational level. Development is characterized by qualitative emergences which are discontinuous in nature.[91]

The OSPD are, therefore, theoretically based on the developmental beliefs of Piaget,[1] which he formulated while observing the psychologic development in his own three children. The designers of the OSPD maintain the view that higher order developmental achievements are derived from but are also qualitatively different from those of a lower order. Psychologic development is conceived as an elaboration of cognitive structures which also have psychologic and emotional significance. These structures develop in the course of repeated and progressively changing perceptual encounters with events, objects, persons, and places. A final view maintained is that one may expect an order within the epigenetic course of each branch of development that may prove to be invariant across individuals.

On the OSPD, no DQ or DA scores are obtained.[88] Instead, the OSPD enable a clinician to determine a child's current intellectual developmental status for educational purposes. The scales permit a comparison of the development of two children in several areas of intellectual achievement relatively independent of their chronologic ages. By comparing the mean ages of infants at successive levels of development, the OSPD can be used to assess the fostering quality of different child rearing regimes. The OSPD can also be used to assess the degree to which development along any given branch is a function of encounters with particular kinds of circumstances. This is done by comparing the average time needed by infants in differing circumstances to move from one step to another on an appropriate scale.

The OSPD consists of eliciting situations initially described by Piaget.[1] The eliciting situations are grouped into six scales spanning the age range of 1 to 23 months.[88] The scales are (1) visual pursuit and the permanence of objects, (2) development of means for obtaining desired environmental events, (3) development of imitation, (4) the development of operational causality, (5) the construction of object relations in space, and (6) the development of schemes for relating to objects. The testing procedures for administering the eliciting situations are generally somewhat flexible permitting the examiner to use varied materials and structures, a notable advantage for testing physically handicapped children.

The current version of the OSPD was developed as a result of a study involving 84 children ranging in age from 1 to 23 months.[88] This sample of children came largely from middle-class families whose parents were graduate students and faculty members at the University of Illinois. The mean percentages of interobserver agreement and the mean percentages of intersession stability for the eliciting situations that comprise the six scales were high (>91 percent and >71 percent, respectively). The intersession stability study was conducted over a time span of 48 hours.

The OSPD are not normed more completely because the authors believe that great plasticity exists in the ages at which infants achieve various developmental milestones.[88] This plasticity exists as a result of varying environmental circumstances encountered by infants and the effect of these circumstances on their development. In addition, an OSPD score for a child does not depend for its meaning upon comparison with the scores of other children, upon the position of the child in some standardized group of children, or upon some rough correlation with age, all of which require extensive standardization studies.

Several validity studies on the OSPD have been conducted. The concurrent validity of the estimated developmental age (EDA) placements assigned to the individual eliciting situations and the estimated mental age (EMA) derived from them were examined in a study of 36 handicapped and at-risk infants and toddlers.[92] The mean chronologic age of the subjects was 14 months while the mean estimated mental age was 9 months. The mean general intelligence quotient obtained from the Griffiths Mental Developmental Scales scales was 77. The scores on the OSPD and the Griffiths scales correlated significantly both within and across scales. In terms of concurrent validity, these results suggest that estimated developmental ages are good indicators of a handicapped or high-risk child's overall quantitative level of development.

Wachs[93] conducted a study assessing the predictive power of the OSPD. The OSPD were administered to a small sample of children at 3-month intervals between the ages of 12 and 24 months. The Stanford-Binet was then administered to all subjects at 31 months. At 12 months, only the visual pursuit and permanence of objects score was significantly correlated with Stanford-Binet scores. By 24 months, all scales except the means for obtaining desired environmental events were significantly correlated with Stanford-Binet performance.

Summary

Even if a physical therapist in a multidisciplinary clinical setting is not responsible for administering certain tests, for example, the Bayley Mental Scale, he or she should be aware of the development, design, and purpose of the tests in use. This can facilitate multidisciplinary communication and function and may also facilitate communication between parents and team members. A physical therapist can also contribute to deciding which tests are appropriate for a specific child or a specific clinical population and/or setting.

A therapist should be extensively familiar with the testing instruments he or she is administering and should keep abreast of the literature pertaining to a specific instrument or similar instruments. It is the author's opinion that a physical therapist involved in the formal testing of children with neurologic dysfunction should periodically test normal children and should periodically have his or her reliability with other testers evaluated.

For a specific child or clinical setting, each test chosen for evaluation will possess certain strengths and weaknesses, for example, cost, reliability, validity, popularity, time of administration, and purpose. These factors require thorough consideration when deciding which test to use. Physicians and other health professionals should not only be provided with test results, but also the interpretation of these results, for example, information regarding long term prognosis, when appropriate. Finally, the results of formalized testing should be used in a combination with other information obtained, for example, posture, range of motion, reflexes, and the quality of movement, in order to produce a comprehensive evaluation of a child with a neurologic dysfunction.

The next two sections of this chapter will present information on assessment of patterns of posture and movement within the overall sequence of motor development. Two perspectives on the evaluation of quality of movement are provided, that of Rood and Stockmeyer, and that of the Bobaths and their colleagues, Quinton and Köng. These frames of reference for assessment of coordination were chosen because they represent the most commonly used approaches in pediatric physical therapy.

THE EVALUATION OF MOTOR DEVELOPMENT FROM A ROOD PERSPECTIVE

For a comprehensive description of Rood's theory and technique the reader is referred to Stockmeyer.[4,94] The material presented in the following sections represents Attermeier's viewpoint based on courses with Rood, Stockmeyer's writing, and her own academic and clinical experience.

The complexity of the conditions encountered in pediatric patients poses considerable problems to the evaluator. Abnormal motor activity must be assessed with respect to some type of "yardstick" in order to make judgments about current status as well as the effects of treatment. For this purpose, measures of milestone attainment based on studies of normal children are of limited value, as they presume normal quality of movement. Detailed descriptions of abnormal movement, while necessary, can result in a deluge of information that needs to be put into perspective in order to be useful. The principles and concepts offered by Rood offer just such a perspective. They are compatible with and complementary to other approaches to evaluation of coordinated movement. In particular, the idea of "central state" and the developmental sequence proposed by Rood contribute a conceptual framework within which information can be organized.

Central State

"Central state" is the term used by Rood[95,96] to describe the overall mental and physical status of an individual at any given point in time. Her ideas on this topic came largely from Gellhorn's extensive review of autonomic-somatic integration.[97] Three basic components comprise central state: autonomic, somatic, and cerebral cortical. Each of these has a range of function that can be assessed clinically. *Autonomic* function tends to be either sympathetic (as indicated by increased heart and respiratory rate, increased blood pressure, and pupillary dilation) or parasympathetic (as indicated by decreased heart and respiratory rate, decreased blood pressure, and pupillary constriction). In order to make judgments about a particular child, one must be familiar with normal age-appropriate expectations as well as the specific patterns exhibited by the child. For information on age-appropriate expectations, the reader is referred to Farber.[98]

TROPHOTROPIC ———————— **ERGOTROPIC**
(Parasympathetic Dominance)   (Sympathetic Dominance)

TROPHOTROPIC	ERGOTROPIC
↓ Heart rate	↑ Heart rate
↓ Resp. rate	↑ Resp. rate
↓ γ outflow	↑ γ outflow

Fig. 2-1. Characteristics of trophotropic and ergotropic states according to Hess.

γ = gamma

The *somatic* component concerns muscle tonus. While the studies cited by Gellhorn measured gamma motoneuron outflow to assess the somatic component, clinically we rely on palpation, response to passive stretch, and observation of posture. Muscle tonus has a normal range from high to low, but neurologically impaired patients frequently exceed normal bounds and exhibit spasticity and/or hypotonia.

The *cortical* component has to do with level of arousal, which can be measured in a laboratory using electroencephalography. Clinically, we note the degree of alertness and emotional state of our patients.

The concept that autonomic, somatic, and cortical functions vary together is based on the work of Hess,[99] who coined the terms "ergotropic" and "trophotropic" (Fig. 2-1). The "ergotropic syndrome" is characterized by sympathetic activity, increased muscle tone, and cortical desynchronization (greater arousal). The "trophotropic syndrome" is characterized by parasympathetic activity, decreased muscle tone, and cortical synchronization (less arousal). These states are not to be thought of as competitive, but rather as cooperating smoothly to provide homeostasis on a moment-to-moment basis. Thus states can be arranged along a spectrum. In a normal individual, deep sleep represents the low end of the trophotropic range, while low-stress activity and feeding (including digestion) are in the high end of the trophotropic range. As the activity or stress level increases, as in exercise, one begins to function more in the ergotropic range, and at the extreme of this range is the "fight-or-flight" state.

The central state concept is useful because it gives a framework for assessing the patient's overall state of readiness for functional activities, and suggests guidelines for altering state if it is inappropriate. The precise nature of the autonomic-somatic-cortical interactions is highly complex and as yet not completely understood. What is clear, however, is that each component can influence the others.[100]

The final common pathway to muscle is influenced by many factors in addition to direct sensory stimulation. The level and patterning of background excitation on the motoneuron pool provides a substrate for voluntary activity and will heavily influence the quality of the motor act. The process of "preparation" for functional activity is familiar to therapists and essentially consists of techniques geared toward balancing the central state of the child before commencing the activity, as well as maintaining the appropriate state during the activity. Neurologically impaired pediatric patients display a variety of abnormalities in central state. Some show extreme trophotropic status (hypotonia with lethargy and consistent parasympathetic bias), while others are excessively ergotropic (hypertonic, overreactive or fussy with too much sympathetic bias). Furthermore, many patients exhibit a disorganized central state, such as combined spasticity and hypotonia with lethargy and fussiness. If for example, a feeding was being evaluated with the disorganized child just described, a combination of preparatory balancing procedures would be used. Muscle tone and fussing would be reduced (made more trophotropic) by using calming, rhythmical input. The parasympathetic functions related to feeding and digestion would thus be allowed to operate. At the same time the child's arousal level would be elevated (made more ergotropic) by presenting alerting stimuli such as the sight and smell of food.

Clearly, these issues are integral to both evaluation and treatment. The point is well illustrated in a recent study that showed an inverse relationship between progression on a behavioral state scale and consistency of reflex responses.[101] The authors supported the recommendation of optimal states for testing[102,103] and urged caution when interpreting test results based on a single examination.

The skill and precision of the therapist's evaluation, then, will be enhanced by careful attention to (1) the child's central state in terms of somatic, autonomic, and cognitive components; (2) the child's response to techniques geared toward state alteration; and (3) the amount of subsequent input needed by the child to maintain an appropriate state.

Overview of Developmental Sequence

Rood has proposed a developmental sequence consisting of "vital" and "skeletal" components. These components interact closely during normal development, and are dealt with concurrently during evaluation and treatment. The vital sequence incorporates the basic life functions of respiration, feeding, and elimination, as well as phonation and speech articulation. The skeletal sequence traces motor development, from a kinesiologic perspective, in four stages (Fig. 2-2):

1. Reciprocal innervation, consisting of flexion and extension patterns
2. Cocontraction
3. Mobility on stability with the distal end fixed
4. Mobility on stability with distal end free (skill) (S-1)

These stages occur in the development of each of the "key patterns" (Fig. 2-3), which develop in time from the neonatal period to independent walking. Key patterns represent the development of mobility and stability, which are then combined to produce dynamic postural control and skilled activity. These key patterns include posture and movement in supine flexion, prone extension, prone-on-elbows, prone-on hands, all-fours, semisquat, and standing.

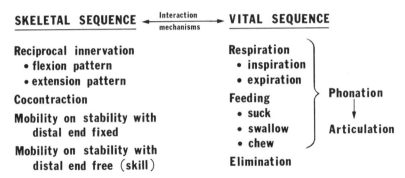

Fig 2-2. Skeletal and vital components of Rood's developmental sequence.

In order to use these patterns effectively, the following should be kept in mind:

1. The key pattern series recapitulates broadly the motor competencies that emerge during the first 12 to 15 months of life. They do not constitute a standardized test and no age norms are attached. The therapist, therefore, must be familiar with developmental expectations at various ages or use formal tests to establish general level of motor development.

2. The key pattern series identifies, in sequence, crucial constellations of motor competencies leading to ambulation. Their value lies in the fact that they allow quick identification of where a child's motor abilities are breaking down, and therefore where treatment should begin. The patterns can be used as a whole or in part, depending on the needs of the child, and can be implemented in a variety of positions. Examination of Figure 2-3 (Key Patterns), however, reveals that the series is not a complete inventory of developmental phenomena (pivoting-in-prone and sitting, for example, are not included). Furthermore, patterns are presented here only as they appear in their fully developed form. Information on lead-up postures as well as transitions between postures must be obtained from other sources. For this the reader is referred to the work of Bly[104,105] (see her section in this chapter, "The Evaluation of Motor Development from a Neurodevelopmental Treatment Perspective").

3. Incorporated into the pattern series are the well-accepted principles of cephalocaudal and proximodistal sequencing, as well as the breakdown of gross into more discreet movement. The more superior and proximal body segments will thus show a more advanced stage of development at an earlier date.

4. Although developmental reflexes are not specifically addressed by Rood, their functions are subsumed within the key patterns. Working on hand-to-mouth patterns, for example, helps minimize the asymmetric tonic neck reflex. Many therapists will choose to include a complete reflex assessment in their evaluation (see later section on reflex assessment). Nevertheless, the

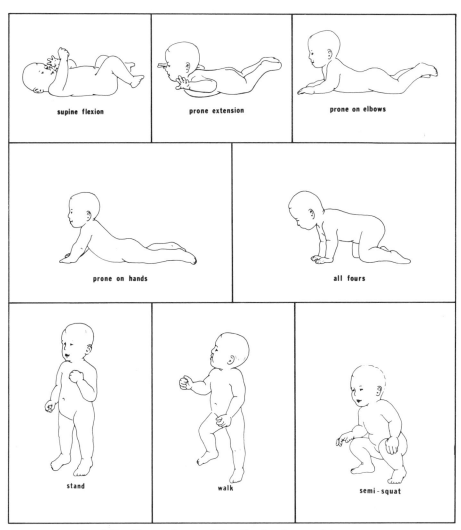

supine flexion

prone extension

prone on elbows

prone on hands

all fours

stand

walk

semi-squat

Fig. 2-3.   Key patterns of Rood's developmental sequence.

importance of viewing reflexes as integral to, rather than separate from, motor performance can hardly be overstated. Milani-Comparetti's[106] work provides further substantiation for this viewpoint.

5.   In addition to observation of the movement patterns themselves, Rood pays considerable attention to which specific muscle groups are producing the movement. Therapists are encouraged to refamiliarize themselves with the location and attachments of muscles and to develop skill in muscle palpation. The addition of this dimension greatly enhances specificity of evaluation and treatment.

The following sections contain a description of normal performance of the key patterns as well as typical deviations seen in patients with high tone, low tone and athetosis.

Normal Performance of Key Patterns

When seen in the light of the "dual systems" theory, the key patterns of supine flexion and prone extension can be viewed as laying the groundwork for further motor developments.

The *reciprocal innervation* stage encompasses the two basic key patterns of supine flexion and prone extension. Rolling is the transitional movement between these two postures, and takes a variety of forms during the developmental period, essentially progressing from being reflexive and nonrotational to voluntary and rotational. The supine flexion and prone extension patterns have characteristics that call to mind the concept of dual (medial and lateral) systems for motor control, as set forth by Lawrence and Kuypers[107,108] and discussed by Buchwald,[109] Stockmeyer,[94] and Perry and colleagues.[110] This proposition contends that the system for maintenance of antigravity posture (carried out by proximal/axial extensor muscles) is relatively separate from and parallel to the neural circuits for limb movement and fine coordination (carried out by distal/flexor muscles). A recent study by Loria[111] lends support to this notion as it relates to reach and grasp. At first glance this idea seems to negate the classical idea of proximodistal developmental trends, but if only antigravity weight-bearing functions are considered, that trend indeed appears to be present.)

To assess *supine flexion*, place the child in supine, sidelying, or a semireclined position. Observe resting posture, vigor and frequency of spontaneous movement, movement responses to toys and food, general response to light tactile stimuli, the extent to which missing components of movement can be elicited using tactile stimuli and any changes in function as a result of placement in the three different positions listed above.

Supine flexion is the basic mobility pattern, though stabilizing components are present. In essence, the pattern involves performance of smooth, reversing limb movements. The trunk, though resting on a surface, is providing the anterior stability which allows antigravity limb movement. It is not expected that a child will consistently perform the patterns described below, but the capability to do so should be present.

The eyes can be stabilized in midline for close vision (roughly arm's length or less) and horizontal tracking is complete and symmetrical. The head can turn smoothly from side to side. The neonate can stabilize the eyes in midline only briefly, but by 4 to 5 months this capability should be well established. The neck is in neutral position, without hyperextension, and the mouth can be closed in a relaxed state. Thorax and abdomen are well-shaped, without flaring of the rib cage. Respiration is relatively shallow with age-appropriate rate. By 6 to 7 months, the child should be bringing the feet to the mouth by lifting the buttocks from the floor.

Both hands can be brought from the side of the trunk to the mouth, in the hand-to-mouth pattern, and returned to the original position. During both phases of the movement, the wrist and fingers can be maintained in extension with the thumb out of the palm. By about 4 months of age, the child should be able to reach accurately into space. All these movements are accompanied by smooth upward rotation, but with very little elevation, of the scapulae. The scapula and humerus do not move as one unit but rather are dissociated during the initial part of the movement.

The hips and knees can be flexed and extended in a balanced, that is, midline, position (babies under 6 months will show more lateral rotation at the hips than older children.) Ankles can be maintained in dorsiflexion with neutral inversion/eversion, toes extended, as the leg is flexed and extended. The ability to perform ankle dorsiflexion with hip and knee extension is of particular importance, as it provides the selective control needed for a heel-strike pattern in gait.[110]

Associated with the skeletal flexion pattern is the ability to perform efficient sucking movements, coordinated with swallowing and respiration. Rood[112] has consistently stressed the importance of sucking/swallowing/breathing, as it provides the first functional integration of autonomic and somatic functions with a trophotropic bias.

Prone extension is the next "key pattern" of the *reciprocal innervation sequence*. To assess, place the child in an antigravity position, either prone on the floor, prone over a ball, or tilted forward while held in your arms. Observe the ability to lift head, trunk, arms, and legs in a symmetrically extended posture, the amount of time the posture can be maintained, and briskness of movement in and out of the posture.

This pattern assesses the critical ability to produce isometric contraction of antigravity postural extensors throughout the body. This is the basic "stability" pattern, though it has mobile features. Extension against gravity develops cephalocaudally over the first 6 to 8 months and during that period has an almost reflexive quality. An alert infant, then, will generally display the extension response when placed prone. On the other hand, an infant who has learned to come independently to sitting on all-fours may require alternate positioning to bring out the extension response. Age, therefore, will be a factor in both the method used to assess the pattern and the conclusion one draws from the response. Described below is the full extension pattern.

The eyes, in addition to being stabilized in midline, can be elevated and can focus on distant objects. The head is lifted so that the mouth parallels the horizon. The spine is fully extended and the thorax elevated; when viewed from the front, the chest is lifted from the surface to the level of the nipples. Spinous processes are obscured by the contraction of deep proximal paravertebral musculature as it acts in concert with the more lateral and superficial erector spinae. The arms are flexed and lifted so that the thumbs are level with the ears. Wrists, fingers, and thumbs can be simultaneously extended. The shoulders are slightly elevated and the scapulae are downwardly rotated and adducted.

The legs are extended at the hips and lifted off the supporting surface. Hips show a slight degree of abduction and lateral rotation; contraction of gluteus medius and maximus muscles can be observed and palpated. At the knees, quadriceps and hamstring muscles are both active and the knees are slightly flexed. Plantar flexion with neutral inversion/eversion of the ankles is present.

Cocontraction is the second stage in the developmental sequence, occurring sequentially in the key patterns of *prone-on-elbows, prone-on-hands, all-fours, semisquat* and *standing*. For assessment, therefore, a child is observed in those positions, with attention to appropriate skeletal alignment. The term "cocontraction" means balanced muscle contraction around a joint, which produces a stable posture yet allows free movement into and out of the position.[113] Normal cocontraction combines the tonic features of the muscle groups developed in the flexion and extension patterns. Cocontraction of the neck and trunk appear first in horizontal alignment, later in upright positions. Limb cocontraction follows a proximodistal and cephalocaudal flow.

In *prone-on-elbows*, cocontraction of musculature in the neck and shoulders can be observed. The child is able to stabilize the neck in a midrange between flexion and extension, as well as lift the head to the vertical position. Support is taken on forearms, with the elbows positioned under the shoulders, forearms parallel, and the hands opened. The scapulae are stabilized against the thorax. Extension of the spine is not as extreme as in the prone extension posture, but paravertebral musculature is active. Legs are extended and rest easily on the floor, though a small degree of hip flexion remains.

The *prone-on-hands* posture is identical to prone-on-elbows except that the arms are fully extended at the elbows and weight is supported on open hands. The transition reflects the proximodistal flow of weight-bearing activity, as the elbows are not stable in cocontraction. The upper trunk is well elevated from the supporting surface and the hips are brought into complete extension.

The assumption of *all-fours* with weight on the knees reflects both cephalocaudal and proximodistal trends in weight bearing. Head and arm positions are as described above. The trunk is horizontal, with both anterior and posterior muscles active. Hips and knees form 90 degree angles, and the knees are positioned directly under the hips. This posture represents appropriate balance of contraction in all hip and knee musculature including hamstrings.

Upright *standing* represents the highest level of the cocontraction sequence, with all neck, trunk, and leg muscles contributing appropriate activity to maintain body alignment against gravity. The head and spine are held erect in midline with slight cervical and lumbar lordosis. When viewed from the side, shoulders, hips, knees, and ankles are in close vertical alignment. Ankles are in a midposition between inversion and eversion, and weight is distributed equally on both feet. Forefeet point straight ahead and the toes are relaxed.

The *semisquat* pattern appears after the child is ambulatory and consists of a strong cocontraction of leg musculature in a midrange position. In this posture, frequently used for play, the trunk is bent forward and hips and knees are held in approximately 90 degrees of flexion. The heels are flat on the floor.

The third stage is *mobility on stability with distal end fixed*, observed in the key patterns of *prone-on-elbows, prone-on-hands, all-fours,* and *standing.* The child is observed in these positions and the presence or absence of weight shifting and oscillating movements is noted.

Having gained the ability to stabilize body parts in midrange weight-bearing positions, the child begins experimenting with movement out of the midranges. The sequence discussed here involves anteroposterior and lateral movement with bilateral weight bearing, though the activities clearly interdigitate with the "skill" patterns described in the next section.

Starting from the *cocontraction* position, weight shift in *prone-on-elbows* beings in a lateral direction. Initially this occurs with a shift of the entire body to one side, with concavity of the trunk to that side. The supporting arm tends to collapse somewhat into flexion and the head is turned to the nonsupporting side. Later, the child can keep the pelvis on the floor during weight shifts, can maintain the original shoulder position, and turn the head in both directions. Muscles on the weight-bearing side are thus being lengthened. Hand postures change as well. Initially the hands are fisted with weight taken on the ulnar border. Later they open and support is taken on the palms. Finally, opening and closing movements of the hand allow play with toys.

The progressions seen in *prone-on-hands* duplicate those seen in prone-on-elbows. At some point during this period, the child also beings to develop locomotor patterns. In addition to rolling, pivoting, pushing backward, and pulling forward emerge.

After the child can assume an *all-fours* posture, the first movement pattern seen is a vigorous forward-backward rocking which takes place in bursts of several seconds duration. This shortly gives way to a less synchronous rocking pattern, which has a more relaxed appearance. At this stage, the child begins to shift weight onto one arm and assume a sitting position by rotating the pelvis backward over the fixed knee.

In free *standing*, vertical oscillations are seen. During these movements, weight is equally distributed on the feet, with the heels flat on the floor. Side-to-side shifts appear shortly thereafter, these being the final preparation for walking.

Mobility on stability with distal end free (skill) is the fourth and final stage. Skill abilities are observed in the key patterns of prone-on-elbows, prone-on-hands, all-fours, and standing/walking. The child is observed in these positions and when walking. The presence and quality of non-weight-bearing trunk and limb movements are noted.

The term "skill," as used by Rood, refers to free coordinate movement of body parts in space (non-weight-bearing). These movements are characterized by being rapid, varied, and well dissociated. The hallmark of skilled movement is the component of rotation. This includes not only trunk rotation but also a variety of diagonal limb movements and postures. Distal movements, including supination and pronation, are superimposed on stabilized proximal body parts. The highest levels of skill are achieved by the most distal and rostral body parts—the eyes, oral musculature, and hands, and, to some extent, the feet. These are the body parts which are most extensively represented in the sensorimotor strip of the cerebral cortex. Skill emerges gradually in the prone, all-fours and upright positions. When a child first assumes a higher level position against gravity, the skill elements previously developed in lower patterns may be lost, but reemerge as the child becomes more secure in the new position.

Having gained the ability to shift weight onto one arm when *prone-on-elbows*, the child begins to free the opposite arm to reach into space. The freed arm is then beginning to function at the skill level, while the supporting arm reverts to cocontraction. The developmental features noted during *mobility on stability with distal end fixed* are repeated during the skill sequence. The first reaching movements are carried out by shifting the entire body to the supporting side, with some collapse of the supporting elbow. The reaching arm extends into the space in front of the body. In the mature pattern, the supporting arm does not collapse; the elbow remains positioned below the shoulder, the humerus is neither medially nor laterally rotated, and the hand remains open. The reaching arm can project to either side, above shoulder level, with elbow, wrist, and fingers extended. The scapula is rotated upward and held firmly on the thorax. Of particular importance is the ability to hold a posture of extension-abduction-lateral rotation at the shoulder, with elbow, wrist, and finger extension. The head should be lifted and rotated in the same direction and the upper trunk rotated on the pelvis so that the muscles on the weight-bearing side elongate. Legs remain in a relaxed extended posture.

The same sequence described above is repeated in the *prone-on-hands* position. During the early phases, one again sees a postural reversion on the supporting arm as the child returns to elbow support. Later, the supporting arm can remain extended during the reach.

Following the rocking phase in *all-fours*, three important skill level activities develop. One is the assumption of sitting, as previously described. Another is the initiation of the creeping pattern. Here the extremities are lifted and advanced while weight is borne on the opposite side. Limbs are first moved hesitantly and kept close to the ground, with limited excursions. Pelvic elevation and depression are prominent as the legs alternately advance. Little or no trunk rotation is present and the child will revert to prone-on-elbows after advancing several inches. In the mature pattern of brisk creeping, contralateral limbs are moved simultaneously and are lifted well off the ground; this involves smooth trunk rotation and increased pelvic stability.

The third skill pattern seen in all-fours is the ability to perform mature reaching with the arms. As in lower level patterns, the arms can be extended above the shoulder in all directions; the ability to reach with extension-abduction-lateral rotation at the shoulder, and extension at elbows, wrists, and fingers is important. Weight is distributed evenly on both knees and the head and upper trunk are rotated on the pelvis.

The weight-shifting movements in *standing* lead naturally to the initiation of *walking*, first sideways cruising, and later walking forward into space. This completes the cephalocaudal and proximodistal flow of weight bearing and locomotion. In early stepping movements, the coordinated, rotational quality present in creeping is lacking. The child uses a wide base of support, holds the arms high and keeps a symmetric trunk position. The feet are lifted rather high and brought down flat. As walking matures, the base of support narrows, the arms lower, and trunk rotation appears. The body alignment described with the standing cocontraction pattern is also observed in walking. The heel-toe gait, which involves rapid dorsiflexion between toe-off and heel-strike, represents the skill level activity of the feet. The hands, eyes, and oral musculature ultimately attain very high degrees of skilled activity. Change in these areas continues well beyond the early developmental period, but by the age of mature ambulation a child should exhibit fine pincer grasp and smooth eye movements (horizontal, vertical, and diagonal) and should be able to articulate simple words.

Pattern Abnormalities Associated with Motor Disorders

Using the description of normal patterns as a basis of comparison, the therapist can observe and record the deviations seen in children with movement dysfunction. The severity of involvement will dictate the extent to which deviations are present. No two children show exactly the same motor patterns, and mixed involvement is common. Nevertheless, the following descriptions of typical abnormalities found in high tone, low tone, and athetoid children can be used as a general guide in evaluation.

High Tone. The first types of abnormalities to be described are those associated with high tone. Within the *reciprocal innervation* stage, observation of the *supine flexion* key patterns will reveal a number of characteristic abnormalities. Superficial, multiarthrodial muscles, such as upper trapezius, sternocleidomastoid, latissimus dorsi, quadriceps, hamstrings, gastrocnemius, biceps brachii, and long finger flexors, are typically overactive. Smooth reciprocal movement and midrange control are deficient.

Horizontal visual tracking is frequently incomplete, jerky and poorly dissociated from head turning. Binocular midline gaze is often impaired. The neck is hyperextended with poor mouth closure. Sucking patterns are often highly abnormal and can be characterized by tongue thrust, poor lip closure, and obligatory biting. Head movements are usually associated with tonic contractions in other parts of the body, and tonic neck reflexes can be observed. A rib cage flattened superiorly and flared inferiorly is associated with poor abdominal muscle tone, particularly in oblique musculature.

Arm movements are characterized by excessive scapular elevation and protraction, forearm pronation, flexion and ulnar deviation at the wrist, and thumb adduction. Wrist/finger extension is deficient during hand-mouth or reaching movements. Leg flexion and extension patterns show lack of balanced midline function. At the hip, lateral rotation is dominant as the leg flexes, medial rotation as it extends. Medial hamstrings frequently show more activity than do lateral hamstrings. Distally, the feet almost invariably dorsiflex with inversion during the flexion phase, and plantar flex with inversion during the extension phase. Furthermore, it is often difficult to move only one leg at a time or to perform selective joint movements.

The overactivity of superficial musculature and underactivity of deep, proximal musculature can be seen clearly when the child with high tone is placed in a prone position to assess a key pattern of extension. Many severely involved children are pulled into flexion and cannot relax enough to initiate extension. In less extreme cases, some lifting of head, trunk, or limbs can be accomplished but superficial muscles dominate movement to a greater or lesser degree.

Head lifting generally takes the form of "stacking," that is, the neck is hyperextended with the occiput often resting on upper thoracic vertebrae. This is brought about by several factors. First, head lifting and stabilizing is carried out by the upper trapezius, a superficial muscle with a wide range of motion. Second, the thoracic spine, due to underactivity of deep paravertebral muscle, either remains horizontal or stays in kyphosis, necessitating cervical and capital hyperextension in order to view the environment. Third, children with poor extension capability frequently have difficulty elevating the eyes, reinforcing the visual need for neck hyperextension.

The lumbar spine will tend to be hyperextended due to the action of relatively superficial erector spinae and overactivity of hip flexors. The underdevelopment of deep musculature is evident when the spinous processes are visible during attempted extension. Even if they are not clearly visible, deep palpation in the area immediately lateral to the spinous processes is recommended in order to establish how well the muscles are contracting.

As flexion/adduction tone predominates in the arms, the lifted-arms posture previously described can rarely be performed. Scapulae are excessively elevated, upwardly rotated, and protracted. Elbow flexion, forearm pronation, and wrist ulnar flexion are excessive. Finger flexion and thumb adduction are common.

The lower limb component of the pattern also shows marked discrepancies from normal. At the hips a slight degree of flexion is usually present along with adduction and medial rotation. Commonly, the knees are fully extended or even hyperextended, and medial hamstrings are more strongly contracted than lateral hamstrings. Ankle plantar flexion is present, but the calcaneus and forefoot are not in midline.

To the extent that deficits are present in the basic flexion and extension patterns, the ability to coordinate muscle groups to produce cocontraction patterns is impaired. The deficits in *cocontraction* generally present as exaggerations of the deficits in those lower level patterns. In most cases, automatic spontaneous cocontraction of postural muscle groups is absent, though this can often be achieved with techniques of physical handling.

In the *prone-on-elbows* key pattern, high tone will interfere with midline, midrange head position. A "stacked" head and open mouth can be frequently observed. The weight-bearing pattern includes excessive elevation, protraction and upward rotation of the scapula, excessive medial rotation and abduction of the humerus, and excessive flexion at the elbow. Wrist flexion with ulnar deviation and finger flexion with adducted thumbs are common. Head turning generally produces a collapse of the arms on the occiputal side as a result of asymmetric tonic neck reflex influence. The trunk and legs show the deficits described with the extension pattern.

If the *prone-on-hands* pattern can be performed, it lacks the midrange, midline position previously described. High tone will produce the same neck, shoulder, wrist, and hand problems as were seen in prone-on-elbows. The elbows are usually hyperextended as stability is achieved by locking the joint in place. This action passively extends the trunk, resulting in further exaggeration of thoracic kyphosis and lumbar lordosis.

As the legs are flexed under the body on *all-fours*, the hips are excessively flexed, abducted, and medially rotated. The knees are flexed to greater than 90 degrees, with medial hamstrings overactive. This posture leads the child directly into the undesirable W-sitting position.

To whatever extent pattern abnormalities are present in the more basic patterns, they will also be present in *standing*, and may be exaggerated due to the stress of working against gravity. In severe cases (e.g., spastic quadriplegia), independent standing is not attained. Hemiplegic children do achieve standing, however, as do most diplegics. Observation of their standing posture from anterior, lateral and posterior perspectives will reveal the same underactivity of deep postural muscles and overactivity of superficial muscles as was seen in all previous patterns. Particular attention should be paid to the weight-bearing position of the feet and the effect that abnormal foot position is having on total posture. Some children will bear weight in an equinovalgus position with knees and hips in flexion and adduction. Others will maintain heels on the floor but hyperextend the knees. This, of course, secondarily influences trunk position.

High tone will interfere with the production of midline, midrange holding contractions necessary to maintain the *semisquat* posture. Attempts to move from standing into semisquat are characterized by excessive medial rotation and adduction at the hips, often to the point that the knees are in contact with each other. The ankles are usually in some degree of equinovarus and weight is borne on the balls of the feet. Children with high tone can rarely maintain the knees at 90 degrees of flexion and will frequently collapse into a W-sitting position.

Patterns of *mobility on stability with distal end fixed* are compromised to the entent that previous patterns are inadequate. Without the ability to assume and maintain midline, midrange cocontraction positions, the child with high tone superimposes weight-shifting and oscillating movements on the postures just described under the cocontraction vital sequence. The range of movement is decreased and lacks a smooth, rhythmical quality.

High muscle tone is associated with stereotypic movement. To whatever extent it is present, therefore, high tone will prevent the varied, differentiated movement characteristic of the "skill" level of Rood's developmental sequence (mobility on stability with distal end free). The active rotational components, which normally emerge in prone-on-elbows, prone-on-hands, all fours, and standing, fail to develop. If ambulation is achieved, lack of heel-strike is almost universal, as the ability to maintain ankle dorsiflexion during hip and knee extension is characteristically impaired.

The fine skill patterns are markedly affected by high tone. Isolated finger movement, thumb opposition, well-articulated speech, and efficient eye control are usually impaired to some degree.

Low Tone. The second types of abnormalities are those characterized by low tone. In general, *reciprocal innervation*, flexion pattern deficits in low tone children stem from proximal instability. Movement patterns of the limbs are not particularly abnormal, although vigor and frequency of movement are decreased. Sucking patterns are often weak and inefficient, with incomplete mouth closure. Lack of proximal stability at the shoulders, anterior trunk, and hips, however, results in characteristic postures. Arms and legs lie flat on the surface in a froglike posture. Early hand-to-mouth behavior is accomplished by head turning rather than antigravity arm movement. Reaching into space, if present, is carried out with shoulder elevation due to insufficient stabilization from inferior scapular musculature. Babies with low tone will sometimes clasp both hands together, possibly to generate increased proximal tone, and reach into space with both arms together. The hips generally show excessive lateral rotation and abduction in movement patterns as well as resting postures. At the feet, it is not unusual to see excessive eversion, possibly the result of pushing into the floor while in a frog-leg posture. Low abdominal muscle tone can cause the belly to protrude, and the lower ribs to flare out. In many cases the infant with low abdominal tone will fail to develop patterns that involve posterior tilt of the pelvis, such as rolling the buttocks up off the surface and grasping the feet with the hands and bringing them to the mouth. Infants with excessive hip mobility, as with Down syndrome, can accomplish the feet-to-mouth pattern without contracting abdominal muscles.

The impaired ability of children with low tone to counter the effects of gravity can be seen very clearly during attempts to perform the extension pattern in the reciprocal innervation sequence. Indeed, it is rare to see the pattern fully present. For assessment purposes, it is important to observe (1) the extent to which the child can generate tonic holding muscle contractions, as opposed to phasic lifting; (2) the extent to which the pattern has developed, and whether it is age-appropriate; and (3) specific positional deviations.

Infants with low tone develop antigravity extension slowly, but the cephalocaudal sequence is generally followed. As the pattern emerges, a phasic rather than tonic quality is seen. Palpation immediately adjacent to the spine will usually reveal that the deep proximal muscles are not sufficiently active. Head lifting often takes the form of "stacking" due to insufficient thoracic extension. Initially spinal extension is diminished in excursion and has a phasic quality. During this stage, the child with low tone will often maintain the hips in extreme abduction and lateral rotation when in prone, just as in supine. Over a period of time this can lead to tightness of the tensor fascia lata muscles and overstretching of hip adductors, further hindering the development of the extension and cocontraction patterns in the legs. Less extreme versions of this posture are often present; therefore, the spontaneous alignment of the legs should be carefully noted.

Often the child will develop an antigravity pattern, which at first glance resembles true prone extension. Closer inspection, however, reveals characteristics that are counterproductive in terms of preparing the child for upright function. Overuse of superficial, multiarthrodial muscles produces neck hyperextension, incomplete thoracic extension, and excessive lumbar extension. At the shoulders, some degree of protraction and medial rotation persists. In the legs, there is insufficient hip abduction and knee flexion. The ankles are plantar flexed but are usually not in a midline position. The excessive eversion seen in supine will often persist. This posture does not strengthen the small, deep musculature, especially in the spine. As a result, when patterns requiring extension in some areas but not others are attempted, antigravity competency is lost. These children will not be competent in sitting or kneeling.

As the child with low tone assumes progressively more advanced antigravity postures, the diminished holding power just described results in deficient joint alignment. Lacking tonic components of the flexion and extension patterns, the child cannot combine those components for joint stabilization.

In the *prone-on-elbows* pattern of the *cocontraction* sequence, the child with low tone will show an inadequately lifted upper trunk, commonly associated with a "stacked" head position and open mouth. Because the serratus anterior and rhomboid muscle groups are underdeveloped for tonic cocontraction, scapulothoracic instability is present in the form of scapular winging or excessive protraction. Likewise, underdevelopment of rotator cuff muscles results in inadequate scapulohumeral stability. The humerus is medially rotated and the elbow is positioned on the supporting surface posterior to the perpendicular projection of the shoulder joint. Leg position varies, but resembles that seen with the extension pattern.

As the child pushes up to *prone-on-hands*, he or she must compensate for instability at the elbows. This is accomplished by locking the joints into complete extension. In cases where joint hypomobility is present, the elbows will be hyperextended.

In *all-fours*, the consequence of trunk instability becomes even more apparent. When viewed from the side, the trunk sags rather than remaining horizontal, and the abdomen protrudes. The combined effect of underactive lower abdominal and hip adductor muscle groups produces an excessively abducted hip posture.

In *standing* position, the child with low tone will compensate at the trunk and legs for deficient cocontraction. Spinal alignment often consists of neck hyperextension and excessive thoracic kyphosis, with variable lumbar posture and abdominal protrusion. The legs are often abducted to provide a wider base of support, with the knees locked into hyperextension. Ankle pronation is almost inevitable and the toes often grip the floor in an effort to maintain balance.

Children with low tone do not generally execute the normal *semisquat* pattern, as it demands strong cocontraction at the knees and ankles. When reaching over to pick up a toy, they usually bend at the waist and keep the knees straight. If they want to play in a squatting position, they lower themselves completely so that their buttocks are almost on the floor.

In the *mobility on stability with distal end fixed* stage, weight-shifting and oscillating movements emerge in prone-on-elbows, prone-on-hands, all-fours and standing, but with decreased vigor. The weight-bearing segments, whether elbows, hands, knees, or feet, are held lateral to the superior joints rather than being positioned directly under them. This limits not only the excursion of weight shifts, but also the emergence of early rotatory components.

Low muscle tone affects the development of skill patterns of the trunk and proximal joints more than it does the finer patterns of eyes, tongue, and hands, although the face may lack expression. The transition from bilateral to unilateral weight bearing is made, but rotational components fail to develop as they normally would, and lateral weight shifting becomes predominant in all positions. Unless very severely affected, children with low tone will go on to develop motor milestones, albeit at a slower rate, in spite of diminished underlying postural competence. The movements and postures, however, have an immature appearance due to wide bases of support and lack of trunk rotation.

Athetosis.   The third types of abnormalities are those characterized by athetosis. Athetosis is an extremely variable disorder in which disorganized movement[114–116] is superimposed on fluctuating muscle tone. Tone can fluctuate between low and normal, low and high, or normal and high.[105] Involuntary distal writhing and intermittent tonic spasms can occur. Movements are characteristically wide-ranging with little midrange control. Children with athetosis are very likely to be under excessive influence from tonic neck reflexes, both symmetric and asymmetric. They can also show poorly modulated responses to visual, tactile, and auditory input.

In the supine *flexion* pattern of the *reciprocal innervation* sequence, midline stability of eye gaze is frequently impaired. Lateral eye movements are often impossible without head turning to the same side. When the head is turned, the influence of the asymmetric tonic neck reflex can be seen, sometimes in the entire body. The reflex can be stronger to one side than to the other; this should be noted, as it can predispose the child to scoliosis.

Arms are moved as a unit in large disorganized arcs; because of poor scapular stability, too much abduction and medial rotation are present at the shoulders. Forearm pronation with wrist flexion and metacarpophalangeal hyperextension are characteristic of athetoid reaching patterns. Grasp/release is deficient, consisting of complete flexion or extreme extension. Children with athetosis experience considerable difficulty maintaining a grasp on an object. Bimanual midline activities and hand-to-mouth patterns are likewise impaired.

Legs show wide-range, rapid, alternating kicking. Due to lack of tonic holding at the trunk, shoulders and hips, athetoids cannot usually tilt the pelvis posteriorly off the floor and bring their feet and hands together.

Feeding problems are virtually universal. Besides the difficulty with hand-to-mouth patterns, oral motor control is disorganized. Further complication is introduced by hypersensitivity to tactile stimuli on the face and hands, as well as to sudden auditory or looming visual stimuli.

Extension pattern ability varies in athetoid children, depending on whether they have predominantly high or low muscle tone. The athetoid with low tone may show little or no ability to extend against gravity with the head in midline, though this child may be able to accomplish some lifting by using the asymmetric tonic neck reflex. Athetoids with increased tone, on the other hand, develop excessive extension, beginning in early infancy. A total-body hyperextension emerges, using primarily superficial, multiarthrodial muscles. The asymmetric tonic neck reflex is likely to be active, detracting from symmetrical midline holding. The neck and trunk are hyperextended. Arm postures vary with the arms frequently being trapped under the body when the child is prone. The legs are often lifted too high from the surface, due to excessive lumbar extension, and the knees are locked into hyperextension. Examination of the athetoid child should include evaluation of the extent to which midline spinal extension can be elicited with the limbs held in flexion. It is also important to assess eye elevation. Many children with athetosis lack the ability to elevate the eyes. In prone, then, they must hyperextend their neck to see objects above eye level. This in itself can contribute to the postural abnormalities described above.

All *cocontraction* patterns are deficient in athetoid children, who move in wide ranges and characteristically lack symmetric midrange stability. In all cases, cocontraction of deep, postural muscles is replaced by fixation of joints in extreme positions.

In *prone-on-elbows*, the head is either insufficiently or excessively extended. The tonic neck reflexes play a role in head lifting, trunk posture, and weight-bearing position of the arms. High tone in the arms will keep them trapped under the chest. Whether tone is low or high, the hands are fisted. The scapulae are unstable and winged. Increased thoracic kyphosis and lumbar lordosis are often present. The legs are stiffly extended in an effort to supply stability.

Prone-on-hands, if it can be assumed, is carried out with stiffly extended arms. The scapulae are protracted and the humerus medially rotated. Elbows are locked into hyperextension and hands are fisted. As thoracic extension is incomplete, the action of pushing up on hands further increases the lumbar lordosis. The legs may remain stiffly extended, or, if the symmetric tonic neck reflex is strong enough, will be flexed under the body with medial rotation at the hips.

The maneuver just described constitutes the athetoid child's approach to assuming an *all-fours* posture. The normal ability to hold the trunk horizontal, with 90 degrees of flexion at shoulders, hips, and knees, is absent. Instead, there is excessive flexion at those joints. The arms remain stiffly extended at the elbows.

Athetoid children have a characteristic standing posture in which joints are mechanically stabilized to compensate for the lack of muscular cocontraction. The hips will be thrust forward and the knees locked into hyperextension. Shoulders and thorax are displaced posteriorly and the head displaced anteriorly. This standing posture is precarious; the child's balance can be easily upset by external forces or even by turning the head.

The athetoid child has difficulty assuming the *semisquat* posture, as it demands good muscular control in midrange. When retrieving objects from the floor, the child's legs often collapse completely and he or she lands in the W-sitting position.

Lacking a stable base of muscular cocontraction, the movements that occur in the *mobility on stability with distal end fixed* patterns are inadequate. In *prone-on-elbows* and *prone-on-hands*, some lateral weight shifting can develop. Because of the influence of the asymmetric tonic neck reflex, however, this shift tends to involve the body as a whole. The supporting arm collapses and the initial stages of thoracopelvic rotation fail to develop. In the *all-fours* position, little true forward-backward rocking takes place, though some oscillating may be done within the excessively flexed leg position. These movements give every appearance of being dominated by the symmetric tonic neck reflex. Their symmetric, midline quality does not give way to the more relaxed rotational movements of the trunk and hips, which permit the child to move into sitting by rotating the pelvis to one side. Nor can the asymmetric pattern of creeping easily develop. Instead, the child with athetosis utilizes symmetric flexion patterns to assume W-sitting and to bunny hop. In *standing*, the normal vertical oscillations do not occur, as they are too threatening to the child's balance, which can be maintained only by locking the joints.

Mobility on stability with distal end free movement, in terms of rotation and dissociation of body parts, does not generally develop, even though the midly involved child may become ambulatory by learning compensatory patterns. The gait pattern has a "prancing" appearance, with legs overflexed during swing phase and hyperextended during stance. The hips remain in some degree of medial rotation during stance. Heel-strike is absent. Fine skill activities of the eyes, hands, and oral musculature are strikingly impaired in the athetoid child, and in many cases involuntary movement is evident.

THE EVALUATION OF MOTOR DEVELOPMENT FROM A NEURODEVELOPMENTAL TREATMENT PERSPECTIVE

According to Bobath,[3,117] assessment and treatment are closely related. An assessment should lead to a logical treatment plan. It should help the therapist determine specific areas to emphasize in treatment, as well as help to select which techniques to use. The assessment should also be a means of measuring progress, or lack of progress in a treatment program.

In Neurodevelopmental Treatment, the emphasis is on evaluation of the whole child. Motor behavior is assessed independently and in relationship to personality and behavioral characteristics, adequacy of basic senses, muscle tone and reaction to stimulation, and musculoskeletal status, which includes range of motion. Assessment of the total child, and his or her family, requires a team evaluation and team coordination to determine the major overall problems and how many overlapping problems can be treated at one time.

Motor behavior is assessed in detail by using a narrative, open-ended, movement assessment form that only outlines positions and movements to be observed in each position. A narrative form is used to enable the therapist to observe and note *how* a movement was accomplished, not just that it was or was not accomplished. In this way, it is hoped that the therapist will become more observant and more cognizant of the specific normal and abnormal movement components utilized during each activity.

Unfortunately, such an open-ended narrative form gives the therapist no guidelines as to what to observe, and no standard by which to measure the quality of accomplishment. Consequently, when such a format is used for evaluation, the resulting narrative description is dependent on that therapist's knowledge, understanding of, and experience in observing normal and abnormal movement patterns and postures.

Although no standardized form exists which measures individual components of movement and postures, Bobath's teachings and writings have given us guidelines from which to observe and evaluate a patient's movement patterns and postures. The standard utilized in neurodevelopmental therapy is that of *normal, age-appropriate* movement patterns, postures, and sequences. The therapist, therefore, must be well informed as to what is normal for various ages and stages of development of the infant, child, and adult. Normal movements of a 4-month-old, a 12-month-old, a 3-year-old, and an adult are significantly different. We cannot measure one age group by the standard of another age group.

Based on Bobath's work,[3,117,118] neurodevelopmental therapy emphasizes the importance of evaluating (1) the postural reactions (the postural reflex mechanism), which include the righting and equilibrium reactions, and (2) the quality of individual movement patterns or components. Included as part of the assessment of movement patterns is the distinction between normal, abnormal, and compensatory components, and the coordination of the components.

To be of real value to the therapist, the information gathered in the assessment must be *analyzed*. It is through analysis that the therapist begins to *understand why* the child moves in a particular way, or *why* he or she cannot move. The analysis should illuminate which specific movement components are normal, which are abnormal, which normal components are *missing* and why, and how *compensatory movements* may have developed. The detailed information enables the therapist to make a valid judgment of the quality of the movement(s).

The following will be a further analysis of what may be considered under the areas of "postural reactions" and "components of movement." For a comprehensive description of neurodevelopmental theory and techniques the reader is referred to the Bobath publications. The following material represents the author's viewpoint based on courses with the Bobaths, Quinton, and Köng, writings by the Bobaths, and her own clinical and academic experiences.

Postural Reactions

Postural reactions of the head, neck, and trunk play a major role in establishing the background movements of all activities. Interaction of the various aspects of postural control enables normal weight bearing with mobility and enhances the variability of movements.[3,117] Postural reactions, therefore, need to be carefully evaluated and analyzed. Normal postural reactions include the following[3,117]: (1) the ability and mobility to move antigravity; (2) the ability to right the head and trunk appropriately when the body moves or is moved; (3) appropriate synergistic fixation of proximal parts to dynamically stabilize distal parts; and (4) the ability of the whole body (head, trunk, and extremities) to respond appropriately and with coordination when the center of gravity is disturbed, that is, equilibrium reactions. Each of these aspects of postural reactions evolve through a developmental process; therefore each can be evaluated sequentially from birth to maturity.

To gain a deeper insight into how each of these aspects of movement can be evaluated, they need to be further analyzed into their individual component parts. The ability and mobility to move antigravity includes normal prone extension, supine flexion, and right and left sidelying lateral flexion. Head, cervical spine, thoracic spine, lumbar spine, pelvis, shoulders, elbows, wrists, fingers, hips, knees, ankles, and toes must be observed. The observation of the whole body during each activity is important because an abnormal or compensatory component in one part of the body will disturb the quality of movement and control in another part of the body. For example, an anterior pelvic tilt during prone extension produces an entirely different quality of extension than does prone extension with a posterior pelvic tilt. An anterior pelvic tilt during supine flexion activities such as hands-to-knees or hands-to-feet also changes the quality of the movement. In the latter, the anterior pelvic tilt inhibits or reduces the activity of the abdominal muscles.

The ability of the head and trunk to right appropriately when the body moves or is moved is dependent upon (1) the normal development of antigravity control and mobility around the body axis, and (2) on the appropriate interpretation of the incoming stimuli. In *Adult Hemiplegia: Evaluation and Treatment*,[117] Bobath's test for balance and automatic protective reactions, although designed for the adult hemiplegic patient, provides a guideline for testing these reactions in neurologically impaired children. The photographs demonstrate the normal reactions and provide very helpful visual guidelines as to what the reactions should be. This test and these photographs are also helpful in evaluating the total body equilibrium reactions.

Appropriate synergistic fixation of proximal parts to dynamically stabilize distal parts is intimately dependent on normal trunk control. The automatic postural reactions provide the background on which more distal voluntary movements are performed. If the postural reactions are inadequate or inappropriate, the quality of the distal movements will not be optimal. For example, when a sitting child reaches out to grasp a toy, the humerus, forearm, wrist, and fingers are moved voluntarily to achieve a fluid coordination of eye and hand for reaching and grasping. During the activity, the trunk and scapula must automatically adjust to and move with the arm. If the child does not have the appropriate trunk (postural) control, the upper extremity reaching pattern will not be fluid. The upper extremity pattern will be altered because the child may need to use the arms to stabilize the trunk, or may need to use scapular adduction to reinforce trunk stability. In each of these cases the quality of the distal components of movement may appear to be poor; however, the child may be able to produce normal distal components of movement if given the appropriate proximal postural control. This is an example of the importance of evaluating the postural reactions first, for they are very often the real source of problems that are manifested with distal symptoms.

Components of Movement

Neurodevelopmental Treatment proponents have stressed the importance of evaluating the quality, or the individual components of movement, used to accomplish milestones, skills, movement sequences, and postures. The Bobaths[3,117,118] continually emphasize the importance of knowing which patterns of movement are normal, which are abnormal, which patterns belong together, and how the patterns are best coordinated. This knowledge and comprehension is gained through an understanding of kinesiology and careful analysis of the movement patterns used by the patient.

To evaluate effectively the components of movement used during a posture or a movement, the therapist must be knowledgeable in kinesiology—the study of human motion. Kinesiology is the science of applying the principles of anatomy and mechanics to determine what movement patterns or sequences are involved in the production of a given skill. It is also concerned with the efficiency of the movements and the understanding of how to improve the efficiency.[119,120]

Therapists of patients with central nervous system dysfunction and developmental delays often neglect to recognize the importance of studying, understanding, and applying kinesiology in assessing the child's motor problems. Most of the assessment scales used to diagnose and evaluate infants and children with developmental problems are designed to measure behavior characteristics. They are not designed to evaluate the kinesiologic components of the behavior skills. Fortunately, most forms do have a space for a brief narrative description of each activity. The information in the narrative, however, is not easy to measure, quantify, or interpret with reliability.

To analyze motor milestones, skills, postures, and movement transitions, the therapist's knowledge of kinesiology should include an understanding of coordinated joint action and coordinated (synergistic) muscle action. How the muscle's actions of agonist, antagonist, and stabilizer are combined or coordinated to produce a movement that is biomechanically efficient or inefficient must be understood. This statement is not meant to imply that muscle testing is appropriate for children with central nervous system dysfunction. The concern is not for individual muscle action, but for appropriate coordination of muscles, and for the flexibility of each muscle to function as an agonist, antagonist, or stabilizer as appropriate to a given skill.

When clinical biomechanics is understood, the quality of movement can be better assessed and the judgment of normal/abnormal can be substantiated. For example, most students of physical therapy would appropriately judge as poor in quality a sit-up accomplished with an anterior pelvic tilt. They would know that the hip flexor muscles were more active than the abdominal muscles. However, how critical is the therapist in analyzing how the milestone of hands-to-feet is accomplished? The normal way for the 5-month-old to bring feet to hands is with a posterior pelvic tilt, hip flexion with slight abduction and neutral rotation, and semiextension of the knee.[121] The abdominal muscles stabilize the pelvis as the iliopsoas flexes and slighly adducts the femur, and the hip adductors contract in synergy with the iliopsoas. In many hypotonic children this milestone is accomplished with a slight anterior pelvic tilt, hip flexion with marked abduction and lateral rotation, and knee flexion.[122] The abdominal muscles are not active. The lumbar extensors are active and provide some stability to the pelvis as the sartorious muscle contracts in isolation. The kinesiology is different than the normal pattern. The quality of the movement is poor when compared to the normal.

The biomechanics of movements can be altered by changes in numerous variables, including muscle tone, range of motion, antigravity muscle control, or reflex actions. During the evaluation, each of these facets must be assessed, examined, analyzed, and synthesized as to its effect on the components of movement. For example, children with hypotonia usually lack the ability to stabilize a proximal part while moving a distal part with synergistic muscle action. In children with hypertonia, the muscles contract inappropriately as antagonists, agonists, or stabilizers. Each of these conditions of abnormal muscle tone markedly alters the biomechanics of normal movements. Conversely, abnormal biomechanics may generate abnormal muscle tone.

Further analysis of the biomechanics of each of the movements utilized by each patient should lead to an awareness of which of the specific components are normal and which are abnormal. The detailed analysis should enable the therapist to determine which normal components of movement are missing. (Facilitation of the missing components should then be part of the treatment plan.) Analysis of the proportion and interrelationship of the normal and abnormal components of movement enables the therapist to judge the overall quality of the patient's movements.

The quality of each specific movement pattern is also determined by the results of its long-term use. In other words, the therapist should be cognizant of the consequences of using specific components of movement over an extended period of time. For example: What are the long-term consequences of an infant's habitual use of head hyperextension and cervical hyperextension in sitting? The consequences are numerous and include[122]: (1) increasing tightness of the capital and cervical extensor muscles; (2) poor mobility and poor muscle development, and thus control, of the capital and cervical flexor muscles; (3) poor development of downward visual gazing because the head is poorly controlled in flexion; (4) poor development of the anterior cervical muscles subsequently provides a poor base of support for normal development of the tongue and jaw muscles leading to poor oral motor control; (5) poor head control in all positions in space, resulting in use of shoulder elevation to stabilize the head; and (6) use of shoulder elevation for head stability leads to poor development of shoulder girdle mobility and thus abnormal upper extremity development.

Major problems in quality of movement become obvious when the long-term consequences of relatively insignificant kinesiologic compensations occurring early in development are analyzed.

In conclusion, if the postural reactions and kinesiologic components of movement are carefully evaluated and analyzed, the child's treatment plan will logically follow. The treatment goals will be to facilitate normal postural tone, the normal postural reactions that are weak or not present, and the normal components of movement that are missing. Simultaneously the abnormal postural tone, abnormal postural reactions, and abnormal compensatory components of movement should be inhibited.

A thorough process of analyzing and synthesizing movement into its component parts is also a valuable tool in helping the therapist to identify subtle changes in coordination. The process also becomes an active and accurate means of measuring progress, or lack of it, in a treatment program.

EVALUATION OF REFLEXES AND REACTIONS

The evaluation of reflexes and reactions is one of many methods used for the analysis of posture and movement in infants, children, and adolescents. This mode of assessment is based on the premise that normal motor coordination is based to a large extent on reflexes and reactions which probably underlie all or most volitional movement in man.[123-125]

The simplest definition of a reflex is that a sensory stimulus transmits information into the central nervous system, which in turn activates a motoneuron to produce a motor response (Fig. 2-4). This motor response may give rise to sensory feedback that elicits yet another motor response so that the cycle is repeated. This classical S → R model is a closed loop paradigm, which is dependent upon afferent input from the environment for the initial response and afferent feedback to maintain or alter the response.

Reflexes may be more complex. Although a reflex is activated from the environment, afferent stimuli are modified by efferent projections from the cerebral cortex and other parts of the nervous system and are even modified via transient or sustained prestimuli.[126] Conclusive evidence exists demonstrating that reflexlike movements are also initiated via central control in invertebrates and some vertebrates.[126,127] Inconclusive evidence suggests that spinal reflexes may be elicited centrally in the human embryo.[128] The final pathway for overt movement is the motoneuron and its efferent projection; thus the motoneuron can be fired from central or peripheral activation. Either

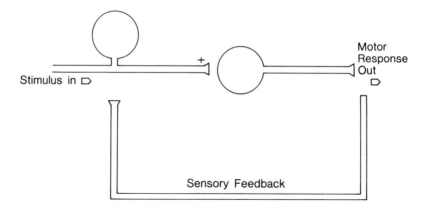

Fig. 2-4. Diagrammatic representation of a simple reflex.

may result in a feedback loop.[123,129–131] The sensory input resulting in a reflex response may, therefore, occur as a result of centrally elicited movement rather than from stimulation in the external environment.

Reflex Components

When evaluating reflexes, the following should be taken into consideration: (1) the adequate stimulus, (2) the number of synapses involved in relaying the afferent input, (3) the number of segments involved in the transmission of the stimulus, (4) the overt movement response, and (5) the function of the reflex.[132]

The earlist reflexes elicitable in the human fetus are exteroceptive in nature.[133–136] Cutaneous sensitivity is restricted to the perioral region at 7.5 weeks gestation. The receptive field spreads as the fetus matures such that, by 19 weeks fetal age, the entire body surface is sensitive to cutaneous stimuli except for the back and top of the head, which remain insensitive until birth.[135]

The first responses elicited by proprioceptive stimulation occur at approximately 8 weeks gestation and consist of slow, local contractions of muscles to a tapping stimulus.[137,138] At 10 weeks gestation, stretch of the biceps brachii and forearm muscles yields arm withdrawal. Tendon reflexes are questionably present at 12 weeks fetal age and are definitely present at 22 weeks gestation.[133] The earliest responses to vestibular stimulation occur at 8 to 9 weeks fetal age when the cristae become functional.[139]

The greater the number of synapses involved in the transmission of afferent stimuli, the more the possible spread of the reflex response. Under normal conditions, responses to proprioceptive input tend to be localized in nature as the number of synapses involved in the transmission of input are few.[133] With central nervous system dysfunction, however, proprioceptive inputs can elicit widespread effects. Reflexes of exteroceptive origin typically consist of circuits having many synapses. Responses to cutaneous stimuli, then, may involve more generalized body responses.[134]

Because of the complexity of the circuitry processing sensory stimuli, the state of the central nervous system is crucial when assessing reflexes in infants, children, and youth. Depending on the receptivity of the nervous system to incoming stimuli, the anticipated motor response may be modified by interneurons, by efferent projections from supraspinal levels, and by the interaction of all inputs on the motoneuron. Not only may the motor response vary, but if the response is completely stereotyped or obligatory in nature, such motor action may be an indication of central nervous system dysfunction.[140–143]

There is evidence, specifically in invertebrates and vertebrates other than man, that early movements are not only elicited by peripheral input but are also evoked by central connections.[123,127–131,144–146] Throughout the central nervous system, there are controlling and organizing centers, rhythmic program generators, which can elicit movement.[123,129,130,145,146] These program generators receive and are driven by sensory stimuli from the periphery as well as from higher centers.[129,130] In the chick, it has been shown that movements generated by spinal centers occur spontaneously from day 3.5 to day 17, independent of afferent input and descending supraspinal input.[123,147] This finding implies that the efferent or motor system begins to function prior to the sensory system. A prereflexogenic period of movement also exists in the pigeon, duck, cat, rat, mouse, and toadfish.[127,128,144] This retrograde sequence of development, which begins with the end organ and ends with maturation of the sensory afferents may be a general feature of neural development.[127,144] Recently, such retrograde progression of development was demonstrated by Okado and associates[128] in the cervical cord of human embryos of 4 to 7 weeks gestational age. These researchers, however, did not study spontaneous movement but only the sequence of structural development. According to Hooker,[133] spontaneous movement and elicited movement occur simultaneously in the human embryo. Thus, with currently available research, it is not known which comes first in human fetal development, the elicited movement or the spontaneous movement, that is, whether the movement was triggered via central or peripheral projections.

A hypothetical model for the control of movement has been theorized that includes rhythmic program generators in the brainstem and spinal cord, which are capable of functioning without peripheral or higher center input. Subsequently, the activity of such generators may be modified via input from higher centers as well as peripheral input. Reflexes initiated from the environment will provide either an additive or subtractive influence on the ongoing activity of the central program generator dependent on concurrent influence from other areas of the nervous system and the relative independence of the generator from these inputs (Fig. 2-5).

Perhaps reflexes play their greatest role during the learning of movement.[148–150] Sensory input to the central nervous system results in local reflex responses. Afferent stimuli also provide input to other centers of the nervous system. These centrally directed processes supply prolonged excitation to

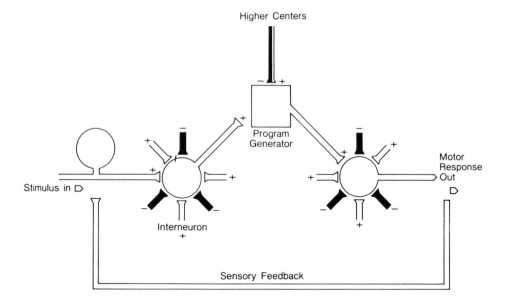

Fig. 2-5. Hypothetical model of reflex control.

many other neurons such that the net result of a sensory stimulus may continue to be elicited long after the original stimulus is removed.[129,130] Cutaneous and vestibular afferents have central processes that terminate on reticular neurons, which in turn participate in producing general arousal.[130,151,152] Stretch reflexes not only provide local reflexive support of movement but also have central axonal processes participating in circuits to the cerebellum and the sensorimotor cortex.[150,153] Vestibular stimuli also are transmitted to the cerebellum and to the sensory areas of the cerebral cortex. The convergence of somatic proprioceptive and vestibular afferents in the cerebral cortex is important for the perception of position and movement.[154,155] Although Taub provided evidence that sensory input is not essential for motor learning in the monkey, such peripheral input is necessary to sharpen and refine movement, especially in the hand, and may speed up the learning process for complex motor skills.[148]

Overt movement elicited via afferent stimuli or triggered by a central program generator can be analyzed with respect to its component parts. Dependent on the age of the child, such movement can be classified grossly as normal or abnormal. When evaluating reflexes, it is not always necessary to use the standard S → R paradigm to determine whether specific reflexes are present, incipient, absent, pathologic, or asymmetric. Instead, the influence of reflexes may be observed during the child's spontaneous movement because this is likely to more accurately reflect the influence of reflexes on functional activities. For example, the neck or body righting reflex can be evoked by the therapist turning the child's head; or it can be elicited when the child turns the head. Because reflexes possess identifiable characteristic components of posture and movement, a reflex assessment can be administered by observing the spontaneous posture and movement of the child. These observations can subsequently be verified, if appropriate, by eliciting the reflex by the standard S → R paradigm.

Reflexes are functional and adaptive to the environment throughout the life cycle.[127] The majority of neonatal reflexes are protective in nature or subserve a survival function.[156] These include the rooting and sucking-swallowing responses, which enable the infant to locate nourishment and feed; and the Moro, crossed extension, flexor withdrawal, and Galant reflexes which protect the infant from noxious environmental stimuli. Spontaneous stepping, crawling, and the neonatal neck on body righting reactions may facilitate positioning the fetus for delivery.[127,144,157] Mature reflexes provide an assistive framework for voluntary movement and exploration in the environment.[156] The righting reactions enable the infant and child to assume the upright erect position, maintaining alignment for locomotion, as the equilibrium reactions provide the necessary responses to maintain the center of gravity when it is displaced such that balance is threatened.

Biologic Substrate

The evolution of reflexes and their relationship to voluntary motor behavior are the subject of quite distinct opinions. Two major theories of development are the continuity theory and the discontinuity theory. The theory of continuity states that development is a continuous progression from infancy to adulthood. Postnatal motor patterns build gradually from simple prenatal movements. These changes are quantitative in nature. Each step in development is dependent on previous steps.[133,158-161]

The discontinuity theory, called ontogenetic adaptation, states that transient adaptations exist at each step of the life cycle, which are unique to that stage, are necessary for that stage of development, and may not be antecedents for another stage or continual development.[127,143,144] Thus development involves fundamental transitions, deletions, regressions, additions, and other discontinuities. The developmental changes are qualitative in nature. This theory, however, does not imply a mutually exclusive process totally independent of antecedent events. Some events may serve immediate as well as influence future goals.

With respect to reflexes, the continuity theory would state that early primitive reflexes are integrated and modified into more complex networks of reflexes; however, the classic theory of reflexology is too global to explain how the transformation of brain mechanisms during development occurs. No scientific evidence exists to support the theory that simple reflexes and S → R associations are the main force in the organization and development of movement.[127,143,144]

With respect to ontogenetic adaptation, the theory predicts that certain reflexes would be present at various stages of development that may not relate to reflexes prior to that stage or have any necessary relationship to reflexes or voluntary movement after that stage. Although there may be no continuity, the reflexes at each stage are uniquely adapted to that stage, that is, they are present for a specific purpose.[127,143,144] How early neonatal reflexes disappear, are suppressed, or are organized or integrated into the expression of voluntary movement are subjects of much interest. Possible mechanisms include the following[143]:

1. Sensorimotor mechanisms simply degenerate or regress.
2. Sensorimotor mechanisms remain intact but come under specific and permanent inhibition from higher centers.
3. Sensorimotor mechanisms change and expand in the composition of neural elements as well as interconnections.
4. Sensorimotor mechanisms become ineffective and are replaced by other sensory channels eliciting the same response.
5. Sensory mechanisms become connected with a different motor system.
6. Two neural mechanisms develop rivalry with each other.

Although the above theoretical explanations are general, one theory that is supported by scientific evidence is active neurophysiologic inhibition.[126,127,144] This phenomenon appears early in all embryos from fish to man and supports the classic concept that the immature brain has many facilitory circuits, but with maturation, develops inhibitory mechanisms. The biologic substrate for this inhibition, however, is not well understood.

Two opposite theories exist with respect to the relationship of reflexes to voluntary motor development. They differ on whether or not reflexes form the biologic substrate for the acquisition of motor milestones.[123–125,162,163,163] Little doubts exists, however, that the nervous system possesses intrinsic properties that provide the basis for voluntary skilled movement, that is, central motor programs.[163] Rhythmic stereotypies are postulated examples of the activity of endogenous pattern generators in maturing neuromuscular pathways that may form the elementary biologic substrate for postural control and coordinated movements.[163–165] Examples of such rhythmic motor behaviors are spontaneous kicking, prone rocking, hands and knees rocking, and bouncing in standing. Obviously, more rigorous and detailed studies are needed to determine (1) the biologic substrate underlying skilled movement, (2) the relationship, if any, of reflexes to the acquisition of motor milestones, and (3) the exact nature of sensorimotor development, that is, whether development is continuous or discontinuous.

Classification of Reflexes and Reactions

A review of the literature yields at least three major classifications of reflexes and reactions: (1) according to levels of the central nervous system, (2) according to function, and (3) according to age of onset, disappearance, or integration into voluntary motor behavior.

Classification of reflexes according to levels of the central nervous system is not appropriate, as such categorization was based on abnormal animal models and brain-injured adults.[143] As the evolution of reflexes and reactions provide a yardstick for the maturation of the infant, and since there is some correlation of reflexes to motor functioning, a classification of reflexes and reactions should be based on age, function, or a combination of both.

The specific evolution of a reflex or reaction has been analyzed by Paine and colleagues,[166] Touwen,[140] Saint-Anne Dargassies,[167] Carter and Campbell,[168] Capute and colleagues[169,170] and Provost.[171,172] From these studies, five general paradigms of the development of reflexes and reactions can be envisioned:

1. Inverted U paradigm: linear increase in the response followed by a decrease, for example, the asymmetric tonic neck reflex
2. N-shaped paradigm: linear increase in the response followed by a decrease and again followed by an increase, for example, the stepping reflex
3. Period of no change in the response followed by a decrease, for example, the Galant reflex
4. No change in a response over time, for example, the deep tendon reflexes
5. Linear increase in response, for example, postural reflexes

By assessing reflexes and reactions in a serial fashion, the clinician acquires a better understanding of the state of the central nervous system of the child and can better predict developmental outcome.[23,173] In other words, the pattern of development may implicate a possible central nervous system dysfunction. For example, the rooting reflex has a developmental course following the inverted U-shaped paradigm, that is, a gradual increase in the complexity of the response from 28 weeks gestational age to 40 weeks, followed by a decline in the response from 6 postnatal weeks to 16 weeks.[42,172] Hypothetically a premature infant could demonstrate the normal developmental course of this reflex from birth to the equivalent of 40 weeks gestation but later exhibit no disappearance or integration of the reflex at the appropriate age, a persistence of the response, which may endanger appropriate development at that age. In other words, initial normal expression of a reflex does not guarantee uneventful development at later points in time. Sequential testing can provide substantial predictability and should be more widely employed by clinicians.[23]

With increasing amounts of research with premature (<37 weeks gestation) infants, many of the reflexes elicited at birth, which later disappear or become integrated, that is, a linear decrease developmental pattern, are being noted to be present prior to 38 weeks gestation. These reflexes often show a developmental pattern of emergence such that with increasing gestational age, the response of the reflex becomes heightened.[167,174,175] Consequently, probably no reflex demonstrates an absolute linear decrease paradigm; rather most follow an inverted U-shaped paradigm in which there is a linear increase in the response prior to 40 weeks gestational age followed by a linear decrease. Ex-

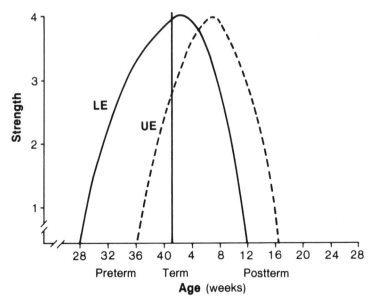

Fig. 2-6.   Asymmetric tonic neck reflex: lower extremities/upper extremities.

amples of this paradigm include the evolution of the rooting reflex, sucking-swallowing reflex, Moro, crossed extension, asymmetric tonic neck reflex, and placing reactions in the upper and lower extremities.[140,171,172,176]

The asymmetric tonic neck reflex is an explicit example of the inverted U paradigm (Fig. 2-6). The reported initial appearance of the asymmetric tonic reflex is variable, as this reflex has not been studied longitudinally in a group of premature infants. St.-Anne Dargassies states that this reflex is observed at 32 weeks gestational age, yet a picture published in the same article shows a 28-week-old infant demonstrating the posture of the asymmetric tonic reflex in the lower extremities.[167] Carter and Campbell[168] observed the evolution of reflexes in one premature infant and noted the presence of the reflex in the lower extremity at 32 postconceptional weeks, the upper extremity at 36 to 37 weeks, and the trunk participating in the response at 41 weeks. Later development of this reflex has been more extensively studied. Coryell and Cardinali[177] indicate that the lower extremities show a maximum response 1 week after birth and decline in overt expression of response to 12 weeks. The overt posture of the arms becomes increasingly apparent until 6 weeks, after which it declines. This was confirmed by Provost,[172] who reported that peak incidence occurred between 4 and 8 weeks of age and integration by 4 months.

Spontaneous stepping and positive supporting reactions follow a three-stage paradigm as do the neck on body and body on body righting reactions. During gestation there is an increase of response followed by a decline which is later modified into a more complex reaction.[140,171,172,176]

From 35 to 40 postconceptional weeks, a general increase in the amount of weight that the child supports when placed in a standing position occurs.[174] This response continues after term and gradually declines until 2 months of age. From 2 to 6 months of age, some children continue to bear some weight, whereas others bear no weight, the so-called physiologic astasia.[178] At variable ages a gradual increase in the amount of weight born when held in standing occurs with the legs assuming a hip and knee extension pattern.[166,172] This is an example of a primitive reflex, neonatal positive supporting reflex in the lower extremity, being modified into a postural reaction, the positive supporting reaction in weight bearing of the lower extremity,[176] or as Milani-Comparetti[106] would state, a primary motor pattern which is being functionally utilized in various ways at different developmental dates.

All postural reactions, including visual placing, protective reactions, tilting reactions, and postural fixation reactions, demonstrate a linear increase paradigm beginning after birth.[9,165,178]

Evaluation

Responses obtained during evaluation of reflexes and reactions depend on the state of the nervous system. Consequently, reflex testing should be administered at times which are optimal for the infant and child and state should be recorded. Because reflexes and reactions may provide the substrate for posture and movement, analysis can be done under two conditions: (1) observing the posture and movement of a child and analyzing components with respect to reflexes and reactions, and (2) providing specific tests in a stimulus-response paradigm.

Each reflex or reaction has specific functions such that use of each is a precise marker of the developmental process from which prognostic clues can be drawn.[106,127,128,132,143,178] For example, Gesell[179] hypothesized that the infant first observes the hand while lying in the asymmetric tonic neck reflex. This has been confirmed in a study of 14 infants videotaped approximately 7 times within the first 12 weeks of life.[180] The authors concluded that the asymmetric tonic neck reflex structures the environment of young infants in such a way that they are likely to see and examine their hands.

The relationship of the traction, palmar, and instinctual grasp reactions with voluntary prehension is another demonstration of the purported importance of reflexes and reactions in development.[163,179–183] If a rattle is placed into an infant's hand, the infant will hold the object because of the traction reflex.[179] As this reflex becomes modified, it is often termed the palmar grasp.[181] This modified reflex allows the child, upon contact with the rattle, to grasp it with a full palmar grasp. Gradually, fractionation of the full grasp along with orientation of the forearm in space makes it possible for the child at 9 months of age to reach for and grasp an object between the tips of the thumb and index finger using a true pincer grasp.[181] This increasingly complex reflex substrata is parallel with voluntary prehension, which also demonstrates a gradual evolution. However, the reflex elements of any form of voluntary grasping can be obtained "experimentally," that is, in a S → R situation prior to the infant's adaptation of its use for functional activities.[182] Because there is an overlap in the developmental evolution of these three reflexes, Prechtl[143] concludes that there is no remodeling of the early grasp reflex into a more complex reaction, but that each reflex exists separately. Also, because Touwen[140] found minimal correlation between the palmar grasp and voluntary prehension, with the exception of the first appearance of the voluntary palmar grasp, Touwen and Prechtl[143] believe that these grasping reflexes do not form the biologic substrate for voluntary prehension. Again, additional research is indicated to determine the exact relationships of reflexes to voluntary motor behavior.

Screening and Evaluation Tools. Milani-Comparetti and Gidoni[184] developed a screening tool to evaluate the relationships between functional motor achievement and the underlying reflexes during the first 2 years of life. This test is divided into two sections: evaluation of motor skills up to the age of attaining a standing position independently; and the assessment of specific reflexes and reactions, which, in their view, provide the underlying reflex substrata for the functional motor skills. For example, they propose that the parachute reaction to sideways movement is needed before sitting up with hand support is possible. Specific reflexes are tested under the S → R paradigm. The original publication provides minimal instructions on how to elicit the response and how to score the motor action. Consequently, specific procedures and scoring criteria were developed by the staff at Meyer Children's Rehabilitation Institute.[185] In addition, the original form was modified by placing reflexive and motor items in the order in which they are administered. The development of this test was based on clinical experience. No data are available on its reliability or validity and no standardization studies have been reported.

The specific testing of reflexes and reactions using the S → R model has been documented in other sources. The most comprehensive book is *The Neurophysiological Basis of Patient Treatment, Volume 2: Reflexes in Motor Development*[176] (Fig. 2-7). This is a programmed test that denotes how to test each reflex and reaction by specifying the position for testing, the stimulus used in the elicitation of the response, and the expected response. In addition this text discusses the function of each of the reflexes in development and describes how the motor developmental process is affected when a reflex is not integrated or a postural reaction does not develop. The material in this text has also been derived from clinical experience.

Other references to reflex testing include Fiorentino,[186] who delineates the position of testing, stimulus, and response and gives the ages at which these reflexes and reactions should be present or integrated. This book does not discuss the relationship of reflexes and reactions to development; however, the book, *Normal and Abnormal Development. The Influences of Primitive Reflexes on Motor Development*,[187] does discuss these relationships. Prechtl's[19] neurologic examination of the full-term newborn has already been discussed. Although this source is limited to primitive reflexes, the ages for demonstration of these reflexes and their developmental importance are reviewed.

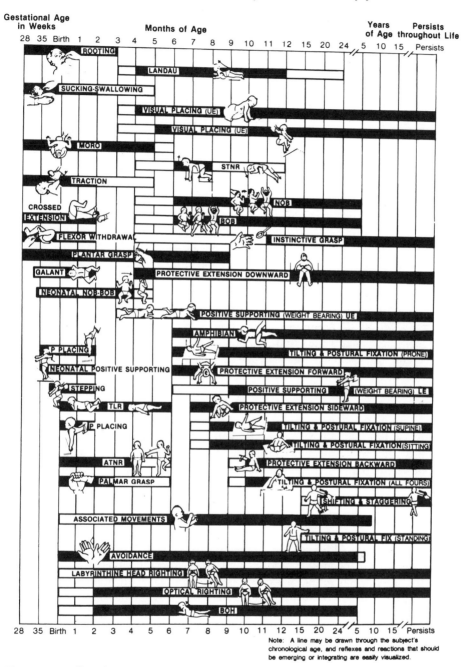

Fig. 2-7. Reflex development. (Barnes MR, Crutchfield CA, Heriza CB: The Neurophysiological Basis of Patient Treatment. Vol. 2; Reflexes in Motor Development. Stokesville Publishing, Morgantown, WV, 1978.)

In each of these tests, the response of the reflex/reaction is scored as present or absent or along an ordinal scale based on the description of the response provided. Two tests have recently been developed that included attempts to define responses of elicited reflexes and reactions in more precise descriptive terms. These are *Primitive Reflex Profile*[188] and *Movement Assessment of Infants.*[189] *Primitive Reflex Profile* describes a coding system for scoring seven primitive reflexes: asymmetric tonic neck reflex, symmetric tonic neck reflex, positive support reflex, tonic labyrinthine reflex in prone and supine, derotational righting reflex (head and body), the Galant reflex, and the Moro reflex. The scoring system consists of a 0–4 scale with 0 being absent and 4 being obligatory. Each reflex response is uniquely described such that each scaled score, that is, 0–4, is specific to the reflex being tested. In addition to the responses being systematically scored, the method of eliciting the response is adequately documented. Each of the seven reflexes are scored separately; no composite score for the total profile can be obtained.

The Movement Assessment of Infants also describes specific testing procedures and a specific scoring system for nine primitive reflexes and the automatic reactions of righting, protection, and equilibrium.[189] Generally the scoring system follows a 1–4 scale with 1 being scored as the reflex being integrated or not elicited and 4 being the dominating response. Again, item descriptions are specific for each reflex and reaction. The reflex items in the MAI do not stand alone, but are part of a more comprehensive test of movement of infants. Administration of the entire test results in a risk score for motor dysfunction; however, data on predictability of the risk score are available only for 4-month-old infants at present.

Although these two sources provide detailed descriptions of reflex responses, data on standardization and validity are lacking. Minimal interrater reliability data was collected on the Primitive Reflex Profile.[188] Four researchers evaluated four children with cerebral palsy, resulting in reliability coefficients of 0.65 for perfect agreement with the mean score, and 0.88 for agreement within 1 point of the mean score. Four researchers also tested four newborns with resultant reliabilities of 0.82 and 0.91. The Primitive Reflex Profile only provides assessment of seven primitive reflexes and does not result in a specific age-related score. Although the Movement Assessment of Infants allows assessment of both primitive reflexes and automatic reactions, a risk score is obtained only when reflexes are administered along with other items. Steps are underway to obtain norms and validate the Movement Assessment of Infants, as well as provide interrater and test-retest reliability information.

Currently, most therapists use a reflex profile with a presence/absence scoring criterion, thus relying on their clinical experience to judge whether the response is normal or abnormal. In addition, most therapy departments have produced their own forms, usually based on one of the above tests, which results in an even greater diversification of testing and scoring procedures as well as dubious reliability and validity. In reviewing eight randomly selected tests of reflexes, Hoskins and Squires[190] noted that all tests were different, and that the most common scoring system was a present/absent criterion.

Why Test for Reflexes and Reactions. Historically, the examination of reflexes and reactions has been an essential ingredient of the analysis of motor development in infants and children.[18,19,25,106,166,178,184,186–188,191–195] Specifically, the evolution of reflexes and reactions provides an index of maturation of the central nervous system as well as the infant's adaptation to extrauterine life.[18,25,106,127,166,184,188] As such, assessment of reflexes and reactions can provide the clinician with a yardstick for the analysis of motor development by yielding the following:

1. An index of maturation of the central nervous system
2. An assessment of muscle strength
3. Identification of motor dysfunction
4. Prognostication of future developmental outcome
5. Establishment of a baseline for treatment
6. Determination of success of treatment
7. Aid in research on motor development

Common areas of significance are as follows:

1. Failure to obtain a response that may indicate general depression of the nervous system or a sensorimotor dysfunction
2. Persistence of a response beyond the expected time of disappearance or integration that may indicate general depression of the nervous system or sensorimotor dysfunction
3. Presence of asymmetries that may indicate[194]
    a. Insult to one side of the brain or unequal injury
    b. Injury to the peripheral nerves of the extremity
    c. Injury to the muscles of an extremity
    d. Muscle weakness
4. Specific clusters of deviant responses that are more predictive of future outcome than a single abnormal response[196]

Research Studies

The most comprehensive studies of the evolution of reflexes and reactions in normal children and those with chronic brain damage were conducted by Paine.[166,197] AT 4 to 6 week intervals 66 normal infants were examined during the first year of life. In a companion study, 129 infants with chronic brain damage (112 with cerebral palsy, 17 with psychomotor retardation) were evaluated at 3-month intervals starting at 6 to 12 months of age and thereafter up to 3 years. In both studies, the evolution of muscle tone, tendon reflexes, and 10 reflex and postural responses were recorded. Results of these two studies indicated that the Moro was rarely retained after 6 months in either group; the placing, positive supporting, parachute, Landau reaction, vertical suspension, and reach and grasp appeared later in the children with chronic brain disorders as compared to the normal children, and the response demonstrated poor qual-

Table 2-2. Primitive Reflexes in Cerebral Palsy and Locomotor Prognosis

Author	Positive Correlation with Nonambulation	No Correlation with Ambulation
Bleck, 1975[201]	Asymmetric tonic neck reflex Extensor thrust (positive supporting— exaggerated) Moro Neck righting (neonatal) Parachute[a]	Foot placement (proprioceptive placing, lower extremities) Symmetric tonic neck reflex
Molnar, 1976[202]	Asymmetric tonic neck reflex Positive supporting (exaggerated) Moro Symmetric tonic neck reflex Tonic labyrinthine reflex Extensor positioning	
Capute, 1978[203]	Asymmetric tonic neck reflex Positive supporting (exaggerated) Symmetric tonic neck reflex Tonic labyrinthine reflex	Derotational neck righting[a] Galant reflex Moro
Effgen, 1982[204]	Plantar grasp	

[a] Postural reactions.

ity of movement. Although the stepping reflex and neck righting reactions were present at later ages in the group with neurologic damage, responses were variable. The asymmetric tonic neck reflex was the most diagnostic sign when persistent beyond the usual time of integration and of an obligatory nature in the children with cerebral palsy. Only 7 of the 17 children with psychomotor retardation demonstrated retention of the asymmetric tonic neck reflex slightly past the time of integration, but the reflex became integrated in all but one child by 9 months of age.

Molnar[198–200] studied the relationship of the attainment of motor milestones with the presence and absence of primitive reflexes and postural reactions: 53 infants and young children with mental retardation and delayed motor development were evaluated on two to six occasions starting at 10 to 23 months of age and up to 20 to 46 months of age. He tested 4 primitive and 10 postural reactions, and then correlated the results with the acquisition of motor milestones. Results indicated that the primitive reflexes were integrated at the normal age but that the acquisition of postural reactions was significantly delayed (5 to 27 months). Once the postural reaction became apparent, the attainment of related motor milestones appeared within one month. This study supports the relationship of postural reactions with the attainment of specific motor milestones.

Several studies have focused on the relationship of reflexes and reactions to locomotor ability (Table 2-2). Bleck studied locomotor prognosis based on the presence or absence of 7 primitive reflexes in 73 nonambulatory children with a diagnosis of cerebral palsy, suspected cerebral palsy, or delayed motor development.[201] These children, aged 10 to 54 months, were examined longitudinally over a period of 15 years. There was 95 percent prediction of nonambulation for children over 1 year of age on the basis of reflexes present. The five most frequently appearing prognostic signs were presence of extensor thrust, absent parachute, and persistent asymmetric tonic neck reflex, Moro, and neonatal neck on body righting reaction.

Molnar and Gordon[202] conducted a longitudinal study to correlate reflex development with later ambulatory status in children with cerebral palsy. A total of 164 children with known cerebral palsy were first seen at or before 12 months of age and were followed from 2.5 to 10 years. At the time of data analysis, 117 children were walking, 47 were not. Six primitive movement patterns were studied in the nonsitters at 12, 18, and 24 months of age. All six were present and obligatory at 12 months of age in 20 out of 21 children who never became ambulatory and in 21 out of 26 children at 18 months of age. At 24 months, these six primitive reflexes were still present in 26 out of 33 children.

Capute and colleagues[203] studied seven primitive reflexes in 53 children with cerebral palsy to correlate their presence with functional levels of ambulation. The children ranged in age from 18 months to 21.5 years. Four of the reflexes were positively correlated with nonambulation (Table 2-2).

Effgen[204] investigated the relationship of a persistent plantar grasp, as tested in the standing position, to presence of independent ambulation. He saw 26 developmentally disabled children initially at a mean age of 6.1 months, and he tested them monthly until they walked independently, or from 3 to 5 years if independent walking was not achieved. Of the 13 children not demonstrating integration of the plantar grasp, 12 did not achieve ambulation.

With the exception of the Effgen study, a cluster of primitive reflexes was important in the prognostication of ambulation or nonambulation in children with cerebral palsy (6 out of the 73 children in the Bleck[201] study initially referred as having cerebral palsy or suspected cerebral palsy were classified as mentally retarded or developmentally delayed at the time of follow-up when no movement disorder was identified). With this exception, the presence of the tonic reflexes (asymmetric tonic neck reflex, symmetric tonic neck reflex, tonic labyrinthine reflex) and exaggerated positive supporting reactions were the reflexes most predictive of future ambulatory status.

Premature infants have routinely been followed in a Premature Follow-Up Clinic at the University of Washington since 1975. In one study the value of the high-risk score of the Movement Assessment of Infants was investigated with 35 infants who were evaluated at 4 months corrected age and again at 12 months.[189] Of these infants, 27 proved to have normal movement at 1 year and 8 were diagnosed as having cerebral palsy. These 8 infants presented with the retention of primitive reflexes, abnormal muscle tone, and some delay in development at 4 months of age. The significant primitive reflexes were the tonic labyrinthine reflex in prone and supine, and the asymmetric tonic neck reflex, exaggerated positive supporting reaction, and the neonatal neck on body and body on body righting reactions.[205]

A retrospective study conducted at the University of Washington included 18 premature infants diagnosed with spastic diplegia at or before 1 year corrected age.[206] These infants were matched retrospectively with 28 control infants. At 4 months corrected age, 12 of the 18 infants with spastic diplegia remained undiagnosed. Of these 12 infants, 6 were believed to have early signs of neurologic abnormality. These signs included the persistence of primitive reflexes (prone and supine tonic labyrinthine reflex and the exaggerated positive support reaction), high muscle tone in different postures, and the inability to bring hands together at midline. None of the control infants demonstrated this triad at 4 months of age. The Moro response and ankle clonus were not helpful in early identification and did not distinguish infants with spastic diplegia from control infants.

Campbell and Wilhelm[207] studied the natural history of motor development in 13 infants at high risk for developmental dysfunction. Three-month scores on the motor portion of the Bayley Scales of Infant Development[48] were predictive of motor outcome at 12 months. The relationship between these 3-month scores and prenatal and perinatal data collected on these same infants and their mothers was investigated. Two variables were identified as related to the 3-month motor score: (1) the mother's score on the historical medical problems list of the Problem-Oriented Perinatal Risk Assessment System, and (2) the total number of abnormal reflex scores on the infant's Brazelton Neonatal Behavioral Assessment Scale[20] conducted as soon as the babies were medically stable and on oral feedings. The medical problem list includes items related to previous pregnancies and other medical problems or risk factors, such as family history, age, and weight. Included on the Brazelton Scale as a screening for central nervous system integrity are 16 reflex items selected from Prechtl's[19] neurologic examination. If left and right are scored separately, 32 responses can be scored. The range of the number of abnormal reflexes was 4–19 with 7 of the 13 infants having scores of 12 and above. Three infants who had the highest number of abnormal neonatal reflexes, 17–19, had the following outcome at 3 years of age[208]:

1. One child with cerebral palsy
2. One child with severe mental retardation but normal motor development
3. One child with mental retardation with more involvement of motor development than mental

Thus early aberrant reflexes may suggest later dysfunction but are not specific in predicting type of motor outcome.

In a precursor study, the reflex performance of the first seven children was described in detail by Campbell and Wilhelm.[209] At 6 months of age, all children demonstrated head righting, with the exception of the single infant in this group who developed cerebral palsy. This pattern also held true for the mature body on body righting reaction. On the other hand, primitive reflexes were present beyond the usual time for integration in many of the children, even those with normal outcome. The authors concluded that delayed postural reactions may be more important than persistent primitive reflexes for identifying high-risk children; however, the presence of persistent *obligatory* prim-

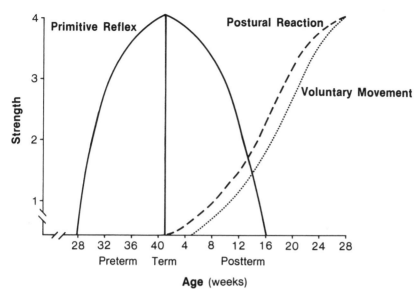

Fig. 2-8.   Hypothetical evolution of voluntary motor behavior on a reflexive base.

itive reflex activity may be significant for differentiating children with central nervous system dysfunction from children with developmental delay.

Of the studies discussed, only four investigations used a descriptive scoring system to score all reflexes.[20,203,205,206] The names given the reflexes varied as well as the details of the scoring system used. Generally, presence of primitive reflexes was predictive of cerebral palsy if these reflexes persisted beyond the usual period of time for their integration or if they were obligatory in nature. Delay in the acquisition of mature righting and equilibrium reactions (protective, tilting, and postural fixation) tended to be significant for the prediction of developmental delay.

From these studies, three paradigms of the evolution of reflexes and reactions and their relationship to developmental disabilities can be theorized. Figure 2-8 denotes the normal relationship among primitive reflexes, postural reactions, and motor development. Primitive reflexes emerge during fetal development and then decline in intensity after birth. These reflexes either disappear, are totally integrated allowing postural reactions to take over the organization of functional motor actions, or are modified into postural reactions thus organizing previous functions to accommodate to a new motor action. Concurrent with this evolution, central programming of movement promotes voluntary control of motor action.

Infants and children with cerebral palsy or other types of neuromotor dysfunction tend to follow a paradigm in which reflexes that emerge during gestation are not integrated nor are they modified into righting reactions. The equilibrium reactions may begin to emerge but are "blocked" by the persistent primitive reflexes and abnormal tone. Motor development is delayed due to the persistent primitive reflexes and the inefficient postural reactions.

Developmental delay can be characterized by either one or two paradigms: (1) the primitive reflexes may be integrated or modified at appropriate times but with a delay in the acquisition of postural reactions and motor action, or (2) primitive reflexes persist but are eventually integrated or modified at a much later than usual time; subsequent to their integration, postural reactions and the attainment of motor milestones occur on a delayed timeline.

Another paradigm can be hypothesized for children with minor neurologic dysfunction. Using clinical observations, Ayres[210] suggested that children with learning disabilities have remnants of primitive reflexes and deficient postural reactions. Two studies lend support to this theory.[211,212] In these studies, 32 reflexes selected from Fiorentino's reflex testing methods[186] were evaluated in a group of 58 children with a mean age of 8 years.[211] Of these children, 38 were considered to be normal and 20 were classified as having learning disabilities. Results indicated a significant increase ($p < 0.02$) in the number of abnormal reflexes present in the children with learning disorders, as compared to the group of children who were normal. In another study,[212] 25 children, aged 3 to 6 years, with minimal neurologic impairment, were compared with 44 children without neurologic impairment with respect to the labyrinthine neck righting and the optical righting reactions. Results indicated that children with minimal impairment showed significantly deficient responses on both righting reactions as compared to the noninvolved children. Although these studies provide some evidence for this paradigm, additional research is needed to determine quantitative and qualitative changes in reflexive responses that occur with age.[213-217]

Conclusion

The concept of a reflex or reaction has changed significantly since first described. Although reflexes and reactions are elicited by afferent stimuli, their overt expression is dependent on all impulses impinging on the motoneurons. As the central nervous system matures from the day of conception, reflexes evolve, disappear, become integrated or modified, and more complex reactions appear. The many studies to date suggest that this evolutionary sequence can be used to document the maturation of the central nervous system.

A dearth of scientific evidence exists to support the implied relationship between reflexes and motor ability. All of the studies on reflexes and reactions have used different tools with their own scoring system; thus, it is very difficult to compare them. Clinicians, too, have developed many evaluation tools. Theories are abundant; now is the time to scrutinize these theories and study the long held concept that reflexes provide the substrate for voluntary movement. In order to do this, universal, standardized tools need to be developed so that clinicians and researchers can adequately discuss reflexes and reactions from a common base.

SUMMARY

The authors of this chapter have attempted to outline for the experienced physical therapist a framework for evaluation of the sensorimotor function of the child with neurologic dysfunction. This framework includes, in order: (1) overall evaluation of the child's general developmental level by the use of formalized developmental assessment tools, (2) detailed observation of posture and movement by the use of less formalized, but comprehensive, assessments of motor development, and also an observation of the impact of reflexes on movement, and (3) a formal reflex test, when needed. For the assessment of movement, the two approaches most commonly used by pediatric physical therapists were presented, that of Rood and Stockmeyer, and that of the Bobaths and their colleagues. Resource information for this framework was provided by the authors.

It is important to consider that the type of evaluations comprising the framework presented in this chapter may be administered by a physical therapist who has specialized training in these areas. On the other hand, these tests and observations may be administered by a multidisciplinary team consisting of a physical therapist, and an occupational therapist or a psychologist. Therefore, this framework for evaluation may be appropriate for a variety of settings where pediatric physical therapists work. Finally, since several of the components of this framework can be done simultaneously, cost effectiveness may be realized.

REFERENCES

1. Piaget J: The Origins of Intelligence in Children. Cook M, Trans. International Universities Press, New York, 1936.
2. Ayres AJ: Southern California Sensory Integration Tests Manual Revised. Western Psychological Services, Los Angeles, 1980.
3. Bobath B: Abnormal Postural Reflex Activity Caused by Brain Lesions. 2nd Ed. Heinemann, London, 1971.
4. Stockmeyer SA: An interpretation of the approach of Rood to the treatment of neuromuscular dysfunction. Am J Phys Med 46(1):900, 1967.
5. Buros OK (ed): The Eighth Mental Measurements Yearbook. Gryphon Press, Highland Park, NJ, 1978.
6. Stangler S, Huber C, Routh D: Screening Growth and Development: A Guide for Test Selection. McGraw-Hill, New York, 1980.
7. Osofsky JD (ed): Handbook of Infant Development. Wiley, New York, 1979.
8. Bagnato SJ, Neissworth JT: Linking Developmental Assessment and Curricula: Prescriptions for Early Intervention. Aspen Systems Corporation, Rockville, MD, 1981.
9. Lewko JH: Current practices in evaluating motor behavior of disabled children. Am J Occup Ther 30:413, 1976.
10. Frankenberg WK, Dodds JB, Fandal AW, et al: Denver Developmental Screening Test Reference Manual. LADOCA Project and Publishing Foundation, Denver, 1975.

11. Knobloch H, Pasamanick B: Gesell and Amatruda's Developmental Diagnosis: The Evaluation and Management of Normal and Abnormal Neuropsychologic Development in Infancy and Early Childhood. Harper & Row, Hagerstown, MD, 1974.
12. Sloan W: The Lincoln-Oseretsky Motor Development Scale. Genet Psychol Monogr 51:183, 1955.
13. Roach E, Kephart N: Purdue Perceptual-Motor Survey. Charles E. Merrill, Columbus, OH, 1966.
14. Thorner R, Reimein QR: Principles and procedures in the evaluation of screening for disease. Public Health Monogr 67 (846), 1961.
15. Frankenberg WK: Criteria in screening test selection. In Frankenberg WK, Camp BW, (eds): Pediatric Screening Tests, Charles C Thomas, Springfield, IL, 1975.
16. Anastasi A: Psychological Testing. 5th Ed. Macmillan, New York, 1982.
17. Magnusson D: Test Theory. Addison-Wesley, Reading, MA, 1967.
18. Prechtl HFR, Beintema D: The Neurological Examination of the Full Term Newborn Infant. Clinics in Developmental Medicine, No. 12. Lippincott, Philadelphia, 1964.
19. Prechtl HFR: The Neurological Examination of the Full Term Newborn Infant. Clinics in Developmental Medicine, No. 63. Lippincott, Philadelphia, 1977.
20. Brazelton TB: Neonatal Behavioral Assessment Scale. Clinics in Developmental Medicine, No. 50. Lippincott, Philadelphia, 1973.
21. Dubowitz L, Dubowitz V: The Neurological Assessment of the Preterm and Full-Term Newborn Infant. Clinics in Developmental Medicine No. 79. Lippincott, Philadelphia, 1981.
22. Parmelee AH, Michaelis R: Neurological examination of the newborn. p 7. In Hellmuth J (ed): Exceptional Infant. Vol. 2: Studies in Abnormalities. Butterworths, London, 1971.
23. Prechtl HFR: Assessment methods for the newborn infant, A critical evaluation. In Stratton P, Chichester J (ed): Psychobiology of the Human Newborn. Wiley, New York, 1982.
24. Prechtl HFR: The mother-child interaction in babies with minimal brain damage. In Foss, BM (ed): Determinants of Infant Behavior II. Wiley, New York, 1963.
25. Beintema DJ: A Neurological Study of a Newborn Infant. Clinics in Developmental Medicine, No. 28. Heinemann, London, 1968.
26. Prechtl HFR: Prognostic value of neurological signs in the newborn period. Proc R Soc Med 58:3, 1965.
27. Prechtl HFR, Dijkstra J: Neurological diagnosis of cerebral palsy in the newborn. In tenBerge BS (ed): Prenatal Care. Noordhoff, Groningen, 1960.
28. Als H, Tronick E, Lester NM, et al: Specific neonatal measures: The Brazelton Neonatal Behavioral Assessment Scale. In Osofsky JD (ed): The Handbook of Infant Development. Wiley, New York, 1979.
29. Als H: Assessing an assessment: Conceptual considerations, methodological issues and a perspective on the future of the NBAS. In Sameroff AJ: Organization and Stability of Newborn Behavior. Monogr Soc Res Child Dev, ser 177 43(5–6):14, 1978.
30. Tronick E, Brazelton TB: Clinical uses of the Brazelton Neonatal Behavior Assessment. In Friedlander BZ, Sterritt BM, Kirk GE (eds): Exceptional Infant: Assessment and Intervention. Vol. 3. Brunner/Mazel, New York, 1975.
31. Divitto B, Goldberg S: The effects of newborn medical status on early parent infant interaction. In Field TM (ed): Infants Born at Risk. SP Medical and Scientific Books, New York, 1979.

32. Goldberg S, Bachfield S, Divitto S: Feeding, fussing and play: Parent-infant interaction in the first year as a function of prematurity and perinatal medical problems. In Field TM, High-risk Infants and Children. Academic Press, New York, 1980.

33. Bakow H, Samaroff A, Kelly P, et al: Relation between newborn and mother-child interactions at four months. Paper presented at the biennial meeting of the Society for Research in Child Development, Philadelphia, 1973.

34. Stengel TJ: The Neonatal Behavioral Assessment Scale: Description, clinical uses, and research implications. Phys Occup Ther Pediatr 1:39, 1980.

35. Horowitz FD, Dunn M: Infant intelligence testing. In Minifie FD, Lloyd LL (eds): Communicative and Cognitive Abilities: Early Behavioral Assessment. University Park Press, Baltimore, 1977.

36. Lancioni GE, Horowitz FD, Sullivan JW: The NBAS-K. 1. A study of its stability and structure over the first month of life. Infant Behav Dev 3(4):341, 1980.

37. Field TM, Dempsey JR, Hallock NH, et al: The mother's assessment of the behavior of her infant. Infant Behav Dev 1:156, 1978.

38. Widmayer SM, Field TM: Effects of Brazelton demonstrations on early interactions of preterm infants and their teenage mothers. Infant Behav Dev 3:79, 1980.

39. St. Clair KL: Neonatal assessment procedures: A historical review. Child Dev 49:280, 1978.

40. Als H, Brazelton TB: A new model of assessing the behavioral organization in preterm and full term infants. J Am Acad Child Psychol 20:239, 1981.

41. Als H, Lester BM, Tronick EC, Brazelton TB: The Assessment of the Preterm Infants' Behavior. In Fitzgerald HE, Lester BM, Yogman MW (eds): Theory and Research in Behavioral Pediatrics. Plenum Press, New York, 1982.

42. Saint-Anne Dargassies S: Neurodevelopmental symptoms during the first year of life. I: Essential landmarks for each key-age. Dev Med Child Neurol 14:235, 1972.

43. Dubowitz LMS, Dubowitz V, Goldberg C: Clinical assessment of gestational age in the newborn infant. J Pediatr 77:1, 1970.

44. Dubowitz LMS, Levene MI, Morante A, et al: Neurologic signs in neonatal intraventricular hemorrhage: A correlation with real-time ultrasound. J Pediatr 99:127, 1981.

45. Graziani LJ, Korberly B: Limitations of neurological and behavioral assessments in the newborn infant. In Gluck L (ed): Intrauterine Asphyxia and the Developing Fetal Brain. Year Book Medical, Chicago, 1977.

46. Casaer P, Akiyama Y: Is body posture relevant for neonatal studies? Acta Paediatr Belg 27:418, 1973.

47. Brazelton TB, Koslowski B, Tronick E: Neonatal behavior among urban Zambians and Americans. J Acad Child Psychiatry 15:97, 1976.

48. Bayley N: Bayley Scales of Infant Development. Psychological Corporation, New York, 1969.

49. Knobloch H, Stevens F, Malone AF: Manual of Developmental Diagnosis. Rev Ed. Harper & Row, New York, 1980.

50. Doll EA: Preschool Attainment Record. American Guidance Service, Circle Pines, MN, 1966.

51. Bruininks RH: Bruininks-Oseretsky Test of Motor Proficiency: Examiner's Manual. American Guidance Service, Circle Pines, MN, 1978.

52. Miller LJ: Get yourself on the map. Totline 8(1):17, Spring 1982.

53. Bayley N: The California First-Year Mental Scale. University of California Press, Berkeley, 1933.

54. Jaffa AS: The California Preschool Mental Scale. University of California Press, Berkley, 1934.
55. Bayley N: The California Infant Scale of Motor Development. University of California Press, Berkeley, 1936.
56. Bayley N: Consistency and variability in the growth of intelligence from birth to eighteen years. J Genet Psychol 75:165, 1949.
57. Werner EE, Bayley N: The reliability of Bayley's revised scale of mental and motor development during the first year of life. Child Dev 37:39, 1966.
58. Bayley N: Consistency and variability in the growth of intelligence from birth to eighteen years. J Genet Psychol 75:165, 1949.
59. Honzik MP, Macfarlane JW, Allen L: Stability of mental test performance between 2 and 18 years. J Genet Psychol 75:165, 1949.
60. Ramey CT, Campbell FA, Nicholson JE: The predictive power of the Bayley Scales of Infant Development and the Stanford-Binet Intelligence Test in a relatively constant environment. Child Dev 44:790, 1973.
61. Honzik MP, Hutchings JJ, Burnip SR: Birth record assessments and test performance at eight months. Am J Dis Child 109:416, 1965.
62. Berk RA: The discriminative efficiency of the Bayley Scales of Infant Development. J Abnorm Child Psychol 7(1):113, 1979.
63. Bayley N, Schaeffer ES: Correlations of maternal and child behaviors with the development of mental abilities: Data from the Berkeley Growth Study. Monogr Soc Res Child Dev 29(6, no 97):1, 1964.
64. Yarrow LF, Pederson FA: The interplay between cognition and motivation in infancy. In Lewis M (ed): Origins of Intelligence: Infancy and Early Childhood. Plenum Press, New York, 1976.
65. Hoffman H: The Bayley Scales of Infant Development: Modifications for Youngsters With Handicapping Conditions. Suffolk Rehabilitation Center, Commack, NY, 1975.
66. Gesell A: Infancy and Human Growth. Macmillan, New York, 1928.
67. Gesell A, Thompson H, Amatruda CS: Infant Behavior: Its Genesis and Growth. McGraw Hill, New York, 1934.
68. Gesell A, Halverson HM, Ilg FL, et al: The First Five Years of Life. Harper & Row, New York, 1940.
69. Stutsman R: Merrill-Palmer Scale of Mental Tests. CH Stoelting, Chicago, 1931.
70. Kirks A, McCarthy JJ, Kirk WD: Illinois Test of Psycholinguistic Abilities. Rev Ed. University of Illinois Press, Urbana, 1968.
71. Roe KV: Correlations between Gesell scores in infancy and performance on verbal and non-verbal tests in early childhood. Percept Mot Skills, 45(3, pt 2):1131, 1977.
72. McCall RB: Toward an epigenetic conception of mental development in the first three years of life. In Lewis M (ed): Origins of Intelligence: Infancy and Early Childhood. Plenum Press, New York, 1976.
73. Knobloch H, Pasamanick B: An evaluation of the consistency and predictive value of the 40-week Gesell Developmental Schedule. Paper presented at the Regional Research Meeting of the American Psychiatric Association, Iowa City, 1960.
74. Doll EA: Vineland Social Maturity Scale: Condensed Manual of Directions. American Guidance Service, Circle Pines, MN, 1965.
75. Doll EA (ed): The Oseretsky Tests of Motor Proficiency. Translation from the Portuguese (adaptation). American Guidance Service, Circle Pines, MN, 1946.
76. Guilford JP: A system of psychomotor abilities. Am J Psychol 71:164, 1958.
77. Cratty FJ: Movement Behavior and Motor Learning. Lea & Febiger, Philadelphia, 1967.

78. Cratty BJ: Perceptual and Motor Development in Infants and Young Children. Macmillan, New York, 1970.

79. Fleishman EA: The Structure and Measurement of Physical Fitness. Prentice Hall, Englewood Cliffs, NJ, 1964.

80. Harrow AJ: Taxonomy of the Psychomotor Domain: A Guide for Developing Behavioral Objectives. David McKay, New York, 1972.

81. Rarick GL, Dobbins DA: Basic Components in the Motor Performance of Educable Mentally Retarded Children: Implications for Curriculum Development (Grant No. OEG-0-70-2568-610). U.S. Office of Education, Washington DC, 1972.

82. Reed H: Test #875. In Buros OK (ed): The Eighth Mental Measurements Yearbook. The Gryphon Press, Highland Park, NJ, 1978.

83. Westman AS: Test #875. In Buros OK (ed): The Eighth Mental Measurements Yearbook, Vol 2. Gryphon Press, Highland Park, NJ, 1978

84. Kimball JG: The Southern California Sensory Integration Tests (Ayres) and the Bender Gestalt. Am J Occup Ther 31:294, 1977.

85. Pauker JD: Test #881. In Buros OK (ed): The Eighth Mental Measurement Yearbook. Vol 2. Gryphon Press, Highland Park, NJ, 1978.

86. Scott DH, Sykes EG: Bristol Social Adjustment Guides. University of London Press, London, 1956–66.

87. Vulpe SG: Vulpe Assessment Battery: Developmental Assessment, Performance Analysis, Individualized Programming for the Atypical Child. National Institute on Mental Retardation, Toronto, 1977.

88. Užgiris IC, Hunt J McV: Assessment in Infancy: Ordinal Scales of Psychological Development. University of Illinois Press, Chicago, 1975.

89. Donahue M, Montgomery J, et al: Marshalltown Behavioral Development Profile. AEA #6, Preschool Division, 1975.

90. Haeussermann E: Haeussermann Educational Evaluation—Inventory of Developmental Levels. Grune and Stratton, New York, 1972.

91. Lerner RM: Concepts and Theories of Human Development. Addison-Wesley, Reading, MA, 1976.

92. Dunst CJ: Validity of scoring procedures for quantifying the sensorimotor performance of infants as measured by the Uzgiris and Hunt Scales. In Dunst CJ (ed): A Clinical and Educational Manual for Use with Uzgiris and Hunt Scales of Psychological Development. University Park Press, Baltimore, 1980.

93. Wachs TD: Relation of infants' performance on Piaget scales between twelve and twenty-four months and their Stanford-Binet performance at thirty-one months. Child Dev 46:929, 1975.

94. Stockmeyer S: A sensorimotor approach to treatment. In: Pearson PH, Williams CE (eds): Physical Therapy Services in the Developmental Disabilities. Charles C Thomas, Springfield, 1972.

95. Rood M: Workshop Lecture Notes, University of Wisconsin, Madison, 1974.

96. Rood M: Workshop Lecture Notes, University of Wisconsin, Madison, 1975.

97. Gellhorn E: Principles of Autonomic-Somatic Integrations. University of Minnesota Press, Minneapolis, 1967.

98. Farber S: Neurorehabilitation: A Multisensory Approach. Saunders, Philadelphia, 1982.

99. Hess WR: Das Zwischenhirn. Schwabe, Basel, 1949.

100. Ginzel KH: Interaction of somatic and autonomic functions in muscular exercise. Exercise Sport Sci Rev 4:35, 1976.

101. Smith S, Gossman M, Canan B: Selected primitive reflexes in children with cerebral palsy: Consistency of response. Phys Ther 62:1115, 1982.

102. Touwen B: Neurological Development in Infancy. Lippincott, Philadelphia, 1976.
103. Prechtl HFR, Beintema DJ: The Neurological Examination of the Full-Term New-born Infant. Lippincott, Philadelphia, 1964.
104. Bly L: The components of normal movements during the first year of life. In Slaton D (ed): Development of Movement in Infancy. University of North Carolina at Chapel Hill, Divison of Physical Therapy, 1980.
105. Connor FP, Williamson GG, Siepp SM (eds): Program Guide for Infants and Tod-dlers with Neuromotor and Other Developmental Disabilities. Ch 5. Teachers Col-lege Press, New York, 1978.
106. Milani-Comparetti A: Pattern analysis of normal and abnormal development: the fetus, the newborn, the child. In Slaton D (ed): Development of Movement in Infancy. University of North Carolina at Chapel Hill, Division of Physical Ther-apy, 1980.
107. Lawrence DG, Kuypers HGJM: Pyramidal and non-pyramidal pathways in mon-keys: Anatomical and functional correlation. Science 148:973, 1965.
108. Kuypers HGJM: The organization of the "motor system." Int J Neurol 4:78, 1963.
109. Buchwald J: A functional concept of motor control. Am J Phys Med 46(1):141, 1967.
110. Perry J, Giovan P, Harris LJ, et al: The determinants of muscle action in the hemiparetic lower extremity. Clin Orthop 131:71, March–April 1978.
111. Loria C: Relationship of proximal and distal function in motor development. Phys Ther 60:167, 1980.
112. Rood M: The use of sensory receptors to activate, facilitate and inhibit motor response, autonomic and somatic, in developmental sequence. In Third Interna-tional Congress, World Federation of Occupational Therapists, 1962: Approaches to the Treatment of Patients with Neuromuscular Dysfunction, Study Course VI. William C. Brown, Dubuque, IA, 1962.
113. Crutchfield, C, Barnes ML: The Neurophysiologic Basis of Patient Treatment. Vol 1: The Muscle Spindle. Stokesville Publishing Company, Morgantown, WV, 1973.
114. Milner-Brown HS, Penn RD: Pathophysiological mechanisms in cerebral palsy. J Neurol Neurosurg Psychiatry 42:606, 1979.
115. Nielson PD: Voluntary control of arm movement in athetotic patients. J Neurol Neurosurg Psychiatry 37:162, 1974.
116. Nielson PD: Measurement of involuntary arm movement in athetotic patients. J Neurol Neurosurg Psychiatry 37:171, 1974.
117. Bobath B: Adult Hemiplegia: Evaluation and Treatment. 2nd Ed. Heinemann, London, 1978.
118. Bobath B, Bobath K: Motor Development in the Different Types of Cerebral Palsy. Heinemann, London, 1976.
119. O'Connell A, Gardner E: Understanding the Scientific Bases of Human Move-ment. Williams and Wilkins, Baltimore, 1972.
120. Kelley D: Kinesiology Fundamentals of Motion Description. Prentice-Hall, En-glewood Cliffs, NJ, 1971.
121. Bly L: The components of normal movement during the first year of life. In Slaton D (ed): Development of Movement in Infancy. University of North Carolina at Chapel Hill, Division of Physical Therapy, 1981.
122. Bly L: Abnormal motor development. In Slaton D (ed): Development of Movement in Infancy. University of North Carolina at Chapel Hill, Division of Physical Ther-apy, 1981.

123. Easton TA: On the normal use of reflexes. Am Sci 60:591, 1972.

124. Kottke FJ: From reflex to skill: The training of coordination. Arch Phys Med Rehabil 61:551, 1980.

125. Capute AJ, Shapiro BK, Wachtel RC, et al: Motor functions: Associated primitive reflex profiles. Pediatr Res 14:431, 1980.

126. Graham FK, Strock BD, Zeigler BL: Excitatory and inhibitory influences on reflex responsiveness. In Collins WA (ed): Minnesota Symposium on Child Psychology. Vol 14. Lawrence Erlbaum Associates, Hillsdale NJ, 1980.

127. Oppenheim RW: Ontogenetic adaptations and retrogressive processes in the development of the nervous system and behavior: A neuro-embryological perspective. In Connolly KJ, Prechtl HFR (eds): Maturation and Development. Clinics in Developmental Medicine, No. 77/78. Lippincott, Philadelphia, 1981.

128. Okado N, Kakimi S, Kojima T: Synaptogenesis in the cervical cord of the human embryo: Sequence of synapse formation in a spinal reflex pathway. J Comp Neurol 184:491, 1979.

129. Thexton AJ: Some aspects of neurophysiology of dental interest. I. Theories of oral function. J Dent 2:49, 1973.

130. Thexton AJ: Some aspects of neurophysiology of dental interest. II. Oral reflexes and neural oscillators. J Dent 2:131, 1974.

131. Evarts EV: Brain mechanisms of movement. Sci Am 421:164, 1979.

132. Marcus E: The motor system and the integration of reflex activity. In Curtis BA, Jacobson S, Marcus EM (eds): An Introduction to the Neurosciences. Saunders, Philadelphia, 1972.

133. Hooker D: The Prenatal Origin of Behavior. University of Kansas Press, Lawrence, 1952.

134. Humphrey T: The relation of oxygen deprivation to fetal reflex arcs and the development of fetal behavior. J Psychol 35:3, 1953.

135. Humphrey T: Some correlations between the appearance of human fetal reflexes and the development of the nervous system. Prog Brain Res 4:93, 1964.

136. Jacobs MJ: Development of normal motor behavior. Am J Phys Med 46:41, 1966.

137. Windle WF, Fitzgerald JE: Development of the spinal reflex mechanism in human embryos. J Comp Neurol 67:493, 1937.

138. Fitzgerald JE, Windle WF: Some observations on early fetal movements. J Comp Neurol 76:159, 1942.

139. Eviator L, Eviator A: Neurovestibular examination of infants and children. Adv Otorhinolaryngol 23:169, 1978.

140. Touwen B: Neurological Development in Infancy. Clinics in Developmental Medicine, No. 58. Lippincott, Philadelphia, 1976.

141. Touwen B: Variability and stereotypy in normal and deviant development. In Apley J (ed): Care of the Handicapped Child. A Festschrift for Ronald MacKeith. Clinics in Developmental Medicine, No. 67. Lippincott, Philadelphia, 1978.

142. Campbell SK: Oral sensorimotor physiology. In Wilson JM (ed): Oral-Motor Function and Dysfunction in Children. University of North Carolina at Chapel Hill, Division of Physical Therapy, 1978.

143. Prechtl H: The study of neural development as prospective of clinical problems. In Connolly KJ, Prechtl HFR (eds): Maturation and Development: Biological and Psychological Perspectives. Clinics in Developmental Medicine, No. 77/78. Lippincott, Philadelphia, 1981.

144. Oppenheim RW: The neuroembryological study of behavior: progress, problems, perspectives. Curr Top Dev Biol 17:257, 1982.

145. Evarts E: The interaction of central commands and peripheral feedback in pyramidal track neurons (PTN's) of the monkey. In Herman RM, et al (eds): Neural Control of Locomotion. Plenum Press, New York, 1976.

146. Keshner EA: Reevaluating the theoretical model underlying the neurodevelopmental theory; Literature review. Phys Ther 61:1035, 1981.

147. Landmesser L: The development of motor circuits in the limb moving segments of the spinal cord. In Herman RM, et al (eds): Neural Control of Locomotion. Plenum Press, New York, 1976.

148. Taub E: Motor behavior following deafferentation in the developing and motorically mature monkey. In Herman RM, et al (eds): Neural Control of Locomotion. Plenum Press, New York, 1976.

149. Burke D: The activity of human muscle spindle endings in normal motor behavior. p 216. In Porter R (ed): International Review of Physiology. Neurophysiology IV. University Park Press, Baltimore, 1982.

150. Stuart DG: Conditional Nature of Spinal Reflexes. Read at the Missouri Physical Therapy Association Fall Meeting, St. Louis, MO, 1981.

151. Brodal A: Anatomy of the vestibulo-reticular connections and possible ascending vestibular pathways from the reticular system. Prog Brain Res 37:553, 1972.

152. Brodal A: Some reflexions on the relations between the reticular formation and the vestibular muscle. Prog Brain Res 37:639, 1972.

153. Scholz JP, Campbell SK: Muscle spindles and the regulation of movement. Phys Ther 60:1416, 1980.

154. Fredrickson JM, Kornhuber HH, Schwarz DWF: Cortical projections of the vestibular nerve. In Kornhuber HH (ed): Handbook of Sensory Physiology. Vol VI, Part 1. Vestibular System, Basic Mechanisms. Springer-Verlag, New York, 1974.

155. Odkvist LM, Ludgren SRC, Aschan G: Cerebral cortex and vestibular nerve. Adv Otorhinolaryngol 22:125, 1977.

156. Moore JM: Sensory Systems in the Developing Nervous System. Read at the Fourth Annual Adaptation Symposium, Denver, CO, 1981.

157. Peiper A: Cerebral Function in Infancy and Childhood. Consultants Bureau, New York, 1963.

158. McGraw MB: The Neuromuscular Maturation of the Human Infant. Hafner Press, New York, 1945.

159. Gesell A: The ontogenesis of infant behavior. In: Manual of Child Psychology. 2nd ed. Carmichael L (ed): Wiley, New York, 1954.

160. Lipsitt LP: Developmental psychobiology comes of age: A discussion. In Lipsitt LP (ed): Developmental Psychobiology. The Significance of Infancy. Wiley, New York, 1976.

161. Brainerd CJ: Piaget's Theory of Intelligence. Prentice-Hall, Englewood Cliffs, NJ, 1978.

162. Zelazo PR: From reflexive to instrumental behavior. In Lipsitt LP (ed): Developmental Psychobiology. Lawrence Erlbaum Associates, Hillsdale, NJ, 1976.

163. Connolly KJ: Maturation and the ontogeny of motor skills. In Connolly KJ, Prechtl HFR (eds): Maturation and Development. Biological and Psychological Perspectives. Clinics in Developmental Medicine, No. 78/78. Lippincott, Philadelphia, 1981.

164. Lund JP: Evidence for a central neural pattern generator regulating the chewing cycle. In Anderson DJ, Matthews B (eds): Mastication. John Wright and Sons, Ltd, Bristol, 1976.

165. Thelen E: Rhythmical stereotypes in normal human infants. Anim Behav 27:699, 1979.

166. Paine RS, Donovan DE, Hubbell JP: Evolution of postural reflexes in normal infants and in the presence of chronic brain syndromes. Neurology 14:1036, 1974.

167. Saint-Anne Dargassies S: Neurobiological Development in the Full Term and Premature Infant. Elsevier/North-Holland, New York, 1977.

168. Carter RE, Campbell SK: Early neuromuscular development of the premature infant. Phys Ther 55:1332, 1975.

169. Capute AJ, Palmer FB, Shapiro BK, Ross A, Accardo PJ: The Primitive Reflex Profile: A new instrument to assess infant motor development. Pediatr Res 16:85A, 1982.

170. Capute AJ, Wachtel RC, Palmer FB, et al: A prospective study of three postural reactions. Dev Med Child Neurol 24:314, 1982.

171. Provost B: Normal development from birth to 4 months: Extended use of the NBAS-K. Part I. Phys Occup Ther Pediatr 1:39, 1980.

172. Provost B: Normal development from birth to 4 months: Extended use of the NBAS-K. Part II. Phys Occup Ther Pediatr 1:19, 1981.

173. Bierman-van Eendenburg MEC, Jurgens-van der zee AD, Olinga AA, et al: Predictive value of neonatal neurological examination: A follow-up study at 18 months. Dev Med Child Neurol 23:296, 1981.

174. Saint-Anne Dargassies S: Neurological maturation of the premature infant of 28–41 week's gestational age. In Falkner F (ed): Human Development. Saunders, Philadelphia, 1966.

175. Saint-Anne Dargassies S: The Development of the Nervous System in the Foetus. Monograph available from the author, 123 Boulevard de Port Royal, 75014, Paris, France. 1968.

176. Barnes MR, Crutchfield CA, Heriza CB: The Neurophysiological Basis of Patient Treatment. Vol. 2; Reflexes in Motor Development. Stokesville Publ, Morgantown, WV, 1978.

177. Coryell J, Cardinali N: The asymmetric tonic neck reflex in normal full-term infants. Phys Ther 59:747, 1979.

178. Andre-Thomas, Chesni Y, Saint-Anne Dargassies S: The Neurological Examination of the Infant. Clinics in Developmental Medicine, No. 1. Lippincott, Philadelphia, 1960.

179. Twitchell TE: Early development of avoiding and grasping reactions. In Locke S (ed): Modern Neurology. Little, Brown, Boston, 1969.

180. Coryell J, Henderson A: Role of the asymmetric tonic neck reflex in hand visualization in normal infants. Am J Occup Ther 33:255, 1979.

181. Twitchell TE: The automatic grasping responses of infants. Neuropsychologia 3:247, 1965.

182. Twitchell TE: Reflex mechanisms and the development of prehension. In Connally KJ (ed): Mechanisms of Motor Skill Development. Academic Press, New York, 1970.

183. Ammon JE, Etzel ME: Sensorimotor organization in reach and prehension. A developmental model. Phys Ther 57:7, 1977.

184. Milani-Comparetti A, Gidoni EA: Routine developmental examination in normal and retarded children. Dev Med Child Neurol 9:631, 1967.

185. A Manual of the Milani-Comparetti Testing Procedures. Meyer Children's Rehabilitation Institute, Omaha, NE, 1977.

186. Fiorentino MR: Reflex Testing Methods for Evaluating CNS Development. 2nd Ed. Charles C. Thomas, Springfield, IL, 1976.

187. Fiorentino MR: Normal and Abnormal Development. The Influences of Primitive Reflexes on Motor Development. Charles C Thomas, Springfield, IL, 1972.

188. Capute AJ, Accardo PJ, Vining EPG, et al: Primitive Reflex Profile. Monographs in Developmental Pediatrics. Vol 1. University Park Press, Baltimore, 1978.

189. Chandler LS, Andrews MS, Swanson MW: Movement Assessment of Infants. Rolling Bay Press, Rolling Bay, WA, 1980.

190. Hoskins TA, Squires JE: Developmental assessment: A test for gross motor and reflex development. Phys Ther 53:117, 1973.

191. Bobath B: The very early treatment of cerebral palsy. Dev Med Child Neurol 9:373, 1967.

192. Bobath K: The Motor Deficit in Patients with Cerebral Palsy. Clinics in Developmental Medicine, No. 23. Lippincott, Philadelphia, 1969.

193. Bobath K, Bobath B: Cerebral palsy. In Pearson PH, Williams CE (eds): Physical Therapy Services in the Developmental Disabilities. Charles C Thomas, Springfield, IL, 1972.

194. Paine RS: Neurological examination of infants and children. Pediatr Clin North Am 7:471, 1960.

195. Illingworth RS: Development of the Infant and Young Child. 3rd Ed. Livingstone, Edinburgh, 1967.

196. Mueller HA: Facilitating feeding and prespeech. In Pearson PH, Williams CE (eds): Physical Therapy Services in the Developmental Disabilities. Charles C Thomas, Springfield, IL, 1972.

197. Paine RS: The evolution of infantile postural reflexes in the presence of chronic brain syndromes. Dev Med Child Neurol 6:345, 1964.

198. Molnar GE: Motor deficit of retarded infants and young children. Arch Phys Med Rehabil 55:393, 1974.

199. Molnar GE: Analysis of motor disorder in retarded infants and young children. Am J Ment Defic 83:213, 1978.

200. Molnar GE: Cerebral palsy: Prognosis and how to judge it. Pediatr Ann 8:596, 1979.

201. Bleck EE: Locomotor prognosis in cerebral palsy. Dev Med Child Neurol 17:18, 1975.

202. Molnar GE, Gordon SU: Cerebral palsy: Predictive value of selected clinical signs for early prognostication of motor function. Arch Phys Med Rehabil 57:153, 1976.

203. Capute AJ, Accardo PJ, Vining EP, et al: Primitive reflex profile. A pilot study. Phys Ther 58:1061, 1978.

204. Effgen SK: Integration of the plantar grasp reflex as an indicator of ambulation potential in developmentally disabled infants. Phys Ther 62:433, 1982.

205. Chandler L: Movement Assessment in Infancy. Read at the Fourth Annual Adaptative Symposium. Denver, CO, 1981.

206. Bennett FC, Chandler LS, Robinson MN, et al: Spastic diplegia in premature infants: Etiologic and diagnostic considerations. Am J Dis Child 135:732, 1981.

207. Campbell SK, Wilhelm IJ: Development of Infants at Risk for CNS Dysfunction. Read at the American Physical Therapy Association Annual Meeting, Washington, DC, June 1981.

208. Campbell SK: Personal communication. October 1981.

209. Campbell SK, Wilhelm IJ: Developmental sequences in infants at risk for central nervous system dysfunction: The recovery process in the first year of life. In Stack JM (ed): The Special Infant—An Interdisciplinary Approach to the Optimal Development of Infants. Human Sciences Press, New York, 1982.

210. Ayres AJ: Sensory Integration and Learning Disorders. Western Psychological Services, Los Angeles, 1972.

211. Rider BA: Relationship of postural reflexes to learning disabilities. Am J Occup Ther 26:239, 1972.
212. Steinberg M, Rendle-Short J: Vestibular dysfunction in young children with minor neurological impairment. Dev Med Child Neurol 19:639, 1977.
213. Parr C, Routh DK, Byrd MT, et al: A developmental study of the asymmetrical tonic neck reflex. Dev Med Child Neurol 16:329, 1974.
214. Parmenter CL: The Asymmetrical tonic neck reflex in normal first and third grade children. Am J Occup Ther 29:463, 1975.
215. Sieg KW, Shuster JJ: Comparison of three positions for evaluating the asymmetric tonic neck reflex. Am J Occup Ther 33:311, 1979.
216. Harris NP: Duration and quality of the prone extension position in four-, six-, and eight-year-old normal children. Am J Occup Ther 35:36, 1981.
217. Zemke R: Incidence of ATNR response in normal preschool children. Phys Occup Ther Pediatr 1:31, 1981.

3 | An Integrated Approach to Treatment of the Pediatric Neurologic Patient

Darcy Umphred

HISTORICAL OVERVIEW

A half century ago Berta Bobath, Mary Fiorentino, Margaret Knott, Margaret Rood, Sarah Semans, and Dorothy Voss were beginning their professional careers. Although these young therapists could not foresee the impact they would make upon their chosen professions, each possessed great sensitivity to other people, keen visual observation skills, and the belief that patient care would be improved if clinicians constantly questioned and critically analyzed their work. Each tried to fit current scientific principles to the treatment protocols found to be successful and to formulate theories and hypotheses that could be shared with their colleagues.

Specific approaches associated with the names of these pioneers became well-known, although these concepts were not generated in close proximity, as their founders were located in distant parts of the United States and in England. In spite of this, each observed normal and abnormal movement patterns and tried to explain their sequential nature, and each tried to use her understanding of the central nervous system, based on available research, and her clinical expertise and translate these qualities into a sound rationale for treatment. Each conceptualized total evaluation and treatment approach for clients with neurologic dysfunction, which differed greatly from the orthopedic

89

approach of employing range of motion and strengthening exercises along with bracing.[1]

Brief summaries of the philosophy and treatment rationale for the various approaches used with children follow, although a summary can never give sufficient credit to the creativity and intellectual effort each founder has put into developing her approach.

Bobath: Neurodevelopmental Therapy

Bobath's initial clinical focus was on treatment of cerebral palsy,[2] but it has been expanded to incorporate management of many adult neurologic disabilities, especially adult hemiplegia.[3] Facilitation of normal movement patterns through various techniques of handling the client is the major approach used by therapists trained in neurodevelopmental therapy. The philosophy is that clients need to experience and learn normal automatic movement in its proper developmental sequence before being asked to carry out a volitional activity. The combination of automatic and volitional patterns occurs naturally in normal children but, to varying degrees, is missing in a child with cerebral palsy. The Bobaths believe that facilitation of the postural, righting, and equilibrium reactions, while controlling and modifying abnormal muscle tone, are the keys to unlocking these natural mechanisms.[4] In order to achieve normal movement, the integration of postural and pure movement-oriented patterns needs refinement. This is accomplished in and through use of all spatial positions in treatment and clearly stresses the rotatory components of movement.

The neurologic rationale used to explain the neurodevelopmental therapy approach has changed over time. Updating a rationale in order to incorporate current research and understanding of brain function in no way negates the clinical value of the approach. Clinical observation and sensitivity to the total needs of the client are important aspects of a neurodevelopmental therapy approach to management of neurologic dysfunction.

Fiorentino

Fiorentino has not developed a specific approach to treatment of cerebral palsy. Instead she has spent her professional career trying to identify reflex behavior, both normal and abnormal, commonly seen in cerebral palsy and how those behavioral responses are integrated into normal development.[5] This philosophy has influenced the evaluation and treatment procedures used by therapists across the United States. Reflex testing has become a common evaluation procedure used with almost all neurologically impaired clients. Fiorentino[6] does not train children to use reflexes; treatment emphasis is placed on integration of reflexes and abnormal tone into functional activities. The study of how these reflexes are triggered gives an important knowledge base to therapists, which then leads to better understanding of the child's clinical problem. Stressing the importance of integrating normal movement into a child's repertoire of behavior by facilitating patterns that naturally control and modify abnormal reflexes is Fiorentino's major emphasis. Incorporating normal perceptual strategies and learning while sequencing normal movement development helps to maintain a focus upon the total needs of the child.

Knott/Voss: Proprioceptive Neuromuscular Facilitation

The proprioceptive neuromuscular facilitation method of exercise is based upon principles of normal motor development. Knott and Voss[7,8] identified the importance of motor learning, which incorporates both the volitional control of a client and some aspects of movement that can be elicited without voluntary effort. These procedures emphasize use of specific spiral and diagonal movement patterns observed in normal motor behavior. Many additional therapeutic procedures such as use of stretch, resistance, traction, and approximation are usually incorporated into the diagonal patterns during treatment to increase facilitation of the proprioceptive system. Both founders believed that this sensory system plays a critical role in normal motor learning. The interweaving of agonist-antagonistic function in normal activity lead to the reciprocal patterns incorporated into the various spiral and diagonal exercise programs. Isometric patterns for joint stabilization, as well as isotonic patterns for functional performance are incorporated into the diagonal patterns during mat and plinth exercises as well as in activities of daily living. The appropriate combinations of diagonal movement, the rate, the specific range, and the degree of volitional effort, are determined by the therapist and based on the specific needs and level of development of the client. The total needs of the client are a major emphasis, and all sensory systems and their integration are intricately intertwined in this method of evaluation and treatment.

Rood

Rood identified a variety of developmental sequences she found to be critical for higher level performance. Her major clinical focus was the evaluation and treatment of children with cerebral palsy.[9,10] Basing her treatment concepts on normal development, she differentiated four general stages: mobility, stability, mobility in a weight-bearing pattern, and mobility in a non-weight-bearing pattern. In order to develop the manipulative and articulative skills required for high level motor function, progression through these stages of development is necessary. Specific treatment procedures, such as use of stretch, resistance, vibration, vestibular stimulation, color, and sound, are selected according to the desired response and needs of the client. Controlled sensory input based on neurophysiologic understanding of input-processing-output control systems is a critical aspect of this approach. Rood used the expression "duality of motor function," emphasized the critical link between posture and movement, and developed treatment procedures whose focus was on one or the other of the two systems. According to Rood, integration of mobility and stability or posture and movement is critical before higher level activities can be achieved. Her emphasis on the total child has helped many therapists to realize that a motor response is a sensory input or feedback for the next aspect of any performance and that awareness of the total sensory environment surrounding the child plays a critical role in facilitating that child's processing of inputs and ultimate response to the world.

Fay/Doman-Delacato: Patterning

Fay, a neurosurgeon, believed that using reflex behaviors would lead to normal processing in lower centers in the brain, which would eventually bring about higher level integration.[11,12] He believed that normal movement was based upon primitive patterns similar to those observed in amphibians, reptiles, and mammals and that neonates and children also exhibit these patterns. Thus Fay believed that by moving children through these patterns, or exercising within them, motor development would improve. Doman and Delacato expanded Fay's procedures and have generalized the treatment protocol to incorporate broader central nervous system organization. Homolateral and cross-diagonal patterns in a variety of spatial positions are included in many of the therapeutic procedures. The term "patterning" is often associated with this approach because of the emphasis placed on passively guiding the child's body parts through certain patterns. Although a trained therapist can use this approach in a clinic, the majority of patterning is done by family and volunteer helpers. More than with other approaches, conflict has developed between the advocates of this method and therapists whose background is in other approaches. Although this controversy, at times, has been very emotional, the fact that many children and adults have shown improvement with patterning would suggest some clinical validity. Analyzing any approach, not just in totality, but also by its component parts, often leads to insight into new and creative methods of successful treatment.

Current Trends

The 1960s brought a new era in the development of these treatment approaches to neurologic disabilities. The founders or their proteges began to congregate at conferences to present their approaches to large groups of people with similar interests and background.[13,14] Additional colleagues such as Jean Ayres also began to present conceptual frameworks for clinical practice. At the conclusion of each of these institutes, an individual or a group of colleagues would summarize the material presented at these meetings and project future trends. Ayres believed in 1962 that the 1980s would bring a unified neurophysiologic approach to treatment of clients with central nervous system dysfunction.[13] The same projection for the future was made in Chicago in 1967.[14] At that time, traditional orthopedic as well as neurophysiologically based techniques were discussed. The question must now be posed as to whether growth has occurred in the projected direction of a unified approach.

The complexity of the brain and our minimal understanding of its function create a salutary climate for numerous explanations of specific behaviors. The rationales used to explain why and how behaviors can be altered are equally numerous. Two trends of thought or separate paths seem to have evolved with respect to neurophysiologic treatment techniques. The first path leading to expanded ideas, since the 1960s, has enticed many therapists to seek comprehensive training in specific techniques based upon one approach derived from one of the previously discussed clinicians. Although many skilled therapists have added to the development of a specific approach, the central core can easily be traced back to one root. This type of growth can lead to advanced clinical competencies; it can also lead to isolationism. Some clinicians may choose this training in a specific approach as a vehicle to project them quickly down the path toward clinical expertise, then pursue their careers with continued eagerness to learn. They use the past as a foundation for future growth and flexibility, always eager to grow in their understanding of the brain and its dysfunction. They become contributors to the intellectual and clinical growth of others yet to come. Unfortunately, other colleagues choose the path for its boundaries. They desire the structure and security of a label and hold tightly to the specific technique, arguing adamantly that their chosen approach has all the answers and that similarities between techniques do not and will not exist. They choose isolationism.

The second clinical trend stemming from the 1960s has led to development of conceptual models, or what are often referred to as integrated approaches to treatment of neurologic disabilities. The term "integrated" does not imply that each previously discussed individual approach is not a conceptual whole. Nor do the proponents of these integrated techniques pretend that all aspects of brain function and dysfunction have been incorporated into the model. *The conceptual framework of this newer philosophy is that commonalities between earlier approaches far outshine differences.* Linking together alternative techniques using neurophysiologic principles creates a stronger, more flexible, approach to client care. A clinician then has the flexibility to select treatment protocols that best fit the client's needs as well as his or her own skills.

Just as the individual techniques developed at similar times, yet in different places, so have these integrated approaches. In any integrated model,[4,15–17] all techniques make up the components of a new end product.

Unlike the earlier clinicians, the proponents of integrated approaches such as Shereen Farber, Eleanor Gilfolye, Anne Grady, Margot Heiniger, Joy Huss, Shirley Randolph, Shirley Stockmeyer, and Darcy Umphred have had the advantage of learning from the founders. Their knowledge and understanding of brain function, behavioral sequencing, and learning strategies have allowed them to start their professional careers at a point farther down the path toward being master clinicians. The new models will in time be components of a larger, more integrated whole, which future therapists will conceptualize.

CONCEPTUAL MODEL

Although some differences exist among the new conceptual models,[15–17] three large content areas can be identified as major components within each model. These areas are (1) normal sequential development, (2) neurophysiologic principles, and (3) the clinical learning environment. The specific emphasis within these areas and how each affects clinical performance is the key to identification of differences between the models. The specific conceptual framework presented in the following sections focus upon these three areas and their interrelationships, but it also represent's my own conceptual framework.[17,18]

Normal Sequential Development

Identification of the stages of normal sequential development has been one important tool for treatment of children with delayed or abnormal behavioral patterns. Therapists have accepted the hypothesis that the potential for normal human behavioral development is under genetic control, resulting in a sequence of observable motor patterns. Environmental factors seem to affect the specific development of perceptual, cognitive, and affective patterns and, in certain instances, even the motor patterns of the child. One can assume that following the normal sequences of motor development would be a good way to help a child with deviant development. Clear understanding of the sequential steps leading to development of any movement pattern would create an important knowledge base for a therapist.

Behavioral sequences are observable during normal development and do have a high degree of ordinality. That is, children learn to lift their heads in horizontal prior to rolling over. This is true for flexion and rotation, or extension and rotation aspects of the neck righting patterns, the pattern used by children when first rolling independently. The fact that these observable behaviors and their sequential nature have a constant order in each normal child's development is a critical element in a conceptual model. This stability gives a strong structural component to the model as well as an integrative thread between isolated techniques. For example, assume a hemiplegic child with cerebral palsy maintains a static posture in the affected upper extremity. Identification of the pattern may result in a verbal description indicating the presence of shoulder adduction, medial rotation, and slight flexion, elbow flexion, and wrist and finger flexion with forearm pronation. The exact tonal characteristics vary slightly with head position and degree of stress. Bobath[2] might state that the behavior is a remnant of the traction response. In order to integrate that response, working in a pattern that facilitates protective extension and maintains inhibition over the spastic pattern would be the treatment choice. A second approach might describe the pattern as the result of release of motor tracts, such as the vestibulospinal and reticulospinal tracts, from higher center inhibition. This results in the production of the observed pattern. One optimal choice for treatment would be to place extreme stretch on the spastic muscles to maintain inhibition through presumed activation of Golgi tendon organs. This stretch should incorporate rotation as well as motions in the cardinal planes to make sure that all spastic muscles participating in the deviant pattern are on stretch. Facilitation of the antagonistic pattern will come not only through externally applied treatment techniques, such as quick stretch or vibration, but

also through r~ ˙ ~al spinal cord circuits such as those activated by Golgi
ten·· ˙ ·ducing facilitation of antagonist muscles. Although the
˙he cause-effect relationship and of the various possible
˙nd extremely different, the pattern all three techniques
˙ulder flexion, abduction, and lateral rotation, elbow
˙ʌ wrist and finger extension with forearm supination. Whether
ʌ is elicited in horizontal, sitting, kneeling, during rolling, or as sec-
ʋnal flexion in proprioceptive neuromuscular facilitation, will depend
˙ʌ the treatment approach used and the therapist's choice, but the observed
behavioral pattern that is the goal for treatment of the upper extremity is the
same. Thus commonalities among techniques exist because the same behaviors
are observed and desired, although verbal description of them may vary dramatically.

This behavior constancy allows therapists to use the patterns of sequential
development in evaluation protocols. Whether a clinician is using reflexes,
specific age-related items, motor assessment, or activities of daily living testing,
each type of assessment incorporates the sequential nature of development of
the central nervous system. For that reason all four types of evaluation procedures should reveal similar information. A reflex test produces an evaluation
of the motor response patterns to specific stimuli. The same stimuli are often
used on age-related items, motor assessment, or activities of daily living tests.
Depending upon the chosen test form, a clinician should be able to extract data
that could then be used to complete any one of the other forms. For example:
assume a strong, dominant, and bilateral asymmetric tonic neck reflex is identified on a reflex test. Any test item that asks the child while turning the head
to perform a task where the extremities need to assume positions contrary to
those of the total asymmetric tonic neck reflex pattern would be impossible.
An age-related item might be prone on extended elbows reaching to the right
in a visually directed activity. An activities of daily living task might be transferring in and out of the tub. Both items require patterns different from the
response of the asymmetric tonic neck reflex; thus the child would fail. On the
other hand, if an activities of daily living form was selected as the primary
evaluation prototype, then a clinician should recognize that the child cannot
transfer in and out of the tub because of the dominant tonal characteristics
observed in the extremities as the head is turned. These patterns would lead
to recognition of the presence of an asymmetric tonic neck reflex.

If an evaluation item is only used to determine whether a child can or
cannot perform successfully on a task, or whether a reflex is present, then
tremendous amounts of pertinent data are lost. Similarly, the time needed to
evaluate thoroughly becomes more demanding if one needs to test each item
on a variety of test forms. Integration means connecting parts into a whole.
Using knowledge of sequential development in an integrated manner leads to
greater flexibility for the therapist with respect to choice of tools as well as
more efficient clinical data collection.

Unfortunately most types of evaluation forms do not easily lead to treatment sequencing. Knowing that a child has a dominant asymmetric tonic neck

reflex does not tell the therapist how best to develop shoulder stabilization. Knowing that a child can perform 6 out of 7 items at a 3-month level, 4 out of 8 at a 6-month level, 2 out of 9 at a 9-month level, and none at a 12-month level is not easily equated to the need to work on a coming-to-sitting-from-prone activity. Nor does knowing that a child can succeed at specific activities of daily living items when some look normal, some awkward, and some bizarre provide significant help to a therapist in how to sequence treatment. Again the integrative link comes with the therapist's ability to take the evaluation data and translate that information into a total framework reflecting all aspects of the child's skills and problems. The ability to do this may require certain cognitive strategies on the part of the therapist, such as the visual-analytical style of holding and rotating images in one's head, or simultaneously overlapping multiple images and summing the net effect. The problem of interpreting evaluation data into usable information is not unique to an integrated model. Yet, more difficulty is present than in isolated approaches because the therapist attempts to incorporate all techniques and alternative approaches into the creation of plans based on the needs of individual children. A high level of problem-solving skill is required.

Several alternative ways to use knowledge of development can be used in treatment planning. First, a therapist can assume that the sequences a child goes through naturally progress from easy to complex and should be presented to a client in that order. For example, when children learn to come to sitting, they first roll to prone, push up to the four-point position and rotate through sidesitting to sitting. Later they rotate to sidelying and push up, using partial trunk rotation. Finally, they progress from a semipartial rotation pattern to an adult pattern of assuming sitting. This is a logical and observable three-step sequence of possible patterns for coming to sitting which seem to go from easy to complex. A second alternative way to use knowledge of normal development would be to consider all possible patterns of muscular coordination used in an activity and determine which developmental factors would assist and which would prevent normal sequencing of the activity. If any of these inhibitory factors are observable in the client, their presence may influence selection of treatment strategies. For example, if a child demonstrates moderate flexor tone in prone with persistence of a symmetric tonic neck reflex, then rolling to prone, pushing up to four-point, followed by rotating into sidesitting may be more difficult than using partial rotation from supine. A therapist using an integrated model would possibly teach a partial-rotation sequential pattern before the prone to four-point pattern. The selection of this sequence does not negate the importance of a child learning to move in space using all three sequential patterns, if possible. It does suggest that the whole is more important than the specific temporal sequencing of any one action. A framework for analyzing activities into component parts is valuable for treatment planning.

This type of activity analysis clarifies the reason for the belief that early sequential behaviors lay the foundation for more advanced skills. As an early behavior, a movement pattern may stand alone as the only component necessary for a movement sequence. When analyzing a more complex movement, that earlier behavior may be only one of many patterns necessary for normal coordination. For example, if a child has not developed the trunk rotation patterns first observed in rolling, then, even though the child can hold the positions of kneeling and half-kneeling, sequencing the transition from kneeling to half-kneeling would be extremely difficult, if not impossible. For the child to advance one step farther, modification of the neck righting and body on body righting responses must be accomplished. The righting is necessary to sequence movement initially from kneel to half-kneel. Modification of the righting is needed to hold the half-kneeling leg in position while the upper body and head rotates back to assume a symmetric trunk posture.

Neurophysiologic Principles

All founders of the original approaches believed that having a sound rationale for any and all treatment procedures was vital for professional validation. Neurophysiology is the basic science for the study of brain function. The founders, as do current clinicians, used this area of study and research to develop the rationales behind the various therapeutic procedures. This science is in a constant state of change as new research uncovers more information regarding brain function. The neurophysiologic rationales of the original approaches do differ and, as a result, some controversies exist among their proponents. Proponents of integrated models avoid the controversies by accepting all approaches as possible treatment alternatives. If treatment strategies can elicit more normal behavior, then a neurophysiologic explanation must exist. Whether that explanation needs modification or even total revision as new research is uncovered should not inhibit the clinician. Just because a once-accepted rationale is no longer valid, the treatment is not necessarily invalid. Clinical research of a controlled nature in which the effectiveness of therapy is investigated is a better way to validate treatment procedures. The combination of better clinical research studies, and updating of the neurophysiologic knowledge used to describe treatment rationales, would be an integrated route toward higher level understanding of clinical results and generation of new treatment rationales based on scientific inquiry and hypotheses based on current neurophysiologic theory.

One way to integrate treatment techniques might be to classify all techniques according to the sensory system to which they are directed.[16] If a response to a certain type of stimulus can be identified, then any technique using a similar stimulus should elicit a similar response. An example of this type of classification scheme is shown in Table 3-1. The scheme identifies the primary input modality for specific treatment techniques; no technique uses only one type of input. The reader can observe that a large number of treatment techniques can use one primary sensory modality, such as somatic proprioception—the muscle spindle. The listed treatment procedures have been advocated by a variety of therapists and used in a number of treatment approaches. If a therapist uses only one approach, then some limitation may exist as to the number of available treatment strategies. If instead, an integrated model ap-

Table 3-1. Classification Scheme

Sensory Modality: Somatic Proprioception Specific Receptor Muscle spindle	Stimuli	Physiologic Response	Treatment Techniques
Ia tonic	Length	Agonist facilitation Antagonist inhibition	1. Quick stretch 2. Sustained stretch 3. Tapping
Ia phasic	Rate of length	Agonist facilitation Antagonist inhibition	4. Reverse tapping 5. Resistance
II's	Change of length	? Most likely same as Ia's	6. Positioning 7. Vibration 8. Electrical stimulation 9. Gravity 10. Pressure on muscle belly 11. Stretch-pressure 12. Etc.
Tendon	Tension		
Joint			
Combined Somatic Proprioceptive Input Spindle and joint Etc.			

proach is used, a clinician should feel free to use any technique. The decision as to preferential selection of any of the techniques then depends upon client needs, client response sensitivity, social acceptability and inherent nature of the various stimuli, allowing tremendous flexibility for the therapist. Knowing a large variety of clinical techniques that may elicit the same response allows the therapist opportunity (1) to change treatment strategies without altering the primary goal, (2) to select and combine additional strategies in order to increase the intensity of the input through spatial summation, and (3) to create novelty for the client, which should promote better learning.

Each specific sensory system can be broken down in a similar fashion as shown in Table 3-1. A therapist must analyze each procedure with respect to the stimuli used to elicit the response, as well as the response itself. Otherwise incorrect classification may occur. For example, quick icing elicits muscle contraction. If a therapist thinks of muscle contraction, he or she may think of proprioception and thus may categorize quick ice under proprioception, rather than the appropriate stimulus category of exteroception through activation of cutaneous receptors.

Once methods of activating specific sensory systems have been identified, techniques that affect multiple sensory systems need to be classified. For example, the technique of sweep-tapping uses a combination of tactile and proprioceptive input. Within the specific approaches to treatment of neurologic problems, techniques are constantly being combined into a complex program of inputs. For that reason, trying to mimic or copy step by step a procedure used by another therapist is almost impossible. By using a common classification system, a therapist has the flexibility to develop individual potential, analyze treatment protocols, and model someone else's talents at a professional-analytical level.

The third area relating to stimulus-response techniques might be called inherent processes, defined as internal neuromechanisms that have been laid down genetically. Reflexes, reactions, synergistic patterns, and learned behaviors can be placed within this system and need classification. In some instances, especially with spinal reflexes, the specific sensory system responsible for evoking a given response pattern has been identified. In others, circuits are hypothetical. Because of the complexity and lack of understanding of brain function, the neural circuits subserving some behaviors cannot be identified at all; indeed, vast numbers of circuits are probably simultaneously involved in any complex activity. Through observation, however, at least three behavioral characteristics inherent to the normal human organism can be identified. The consistency of these characteristics means a neurophysiologic explanation must exist, even if it has not yet been found. Although these inherent processes are identified in normal development, they also relate to children with neurologic impairment who seem to get locked into response patterns that would be considered abnormally dominant and of a lower order. This order does not necessarily reflect structural levels of processing within the central nervous system but rather a hierarchic level of *function*. The three principles relating to inherent processes are as follows:

1. A hierarchic functional relationship of reflexes and reactions exists.
   a. The higher order the reaction, the more complex the response.
   b. Higher order reactions integrate, modify or inhibit lower order reflexes.
   c. Lower order reflexes can block a higher order reaction but cannot otherwise control or modify it.
2. Different types of responses to the same stimulus can occur.
   a. Dominant patterns: if stimulus is present, response is obligate, although postural tone may vary.
   b. Typical patterns are present but not dominant. Stimulus influences tone, but client is not obligated to the pattern of response.
   c. Patterns are modified, integrated, or inhibited from higher centers. Client can inhibit the response or can allow pattern to be expressed, as appropriate to ongoing activity.
3. An interactive relationship of all reflexes and responses exists within the central nervous system.
   a. Two or more potential reflexes or reactions can interact to produce a response whose end product is a combination of patterns.

Although the specific neuronal networks causing these observable trends in stimulus-response reactions are not known, holding in mind a gestalt of the interweaving mechanisms within the many circuits and systems of the central nervous system is important when using these principles in treatment.

Principle 1 (hierarchic relationships) is presented in Figure 3-1. The hierarchic nature of behavior helps a therapist identify relevant treatment sequences. For example, assume a child has a dominant asymmetric tonic neck

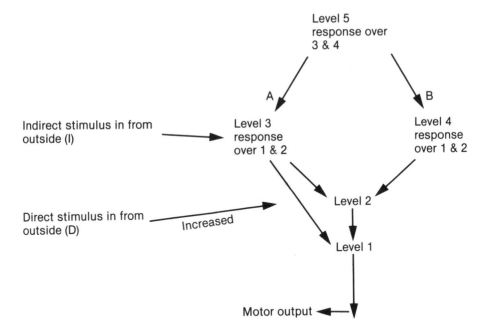

D = direct stimulus from outside which naturally elicits a reflex or response
    pattern in man

I = indirect stimulus such as vision, audition, or intentional motor planning which
    elicits a stimulus. That stimulus normally facilitates motor response.

Level	Stimulus	Response – Motor Output
1.	Therapist rotates head to right (D)	Child goes into ATNR
2.	Therapist rotates head to right (D)	Child rolls over to right
3a.	Therapist rotates head to right (D)	Child inhibits both ATNR and NR (inhibits level 1 and 2 responses)
3b.	Therapist increases rate/amount of stimulus (D)	Child rolls over (facilitates level 2 due to increased stimulus)
4.	Child turns head toward a stimulus (I)	Child rolls over (facilitates level 2)
5a.	Child turns head toward a stimulus (I)	Child inhibits body righting after the head (inhibits 1 & 2)
5b.	Child turns head toward a stimulus (I)	Child intentionally rolls toward the target
5c.	Therapist rotates head with high velocity/intensity of stimulus (D)	Child inhibits response: controls environment

Fig. 3-1. Hierarchic behavioral relationship of asymmetric tonic neck reflex, neck righting, and higher order patterns.

reflex to the right. Figure 3-1 suggests a clear treatment sequence. If a dominant asymmetric tonic neck reflex is present to head turning, then modification of that reflex will be important in order for the child to gain normal neck righting and rolling patterns. If the typical pattern elicited is at stimulus-response Level 1 (a dominant reflex), then asking for control and modification of that response (Level 5), especially with a rapidly applied stimulus, would be an extremely difficult, if not impossible, task for the child. Such a demand would require tremendous conscious energy not then available for other, higher level, tasks. Identifying which reflexes and reactions have this hierarchic nature with typical responses at Levels 1 and 2 is important in understanding the abnormal central nervous system. Realizing that a child can inhibit a response at about the same time developmentally that the child will automatically demonstrate the response is important. Knowing that at least two internal systems exist for control of behavior, one facilitory and one inhibitory, helps the therapist to identify which mechanisms are functioning, at what level, and whether the child has control over both. Obviously a primary treatment objective is the child's independence and flexibility when dealing with the environment, a Level 5 response to all incoming stimuli.

Principle 2, that different types of responses can occur to the same stimulus, also gives important clinical information. The central nervous system is set up to produce and modify output response according to incoming sensory data and internal control signals. The resulting control is not an "all or none" mechanism but rather on a gradient from facilitating maximal response to off. The off end of the spectrum would mean no observable response, although neuroexcitation in central circuits may still be present. This second principle tells a therapist that if a child is limited to a dominant pattern distribution of abnormal tone, whether labeled a reflex or a synergistic pattern, development of control over that tone will follow a specific order or treatment sequence. Unless spontaneous return occurs, the child will not go from dominant tone directly to controlled tone. The therapist may first need to modify the tone via techniques such as handling to modify postural set and then begin to demand in an activity that the child take over more control as he progresses. The purpose of the therapist-controlled activity is to provide normal feedback to the child's central nervous system to assist that child in gaining a higher and more normal level of function.

The third principle, that of an interactive relationship of reflexes and reactions, causes more frustration for therapists in the clinical setting than any other. As students we learn to recognize behaviors in pure form. We verbally rehearse the behavior and construct a visual image of its appearance. The exact image created in the mind of the clinician may not match the specific pattern observed in the child. Even if the therapist has a flexible mental image of a reflex pattern that incorporates a large number of variations of response patterns, the child's motor responses to various stimuli may not be what the clinician expects to see. The child, however, may still have dominant reflex behaviors that incorporate the specific pattern the therapist was trying to test and observe. The primary reason for the discrepancy is related to principle 3. The concept of an interaction of responses means that a vast number of possible spatial patterns of posture and movement are possible; the more flexible the central nervous system, the greater the variety available. The potential for these interactions always exists if adequate stimuli are present. Higher centers must control and modify these interactions to avoid the production of stereotyped dominant patterns.

Neurophysiology helps to explain the reasons why events do or do not occur in the client-therapist interaction. Maintaining a high level of understanding through study is a constant challenge.

The Clinical Learning Environment

The third and major area within an integrated model might be labeled the clinical learning environment and may be the key to the art of therapy. All clinicians elicit responses, ask the client to help, provide success, allow failure, stop to give the child a hug, or are stern and demand that the child respond. A gifted few seem to know just the correct time to do any one of those activities in order to facilitate optimal responses from the child. Some therapists never know the correct time and probably stop treating children. Most of us fall somewhere along the spectrum between the former and the latter. We also seem to be more successful with some children than with others. The question arises as to what behaviors gifted therapists use that explain their success. Undoubtedly many variables interact to create that high level of talent. If analysis is made of the interactive environment, however, some answers can be found.

Four major environmental categories affect the total therapeutic setting: the external and internal environments of the child and those of the clinician. The focus of therapy is generally upon affecting the internal mechanism of the child with little focus placed upon the other three components. The problem with that approach is that the external environment bombards the child with millions of stimuli per second. The intensity and the duration of this stimulation will affect many processing and response patterns within the central nervous system of the child, irrespective of the presence of dysfunction. The processing and responses affect perception and learning and thus the attention to and processing of future stimuli. For example, if the child is emotionally upset because of personal interaction in the external environment, then his or her internal environment has been altered. The child's response to the treatment procedures will be different than if the emotional factors were not present. The therapist, being part of the child's external worls, also has the ability to alter the child's internal environment. How that is accomplished depends in turn upon the therapist's internal processing system, which is being affected by his other external environment (Fig. 3-2). No matter which specific approach a therapist may use, all are trying to help the child learn a more efficient way to deal with the external world. They do this by altering the external environment in ways that enhance learning better motor control. In fact, the clinician might be considered a huge biofeedback system. The more efficient that system is at

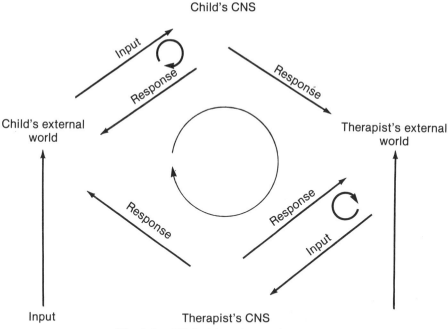

Fig. 3-2. Clinical learning environment.

regulating input, the better the response of the child. Thus, the child's central nervous system may not be the crucial element, but rather that of the clinician. The gifted therapist maintains a sensitivity to multiple stimuli coming from the child while focusing upon facilitating a desired response pattern. The therapist continues treatment or input to the child's output, then alters treatment slightly in order to regain the desired response. The thought process used by the therapist appears to have a strong spatial component. The clinician is holding mentally a huge number of simultaneous visual and kinesthetic inputs that require simultaneous and sequential processing. Perhaps those who are gifted therapists possess a high level of spatial-analytical ability. These cognitive strategies are not generally taught in school; thus the therapist's gift may be innate. This hypothesis does not state that these learning styles make a gifted therapist or that they cannot be taught to most students. It does suggest that this strategy may be an important element in the child-therapist learning environment.

Another factor leading to the high success of some colleagues may stem from their ability to identify the primary learning styles of a child and adapt their instruction to match that style. In order to do this, a therapist would not only need a large repertoire of accessible instructional strategies, but also the flexibility of shifting strategies according to the needs of the child.

Before we can find answers we sometimes need to pose more thoughtful questions. What those questions are will depend upon future therapists and their skill in uncovering critical attributes of the clinical interaction. As more is learned about the normal learning environment, its application to the clinical environment must also be integrated into the therapeutic model.

CONCLUSION

Development of an integrated model does, however, reflect a change. That change veers away from the philosophy that individual approaches (1) need to be followed explicitly, (2) cannot be interchanged, and (3) if combined, may harm the child. This does not mean that some techniques are not more appropriate at times, nor does it mean that those who use one approach are narrow, inflexible, or unwilling to accept new ideas. Using an integrated model as a philosophical base does not make the task of the therapist any easier. In reality, it may be more difficult, for it requires the clinician to be flexible, analytical, and willing to accept all approaches as possible treatment alternatives.

REFERENCES

1. Pinkston D: Analysis of traditional regimens of therapeutic exercise. Am J Phys Med 46:713, 1967.
2. Bobath B: Abnormal Postural Reflex Activity Caused by Brain Lesions. Heinemann, London, 1971.
3. Bobath B: Adult Hemiplegia: Evaluation and Treatment. Heinemann, London, 1978.
4. Bobath K, Bobath B: Cerebral palsy. In Pearson PH, Williams CE (eds): Physical Therapy Services in the Developmental Disabilities. Charles C Thomas, Springfield, IL, 1972.
5. Fiorentino MR: Normal and Abnormal Development. Charles C Thomas, Springfield, IL, 1972.
6. Fiorentino MR: A Basis for Sensorimotor Development—Normal and Abnormal. Charles C Thomas, Springfield, IL, 1981.
7. Voss DE: Proprioceptive neuromuscular facilitation: The PNF Method. In Pearson PH, Williams CE (eds): Physical Therapy Services in the Developmental Disabilities. Charles C Thomas, Springfield, IL, 1972.
8. Knott M, Voss DE: Proprioceptive Neuromuscular Facilitation: Patterns and Techniques. Harper & Row, New York, 1968.
9. Stockmeyer SA: An interpretation of the approach of Rood to the treatment of neuromuscular dysfunction. Am J Phys Med 46:900, 1967.
10. Stockmeyer SA: A sensorimotor approach to treatment. In Pearson PH, Williams CE (eds): Physical Therapy Services in the Developmental Disabilities. Charles C Thomas, Springfield, IL, 1972.
11. Fay T: The neurophysical aspects of therapy in cerebral palsy. In Payton OD, Hirt S, Newton RA (eds): Scientific Bases for Neurophysiologic Approaches to Therapeutic Exercise: An Anthology. Davis, Philadelphia, 1977.
12. Page D: Neuromuscular reflex therapy as an approach to patient care. Am J Phys Med 46:816, 1967.

13. Third International Congress—World Federation of Occupational Therapists: Approaches to the Treatment of Patients with Neuromuscular Dysfunction. William C. Brown, Dubuque, IA, 1962.

14. Proceedings: An exploratory and analytical survey of therapeutic exercise. Am J Phys Med 46, 1967.

15. Heiniger M, Randolph S: Neurophysiological Concepts in Human Behavior: The Tree of Learning. Mosby, St. Louis, 1981.

16. Farber SD: A multisensory approach to neurorehabilitation. In Farber SD (ed): Neurorehabilitation: A Multisensory Approach. Saunders, Philadelphia, 1982.

17. Umphred DA: Conceptual model: A framework for clinical problem solving. In Umphred DA (ed): Textbook for Physical Therapy. Vol III. Mosby, St. Louis, (in press).

18. Umphred DA, McCormick G: Classification of common facilitory and inhibitory treatment techniques. In Umphred DA (ed): Textbook for Physical Therapy. Vol III. Mosby, St. Louis, (in press).

4 | The Neurologically Suspect Neonate

Irma J. Wilhelm

WHO IS THE HIGH-RISK INFANT?

The term "high-risk infant" has many meanings, often dependent on the professional background of the user. To the obstetrician, an unborn fetus is considered to be a potential high-risk infant if the mother is considered high-risk for obstetric casualty. To the pediatrician or neonatologist these factors are also important, but the newborn infant's risk status is evaluated initially as it relates to that infant's risk of neonatal death. Finally, to those concerned with the long-term care of infants and children (e.g., therapists, educators, psychologists) the high-risk infant is a baby who, for whatever reason, is likely to have significant developmental deviance, including mental retardation, neuromuscular dysfunction, learning disability, psychiatric disorders, or social/emotional problems.

For the purpose of this discussion, the definition of the high-risk infant must be limited so as to maintain a focus useful to the reader and to avoid overlap with other topics in this volume. A definition provided by Parmelee and Haber[1] will be used as a framework. They considered a risk infant as "any newborn or young infant who has a high probability of manifesting in childhood a sensory or motor deficit and /or mental handicap."

Although they fit our definition, infants with recognizable or diagnosed congenital anomalies known to affect later development will not be discussed in this chapter because these conditions are treated elsewhere in this volume. We will concentrate on newborn infants at high risk for central nervous system (CNS) dysfunction (especially neuromotor dysfunction) as a result of certain perinatal events known to increase that risk.

For physical therapists, working with high-risk infants involves a set of circumstances very different from those to which they are accustomed in several basic ways. First, the high-risk infant is just that—*high-risk*—and may never be diagnosed as having any condition for which physical therapy is traditionally considered helpful. Second, the high technology nursery settings in which these infants are initially cared for are relatively unfamiliar to those physical therapists who work most with children (i.e., pediatric therapists involved with older children with central nervous system dysfunction) but also to those therapists more familiar with acute care settings, but who usually care for adults (i.e., physical therapists in general hospital work). Third, the immediate goal for these infants is usually survival with relatively less emphasis, of necessity, being placed on long-term considerations (e.g., the quality of motor functioning) with which therapists are ultimately concerned. Fourth, the infant patient is afflicted with, or recovering from, a variety of conditions with which the average physical therapist has little familiarity either through clinical experience or basic education. Finally, the physical therapist is working with a number of other specialists who have not before been close colleagues in the more traditional hospital or rehabilitation setting (e.g., neonatologists and special care nurses); as well as with families in a special kind of crisis situation.

Given these unique circumstances, the physical therapist planning to enter this field of work is obligated to consider a number of important questions:

1. Does (or should) a physical therapist have a unique contribution to make to the management of an acutely ill neonate whose eventual neurologic outcome cannot be accurately predicted?

2. To which infants can the physical therapist contribute most, regardless of when the physical therapy involvement is begun?

3. What must the physical therapist do to become prepared to contribute to the care of high-risk infants?

4. What physical therapeutic theories and techniques will enable the physical therapist to contribute most effectively to the total management of high-risk infants?

The following discussion has a number of purposes related to the special circumstances previously described and to the questions posed. The first aim is to provide the reader with some background information about high-risk infants, the current status of the care they receive, the settings in which this care is delivered, and what is known about their neurologic outcome. A second purpose is to review critically the research on assessment and intervention with high-risk infants with the aim of gleaning from it some general principles and rationales the physical therapist might apply in developing programs to enhance motor functioning in these infants. Finally, some suggestions will be presented for physical therapists to consider in preparing for, developing, and evaluating therapeutic programs for high-risk infants.

PERINATAL EVENTS CONTRIBUTING TO RISK FOR CENTRAL NERVOUS SYSTEM DYSFUNCTION

The therapist involved with high-risk neonates will rarely be in a position to provide services to every infant entering a special care nursery. Logic would dictate, therefore, that consideration be given to those infants whose problems are most likely to result in later developmental dysfunction. A number of these problems have been studied extensively and will be reviewed here. The reader must remember, however, that very rarely can a single perinatal event be shown to contribute directly to later developmental dysfunction. Most likely clusters of perinatal problems, in combination with suboptimal environmental conditions in infancy, contribute most to poor long-term developmental outcome.

Very Low Birth Weight (VLBW)

Infants born prematurely or who are small for gestational age (SGA) are broadly classified by birth weight into two major groups: low birth weight (LBW), between 1501 and 2500 grams, and very low birth weight (VLBW), 1500 grams or less. This discussion will concentrate on VLBW infants, because recent reports indicate that LBW infants have relatively good prognoses for both survival and neurologic outcome, if they are otherwise basically healthy.[2-4]

The etiology of VLBW is, in many cases, still unknown, but it is highly associated with a number of maternal factors such as age (<15 or >44), chronic illness (e.g., hypertension), poor nutrition, smoking, low socioeconomic status, multiparity (>5), and past reproductive problems (e.g., habitual spontaneous abortion).[5]

VLBW infants represent only about 1.0 percent of live births in the United States, but this means that about 35,000 are born each year. They form the largest single group found in neonatal intensive care units (NICU) and follow-up clinics and are at increased risk for neonatal and postneonatal mortality and morbidity and for poor neurologic outcome.[5]

The actual fact of low birth weight is probably not the major contributor to later handicap, rather, the VLBW infant is particularly susceptible to a number of other neonatal conditions that may be exacerbated in an immature infant. Sostek and associates[6] list intraventricular hemorrhage, asphyxia, and meningitis among the major risk factors with potential to affect the central nervous system of the preterm infant; and birth asphyxia, sepsis, and meningitis as major problems in the term infant. Although general agreement exists that these are the major factors that place an infant at risk for central nervous system dysfunction, the degree of risk attributable to each is not known. Very likely the greatest risk occurs when, as is often the case, these factors become cumulative.[1,6]

Hypoxic-Ischemic Encephalopathy

The major etiologic factor in producing hypoxic-ischemic encephalopathy is perinatal asphyxia, which may occur in utero and produce respiratory failure at birth, or postnatally as a result of severe respiratory distress syndrome or apnea or from severe right-to-left shunting as a result of cardiovascular disease or persistent fetal circulation. About 90 percent of the cases are the result of intrauterine asphyxia.

Clinically the syndrome begins soon after the insult with the infant becoming stuporous and unresponsive. Seizures and apnea frequently begin during the first 24 hours of life. The infant who survives this period of about 72 hours usually goes on to show hypotonia and disturbance in sucking and swallowing. The rate of improvement is variable.[7]

The prognosis for survival and outcome is dependent on the location of the lesion and severity of the insult, both of which are difficult to assess clinically. Sarnat and Sarnat,[8] however, have identified three stages of postanoxic encephalopathy, the severity and duration of which was predictive of later status in 21 full-term asphyxiated neonates. Stage 1, when it occurred, lasted less than 24 hours and was characterized by hyperalertness, low threshold Moro responses, and stretch reflexes, but normal muscle tone, no seizures, and a normal electroencephalogram (EEG). Stage 2 was exhibited by all the infants and lasted about five days. It is characterized by lethargy or obtundation, mild hypotonia, strong distal flexion, hyperactive stretch reflexes, weak suck and Moro, strong tonic neck reflex, and multifocal seizures. Improvement in the EEG preceded improvement of clinical signs. Stage 3, or stupor, consisted of flaccidity alternating with intermittent decerebrate posturing, absent reflexes, response only to strong noxious stimuli, rare seizures, and an isopotential EEG. This stage lasted from a few hours to four weeks. Infants who never entered Stage 3 and recovered from Stage 2 within 5 days had good outcomes. Persistence of Stage 2 for over 7 days or failure of the EEG to revert to normal was associated with later neurologic impairment or death. In another study with 95 full-term asphyxiated infants,[9] the Sarnat and Sarnat system[8] was used to grade the degree of hypoxic-ischemic encephalopathy. Significant relationships with handicap or death were found for low 5-minute Apgar scores (0–3), seizures within the first day of life, Stage 2 or 3 hypoxic-ischemic encephalopathy or suppressed EEG. All children with Stage 3 hypoxic-ischemic encephalopathy had moderate or severe handicap or had died.

The majority of the studies of outcome in hypoxic-ischemic encephalopathy are of asphyxiated full-term infants and report mortality rates ranging from 7 to over 30 percent.[9–15] When VLBW or premature infants are included in study samples, the mortality rate is usually close to 50 percent overall and as high as 80 percent in the smallest infants.[12–14,16] Criteria for assessing long-term outcome in these studies vary, but most reports note rates of 2 to 25 percent of cerebral palsy in full-term survivors or mixed groups of full-term and preterm infants (although in most reports, the majority of VLBW infants did not survive to participate in the follow-up). Few data are available on the outcome of severely asphyxiated VLBW survivors, but theories are that the preterm infant who suffers asphyxia may develop more severe respiratory distress syndrome and be more likely to have brain hemorrhages, particularly in the periventricular area where many hypoxic-ischemic encephalopathy lesions occur. The severe respiratory distress syndrome probably occurs as a result of inhibition of surfactant synthesis.[16,17]

Intracranial Hemorrhage

Periventricular and intraventricular hemorrhage are the most common forms of intracranial hemorrhage in patients in the neonatal intensive care unit. Their incidence is inversely related to gestational age, and recent use of computed tomography (CT) has shown that 40 percent or more of VLBW infants demonstrate periventricular and intraventricular hemorrhage.[7]

In the preterm infant, hypoxia and intraventricular hemorrhage are intimately related; the latter typically follows an hypoxic-ischemic event. The site of initial bleeding is from the fragile capillary bed in the subependymal germinal matrix. The exact pathophysiology of intraventricular hemorrhage is still a matter of debate, but much more information is becoming available.[7,18–20]

Initially, periventricular hemorrhage ruptures into the ventricular system in about 80 percent of the cases and progresses into the posterior fossa where, after a time, arachnoiditis may develop, obstructing the cerebrospinal fluid flow and producing hydrocephalus.[7] The hemorrhage may also extend into the cerebral white matter, resulting in an intracerebral hematoma, which may then evolve into a porencephalic cyst.[21,22] Four grades are used for describing intraventricular hemorrhage in computed tomography and ultrasound scans or postmortem examinations: Grade I, isolated subependymal hemorrhage, Grade II, intraventricular hemorrhage without ventricular dilatation; Grade III, intraventricular hemorrhage with ventricular dilatation; Grade IV, intraventricular hemorrhage with ventricular dilatation and hemorrhage into the brain parenchyma.[23] Clinically, intraventricular hemorrhage is characterized either by a catastrophic deterioration that often results in death, a less dramatic sequence involving alterations of consciousness and mobility from which the infant eventually stabilizes, or an almost clinically silent presentation.[7] Because most early studies were based on autopsy data, the assumptions were that intraventricular hemorrhage was almost always fatal or, if not, survivors had uniformly poor prognoses for developing normally and the development of posthemorrhagic hydrocephalus was inevitable.[22,24] This was most likely because of the difficulty in diagnosing any but the most severe hemorrhages clinically, resulting in underestimates of true incidence and no knowledge of the range of severity of hemorrhages.[25]

Since the advent of computed tomography and ultrasound brain scanning, some of these assumptions have been challenged. The mortality from intraventricular hemorrhage is high, but the outcome is not as hopeless as was once thought. In several reports comparing VLBW infants with and without intraventricular hemorrhage, the mortality rates are between 50 and 60 percent in those who have this disorder, compared with 7 to 32 percent in the infants who do not.[25–27] With these methods of diagnosis, the incidence of intraventricular hemorrhage in survivors has been shown to range from 30 to 70 percent in VLBW infants.[24–30] The major factors associated with increased incidence of intraventricular hemorrhage, the mortality resulting, and poor outcome are the extent of the hemorrhage, the development of posthemorrhagic hydrocephalus, low birth weight and prematurity, and the general medical condition of the neonate. Handicap in survivors ranges from 20 to 35 percent, but can be as high as 40 to 50 percent in infants who develop hydrocephalus. Continuous seizures and delayed (>24 hours) neurologic recovery are prognosticators of poor outcome.[22,24–26,28,31–33]

Sepsis Neonatorum

The pathogens responsible for neonatal bacterial diseases constantly change for unknown reasons. The most common organisms now encountered are *Escherichia coli* and Group B streptococcus, which account for about 60 percent of the infections in North American nurseries. The blood stream is the primary site of infection, which occurs in 1 to 10 percent of live births (dependent on the maternal condition, degree of prematurity and need for postnatal life-support procedures). The majority of infections are transmitted from mother to infant during delivery, with increased risk in those with amniotic fluid infection, and even more if the infant is premature and membranes are ruptured >24 hours before delivery. About 25 percent of infections spread to the meninges.[34]

Group B streptococcal meningitis is frequently (in 65 to 90 percent of cases) associated with ventriculitis. The presence of ventriculitis contributes to poor response to antibiotic therapy and sequelae related to obstruction of cerebrospinal fluid flow. Poor prognosis is, therefore, directly related to the presence of ventriculitis and the persistence of positive cerebrospinal fluid cultures. Mortality rates range from 20 to 75 percent or more, and a substantial proportion of survivors have neurologic handicaps.[34,35]

Neonatal Seizures

"Seizures in the neonatal period are usually the clinical manifestation of serious underlying neurological disease."[7] These underlying causes include hypoxic-ischemic encephalopathy, intracranial hemorrhage, and intracranial infection. In newborn infants, and especially in premature infants, seizures are difficult to recognize because the immature nervous system does not allow propagation and maintenance of generalized tonic-clonic seizures. They are more readily propagated in structures with limbic, diencephalon, and brainstem connections, which in the neonate are relatively more mature than cortical structures, and thus may be evident in the form of apnea, oculomotor disturbances (horizontal eye deviations, repetitive fluttering of eyelids), or oral motor movements (drooling, sucking). The premature infant may also have seizures involving tonic extension (as in decerebrate posturing) and jitteriness. In all cases, metabolic imbalances must be considered as an etiologic factor, as jitteriness and frank seizures are frequently caused by hypoglycemia and hypocalcemia, as well as postnatal infection. The EEG will aid in the diagnosis of neonatal seizures, but, at least in the premature infant, has little prognostic value. In the term neonate, however, a normal interictal EEG carries a good prognosis, while flat, periodic, or multifocal patterns have poorer prognoses for normal development. The best prognosticator is the underlying neurologic condition. When seizures are related to metabolic imbalance, the prognosis for normal development is better (depending more on other factors, if treated promptly) than when they are the result of perinatal asphyxia, intraventricular hemorrhage, or intracranial infection.[7]

MEDICAL CARE

Since the 1960s, high-risk neonates are being cared for in modern perinatal care networks in most developed countries. These regionalized networks involve three levels of care: primary care facilities are equipped for normal newborn care, transitional care for high-risk newborns awaiting transfer, and risk assessment; level II nurseries provide care for moderately ill neonates or those treated initially in a higher level facility who are now stable; while a tertiary level unit provides neonatal intensive care and maternity care of the highest sophistication in life-support systems, specialized perinatal and maternal care personnel, and access to all necessary subspecialty personnel. The tertiary facility is noted for its low doctor and nurse to patient ratio.[5] These facilities are linked by a variety of transport systems with units designed to treat, not just to maintain, the infants while in transit or to transport the infant in utero in the case of high-risk pregnancies. Often regional communications networks are also involved to assist in the location of available NICU beds.

Evaluating the actual effect of this system of care on the mortality and morbidity of high-risk infants is difficult, as a number of other factors have been operating at the same time, which might tend to improve infant outcomes; for example, a general rise in the standard of living, easier access to family planning information, legalization of abortion on demand, and general improvement in health among prospective parents.[36]

Nevertheless, a decline in birth weight-specific neonatal mortality has certainly accompanied the increase in attention to mothers and neonates in the form of modern techniques of perinatal medicine.[37] This has been demonstrated in studies of a number of aspects of the perinatal care system.[3,38]

Similar declines are also cited in immediate and long-term morbidity for the survivors of modern neonatal intensive care programs when compared to reports from the 1950s and 1960s. Since then, some of the iatrogenic hazards of neonatal intensive care have been recognized and eliminated, and a better understanding of the physiologic needs of high-risk infants has contributed to their improved neonatal care, and presumably, to improved long-term outcome.[39]

In spite of this optimism, Sinclair and colleagues[36] remind us of the need for further evaluation of the efficacy, effectiveness, efficiency, and availability of neonatal intensive care services. They cite that few evaluations have gone beyond the referral centers to assess the total populations served. Few, if any, have used controlled experimental designs, and little information is available as to the cost effectiveness of these programs.

Two such studies are currently underway. In North Carolina, preliminary analysis of the developmental status of infants born in a five-county region receiving large amounts of federal and state aid for the purpose of improving perinatal care demonstrated few significant differences from babies born in a control group of counties.[40] A larger study, such as that being conducted on the eight regional networks funded by the Robert Wood Johnson Foundation, may be necessary to reveal significant effects of improved medical care on the total population of a region.[41]

Routine Medical Care of the High-Risk Infant

As was implied earlier, a better understanding of the physiologic needs of high-risk infants has been translated into routines of care aimed at controling many of the perinatal and neonatal risk factors commonly associated with poor immediate and long-term outcome, especially in very low birth weight, premature, and asphyxiated neonates. Some of these routines are preventive, some are diagnostic, and others are treatment-oriented. They include prenatal identification of high-risk mothers, fetal monitoring during labor, and performance of Cesarian sections when vaginal delivery is judged to be an additional risk factor. Premature labor can sometimes be stopped, or, if preterm delivery seems inevitable, glucocorticoids can be given to decrease the risk of respiratory distress syndrome in the neonate.

When the high-risk infant is born, the physiologic parameters are routinely monitored electronically and through laboratory analyses to enable prompt intervention should they show abnormalities. Routine care also includes the use of prophylactic antibiotics, prompt initiation of intravenous feeding, respiratory support and control of metabolic imbalances.

As the condition stabilizes, the infant is monitored closely for weight gain, begins oral feedings, and is weaned from ventilatory support, supplementary oxygen, and automatic temperature controls.

The results of this impressive armamentarium of care are generally equally impressive, but the care itself is not without risk. In fact, some of the problems high-risk infants develop are the result of the efforts aimed at insuring their survival.

Umbilical catheterization, necessary for vascular access for blood analyses and administration of fluids and medications, carries the risks of tearing of the vessels, hemorrhage, and thromboembolic complications. Thromboembolic complications are implicated in the development of lower extremity cyanosis ("cath feet") and necrotizing enterocolitis; catheters are also frequent sites of local infection which may progress to generalized sepsis.[42]

Respiratory support also has inherent risks, largely related to increased pressure to the lungs and blood vessels, and to increased concentrations of oxygen. Continuous distending pressure or positive end expiratory pressure therapy greatly increase the risk of pneumothorax. Both high airway pressure and prolonged oxygen therapy at high concentrations are associated with the development of the chronic pulmonary condition known as bronchopulmonary dysplasia. Oxygen is also toxic to the retina if the arterial oxygen tension is allowed to go too high, and produces the condition known as retrolental fibroplasia.[42]

The use of phototherapy for reducing serum bilirubin levels may also have some side effects, such as diarrhea, abdominal distention, hypocalcemia, and increased insensible water loss, which require close monitoring; phototherapy, therefore, should not be considered a "routine" procedure for minor elevations of bilirubin.[42]

Finally, the NICU environment itself, may place an infant at increased risk. Lucey[43] suggests that hypoxemia (which may contribute to right-to-left shunting) occurs frequently in infants in the neonatal intensive care unit, often in response to disturbing the infants via loud noise, handling, and invasive procedures during routine care (e.g., respiratory setting changes, blood transfusions and samplings, and events which cause crying). He hypothesizes that this may contribute to opening or reopening of the ductus arteriosus.

The neonatal intensive care unit environment is one of excessive noise (from machinery and personnel) averaging between 70 and 80 dB, which fluctuates continuously, and monotonous brilliant illumination. The stimulation received is unorganized and little diurnal rhythmicity is evident.[44] Although the long-term effect of this experience is not known, investigators speculate that it may contribute to deficits in processing sensory information.

A number of the exciting innovations in medical care have been developed as the result of the recognition of some of the hazards of neonatal intensive care and the desire to minimize the numbers of invasive procedures necessary to diagnose, monitor, and treat sick neonates.

Visualization of Intracranial Pathology

Since hypoxic-ischemic encephalopathy, intracranial hemorrhage and postmeningitic encephalopathy are among the leading contributors to poor immediate and long-term outcome, especially in VLBW infants, the ability to diagnose, monitor and observe the results of therapeutic management in these conditions is imperative. Until very recently these functions had to be performed indirectly through clinical observation, laboratory analyses of various body fluids, and general monitoring of the infant's vital signs.

With the advent of computed tomography (CT) and, more recently, ultrasonography, the brain of the neonate can be visualized directly and in a relatively noninvasive way. A number of studies have established that CT is more accurate than either prediction from clinical signs or analyses of cerebrospinal fluid in the diagnosis of intraventricular hemorrhage. The major reasons for this are probably that a number of intraventricular hemorrhages are clinically "silent"; the signs, when detectable, may not be specific for intraventricular hemorrhage; and many lumbar taps are unsuccessful or traumatic. Probably only the more severe hemorrhages accompanied by dramatic clinical deterioration or frankly bloody cerebrospinal fluid are detectable by indirect methods.[45,46] Although CT has been very useful in documenting the incidence and severity of intraventricular hemorrhage, it is less useful in monitoring the course of the condition. The danger of excessive ionizing radiation limits the numbers of serial scans that can be performed, and the need to transport extremely ill neonates for CT scanning adds to the risk of iatrogenic problems if the infants are separated from life-support systems. CT is also not able to demonstrate periventricular infarction in the early stages of hypoxic-ischemic encephalopathy as readily as it shows early periventricular hemorrhage. Only later in the course of hypoxic-ischemic encephalopathy will CT demonstrate large cavitating lesions.[22]

Ultrasonography shows great promise for overcoming these limitations of CT. The accuracy of ultrasound diagnosis of intraventricular hemorrhage when compared with CT appears to be excellent,[47,48] and it may increase the accuracy of diagnosing early ischemic lesions.[22] Ultrasound is also being used to visualize abnormal intraventricular structures thought to be associated with ventriculitis in cases of neonatal bacterial meningitis, as well as the progressive ventricular enlargement that often follows.[35] Since the apparatus is portable, scans can be performed without transporting the neonate and with minimal disturbance of the ongoing therapy and life support. Since ultrasound involves no ionizing radiation, scans can be repeated frequently to monitor the progression of the condition and the response to therapy[22,47,48]; nevertheless, experience with use of ultrasound is too limited to guarantee that no untoward effects result from repeated exposure.

Ultrasound may also be valuable for predicting survival and risk for poor eventual neurologic outcome. Thorburn and associates[49] have demonstrated, in preterm infants of less than 33 weeks gestation, over 50 percent mortality in infants with abnormal ultrasound scans, compared with less than 12 percent in those with normal scans; and over 25 percent major neurologic handicap in survivors who had abnormal ultrasound scans, compared with less than 5 percent in those with normal ones. They identify four major implications for the increased routine use of ultrasound, especially in very premature and VLBW neonates: (1) early identification of the presence and extent of an intracranial lesion; (2) monitoring controlled trials of medical intervention, such as those aimed at preventing intraventricular hemorrhage and the progression of posthemorrhagic hydrocephalus; (3) early identification of infants at highest risk for poor outcome; and (4) early identification of hopelessly damaged infants for whom ethical withholding of heroic efforts at sustaining life might be justifiably considered.[49]

Transcutaneous Monitoring

A number of transcutaneous, noninvasive techniques are now available for monitoring blood gases. The most widely used to date is transcutaneous monitoring of blood oxygen tension ($tcPo_2$). The basis of the technique is that oxygen can diffuse through intact skin and, if the region to be monitored is hyperfused sufficiently, the skin blood can be arterialized and Po_2 can be monitored transcutaneously. The local hyperemia is produced with an electrode that heats the skin underlying it.[50] Arterial blood Po_2 (Pao_2) and $tcPo_2$ are not identical, but have been shown to correlate closely in trials with normal neonates ($r = 0.97$), with preterm infants on assisted ventilation ($r = 0.94$),[50] and with infants with severe respiratory distress.[51] The most accurate correlation is in the range of 30–100 mmHg, the most critical range for neonatal monitoring.[51,52] Inaccuracies occur primarily in conditions that greatly reduce peripheral circulation (e.g., shock, very low temperature).[52,53] The major advantages of $tcPo_2$ monitoring over available methods relate to its continuous and noninvasive characteristics. When monitoring is done by blood sampling, it is discontinuous and the trauma involved in taking the sample may invalidate the readings. When monitoring is done continuously through indwelling catheter, the risks associated with prolonged catheterization are encountered, as well as the potential of abdominal aortic Pao_2 not accurately assessing Pao_2 in the brain circulation.[50,52] Some authorities, nevertheless, recommend use of an intravascular electrode during the acute stage of illness, when access to the blood through umbilical catheterization is needed for other reasons (e.g., $Paco_2$, pH, and electrolyte monitoring and infusion of medications).[51]

PHYSICAL THERAPY EVALUATION

In the preceding sections some beginning points for evaluation have been discussed. Whether the objects of assessment are high-risk infants or patients with other conditions, the process of evaluation consists of a number of steps. In the broadest sense, five steps appear to be essential.

First, one must decide *who* to assess. This involves a selection process that may be one of the more unique parts of evaluating high-risk infants.

Second, the therapist must determine *when* to evaluate. At what points in the course of the infant's recovery from perinatal problems, will physical therapy evaluations provide the most useful information upon which to base future action?

Third is the question of *what* to evaluate. Physical therapists know a great deal about the neuromuscular functioning of the human organism. What portions of this knowledge can best be applied to evaluation of the high-risk infant?

Fourth is the consideration of *how* to assess, or the selection of the best evaluation tools for use with the neonate and infant at risk for central nervous system dysfunction.

Finally, one must consider what options are available for *action* following analysis of the results of evaluation.

These steps will be discussed in order with consideration of the information already presented as well as additional information pertinent to each.

Selection of Infants in Need of Evaluation

In order to function smoothly in the special care nursery setting, the physical therapist must establish, in collaboration with his or her colleagues in neonatal medicine and nursing, which high-risk infants should be candidates for physical therapy evaluation. This implies that the physical therapist must be very knowledgeable about the perinatal conditions known to place an infant at increased risk for poor neurologic outcome. Since an actual diagnosis of developmental problems will rarely be possible, the therapist cannot rely on that for selection purposes. Selection of infants for evaluations is, therefore, similar to a screening process. Like any good screening process, it should attempt to minimize the numbers of infants evaluated who do not need it while maximizing the numbers evaluated who are in need of later physical therapy or related services.

Evidence from the preceding sections would strongly suggest that the neuromuscular functioning of all VLBW infants, especially if the perinatal or neonatal period was complicated by documented asphyxia, intracranial hemorrhage, or major infection, should be assessed. The same criteria would be true of the full-term infant with these conditions.

If some of the recent innovations in diagnosis and monitoring of these conditions are in use in a particular setting, the therapist may wish to narrow these criteria even further. For example, if CT or ultrasound evidence of moderate to severe hemorrhage, defined hypoxic-ischemic encephalopathy lesions, posthemorrhagic or postmeningitic hydrocephalus is available, the selection process may be even more precise. Evidence from $tcPo_2$ monitoring of significant episodes of hypoxemia may also enter into consideration. Lacking this more definitive evidence, selection must be based on judicious assessment of clinical and laboratory data such as neonatal seizures documented by abnormal EEG, grossly bloody cerebrospinal fluid in lumbar taps, documented sepsis, episodes of severe cardiopulmonary deterioration, and the like.

The therapist may also want to assess the risk associated with maternal factors and document these and the neonatal risk factors in a semiobjective way. Several systems are available in which antepartum, intrapartum, and neonatal risk factors can be assigned scores in an additive fashion as an aid in selecting infants for careful follow-up. These include the Problem-Oriented Perinatal Risk Assessment System developed for obstetricians following women with complicated pregnancies,[54] the Obstetric and Postnatal Complications Scales developed as part of a cumulative developmental assessment system to predict cognitive and affective performance,[55] and the "optimality" concept developed by Prechtl[56] to assess the events of pregnancy and delivery. Much of the groundwork for determining who should be evaluated can be done through consultation with the medical and nursing staff and through perusal of the medical record. In a number of centers, this has resulted in the establishment of a protocol that includes referral or blanket permission for physical therapy evaluation of infants meeting the defined criteria.

Timing of Evaluation

As in many other acute care situations, the timing of any events that might disrupt the recovery process is critical. If the physical therapy evaluation is to be of benefit to the high-risk neonate or infant, it certainly should not contribute to that infant's risk for mortality or morbidity. In the same view, if the evaluation is to provide the physical therapist with useful information about the infant's eventual need for physical therapy, it certainly should not be done at a time when that infant is either too ill or unstable to respond or at such an early stage of recovery that present status is totally unreflective of his or her later condition. The latter point does not imply that serial evaluations which may serve to document the degree of recovery are not useful, rather that the timing of the initial evaluation is critical, as is consideration of the infant's condition prior to any repeated evaluation.

To assist in determining when best to initiate evaluation procedures, some understanding of the developmental course in high-risk (especially premature) infants and the effects of handling is necessary. Als[57] conceptualized a hierarchical model of newborn neurobehavioral organization incorporating a number of levels of organization in which each level is a prerequisite for the next. The earliest level to be achieved, and the primary developmental agendum for the premature and the very stressed full-term neonate, is to achieve homeostasis of physiologic functions, including cardiorespiratory and temperature control functions. Gorski and associates[58] postulate a similar level in a three-stage model of behavioral organization in the high-risk neonate, which they term the "physiologic stage" or stage of "in-turning." A stressed infant, during this stage, may be unable to participate reciprocally with caregivers, needing first to develop sufficient physical integrity and internal stability. Only after this physiologic homeostasis is achieved, can the high-risk neonate demonstrate some progress in the second level of increasing motor control and motor differentiation.[57] In contrast, the healthy full-term infant is capable shortly after birth of demonstrating integration of physiologic homeostasis and motor control, and is, in fact, beginning at the third level proposed by Als,[57] that of increasing behavioral state differentiation and capable of moving into the fourth level of social interactive capacity.

Coupled with this information is the need to consider the direct effect on the neonate should an evaluation procedure be carried out with a physiologically unstable, motorically uncontrolled neonate.

Speidel,[59] using continuous umbilical artery Pao_2 monitoring, demonstrated frequent sharp drops in Pao_2 following even minor disturbances associated with routine nursing and medical procedures, especially when such procedures followed in close succession. Long and associates[60] studied three equivalent groups of LBW, premature (≤ 36 weeks GA) infants as to the amount of hypoxemia and hyperoxemia experienced during the first several days of life, the relationship between oxygenation abnormalities and intensive care procedures, and the degree to which these abnormalities could be reduced by modifying the procedures. One group had only conventional cardiorespiratory (heart rate and "apnea") monitoring; a second group had conventional monitoring and tcPo$_2$ monitoring (but nursery staff was uninstructed in interpreting the tcPo$_2$ monitor findings); while a third group had the same monitoring, but the nursery staff were instructed in ways to interpret the tcPo$_2$ output. The results showed that the first two groups did not differ from each other, but differed significantly from the third group. Comparisons between the two tcPo$_2$ groups showed that the third group had over five times less time in which tcPo$_2$ was <40 mmHg (range of hypoxemia) or >100 mmHg (hyperoxemia) and about four times fewer times when tcPo$_2$ fell >20 mmHg within a 1-minute time period. Seventy-five percent of the undesirable time (hypoxemia or hyperoxemia) experienced by both groups was associated with caregiving disturbances, but the total undesirable time in group two was 325 minutes and in group three was only 5 minutes. Undesirable time was greatly reduced in the group in which tcPo$_2$ monitoring was interpreted and used to monitor procedures (group three). Another important finding in this study was that the conventional monitors detected only 5 percent of the undesirable time. Among the procedures which produced hypoxemia in these infants were neck flexion or hyperextension, hand-under-jaw feeding, crying, airway suctioning, and rough handling.[53]

The initial evaluation of a high-risk neonate, therefore, may consist mainly of assessing the infant's readiness to be evaluated. One should consider strongly requesting the use of a tcPo$_2$ monitor during an evaluation and, of course, be thoroughly instructed in its use and in ways to modify procedures so as to minimize physiologic stress. Even if the neonate demonstrates some degree of physiologic stability, evaluation of motor functioning (Als' level 2) may be misleading. Premature infants are frequently unable to inhibit their motor responses which tend to be tremulous and jerky, may spread to involve the entire motor system from a single stimulus, and often are repeated over and over until the infant is exhausted. On the other hand, the musculature may be so weak that a response is inadequate or greatly delayed. Either of these responses can occur in an *intact* preterm infant.[61]

In the motoric system, these types of responses may alert the evaluating therapist to the fact that the infant is still in one of the two extremes of preterm infant functioning described by Als and associates.[61] These are (1) the hyperactive infant who is at the mercy of internal and external stimuli, being unable to shut these out and regulate behavior, and (2) the lethargic, depressed infant who preserves autonomic regulation by not responding to any stimulation.

The initial evaluation may, therefore, have questionable value for future prediction, but does serve to assess the current status of the infant and as a baseline upon which to judge recovery upon subsequent evaluation.

Scope of Evaluation

Assuming that these two steps provide a pool of infants in need of evaluation, the question arises as to the areas of functioning which the physical therapist is best equipped to assess.

Ideally, the neonatal evaluation should serve *three* major purposes: (1) to measure the process and extent of the infant's recovery from perinatal stress; (2) to assess the current state of central nervous system organization; and (3) to predict future functioning.[62] From these purposes can be derived several principles of neonatal assessment. One is that assessment must be repeated at a number of points in time to document the recovery process; another is that assessment instruments should be sensitive enough to allow discrimination of neurobehavioral deviations from individual differences in normal behavior and to detect those deviations most likely to result in significant impairment of future functioning.

In applying these principles to physical therapy assessment, we must also consider the areas of function in which the physical therapy assessment can contribute most to both the overall plan for the infant's present and future management and the specific habilitation plan for therapy if this is indicated.

In the neonatal period the physical therapist would seem uniquely qualified to assess neuromuscular maturation and motoric functioning, identify musculoskeletal abnormalities in need of immediate attention, evaluate oral motor function, and assess the need of the infant for therapeutic intervention or long-term evaluation. As the infant matures, the physical therapist will provide on-going expertise in assessing the level and quality of neuromuscular development as well as the need for initiation, continuance, or termination of therapeutic intervention.

NEONATAL ASSESSMENTS

Given these qualifications, the next step in the evaluation process is the selection of assessment methods and instruments that will contribute most to meeting the ideal goals of assessment. A number of the available instruments and strategies are thoroughly discussed in Chapter 2 by Stengel and associates. These include neurologic[63-67] and neurobehavioral assessments.[68-70]

Saint-Anne Dargassies has undertaken the most extensive descriptive study of the premature infant's neurologic development utilizing the principles of examination of the French neurologists. Her classic descriptions of sensory responses, neurovegetative responses, primary reflexes, muscle tone and mobility characteristic of premature infants born at or attaining various gestational ages are the nearest thing we have to norms for the prematurely born infant and should be thoroughly studied by therapists evaluating these infants.[71,72]

Some of the descriptive findings of characteristic postures and mobility at various gestational ages reported by St.-Anne Dargassies, have not been confirmed in a group of low-risk preterm infants studied by Prechtl and associates.[73] They did not find patterns or preference postures nor some of the mobility patterns described by St.-Anne Dargassies. Some reasons for these discrepancies may be major differences in methods of recording data (anecdotal vs. quantitative), or differences in infants' health status based on sample selection or methods of routine care.

The French methods[63,71,72] and those developed by Prechtl and his colleagues[66,67] in the Netherlands form a kind of transition between the standard neurologic examinations and the neurobehavioral assessments, such as the Brazelton Neonatal Behavioral Assessment Scale (BNBAS).[70] Two of the major contributions are (1) the emphasis on observing and recording the quality and intensity of responses (as opposed to mere presence or absence); and (2) the recognition that the behavioral state of the infant must be considered as a major component of and contributor to the infant's performance.

A single neurologic or neurobehavioral test, may never satisfy the needs of the physical therapist for assessing high-risk infants (until, perhaps, a physical therapist develops, standardizes, and validates one). The functions of the two major types of tests differ greatly, reflecting the different goals of their developers. Neurologic tests generally function to identify abnormal neurologic signs and syndromes in the neonate which may require immediate medical intervention or may be predictive of future neurologic dysfunction. Behavioral tests generally are designed to detect individual differences among neonates, with such information being used to educate parents about the behavioral style of their infant. To the extent that these differing goals are shared by the physical therapist, these tests can be useful, but neither type of test can serve both purposes.

Regardless of the tests selected, therapists should beware of the tendency to select from a test certain items or to abbreviate the test by omitting items. Much of the value of these tests for use in diagnostic or planning activities is lost if the sequence of administration is altered. Once assessment tools are selected, they should be used intact, as originally described in their respective manuals.

Oral Motor Assessment

Oral dysfunction in high-risk neonates may result from deficient oral experiences secondary to the medical care necessary for the infant's survival or from the immaturity of the neuromotor mechanisms controlling oral functions.[74] High-risk neonates with histories of perinatal distress have aberrations in sucking patterns when compared with healthy infants, yet no evidence indicates that sucking aberrations during infancy are predictive of later neurologic problems.[75,76]

In order to assess the adequacy of the high-risk neonate's oral functioning, the therapist must have a thorough understanding of normal oral functioning in infancy and the development of oral functions during pre- and postnatal life. A discussion of these topics is beyond the scope of this chapter, but a number of excellent resources are available for the interested reader.[74,77,78]

The oral motor evaluation must include assessment of the tactile responsiveness of the facial area, breathing pattern, oral reflexes, tongue mobility, coordination of sucking and swallowing, jaw stability, and facial musculature balance.[78-80] This evaluation is best done in the context of a feeding situation, as it also includes assessment of the infant's response to handling and positioning for feeding, the amount of nourishment ingested, and an estimate of the energy required to complete a feeding.

Other Evaluations

Other evaluations must include assessing the needs of infants with pulmonary problems for bronchial drainage and the need for positioning of infants who have long periods of immobilization. Attention to positioning can minimize the typical deformities associated with long-term confinement such as elliptical deformity of the head or torticollis from resting laterally on the bed, and positional disorders of the limbs (abducted and externally rotated hips and shoulders) from the effect of gravity on the immobile, hypotonic neonate lying in supine or prone positions.[5]

The final stage of evaluation, that of determining what action should occur as the result of the assessments, may lead to a number of options for subsequent action. As a means of summarizing this discussion of evaluation, we will consider three of these options as they relate to the high-risk neonate during the hospital stay.

Option one might be to delay extensive evaluation until a later time. This option would be appropriate in situations which might be considered as representing the two extremes of the high-risk infant group being managed. The first would be the infant who, although meeting selection criteria for evaluation, is so ill or physiologically unstable as to make testing meaningless or even dangerous to the infant's well-being. The second is the infant who does not meet selection criteria for evaluation at any time during the hospital course. Although the option to delay evaluation is the same in these two cases, the timing of the eventual evaluation is not necessarily the same. The first infant should receive an evaluation as soon as survival is considered fairly sure and physiologic instability is either resolved or easily managed through judicious monitoring and handling. The second infant might receive an extensive evaluation either immediately preceding hospital discharge, at first return visit following discharge, or at the earliest opportunity at an outside agency which will be overseeing his or her future care.

Option two might be to plan for a series of later evaluations once an initial evaluation is accomplished. This option would seem appropriate in a number of instances. One might be an instance where the initial evaluation was, in some way, inconclusive or unsatisfactory. Perhaps the initial evaluation could not be completed or the infant did not appear to function at optimal capacity. Second, the infant who demonstrated some questionable responses on initial testing should be reassessed to determine the quality and rate of recovery or the resolution of or persistence of the questionable areas of functioning. Finally, an infant who demonstrates no questionable functioning on initial evaluation should be reassessed if subsequent events occur during the neonatal period which would again place him or her at increased risk for central nervous system dysfunction.

Finally, *option three* might be to initiate an intervention program, following a series of appropriate evaluations. The need to precede this decision with a number of evaluations should be obvious at this point in this discussion. Those infants who are selected for initial evaluation, show cumulative medical, neurologic, and neurobehavioral evidence of deviant maturation or function may benefit from therapeutic intervention aimed at enhancing the recovery process and preventing or minimizing some of the sequelae of perinatal or neonatal complications.

THERAPEUTIC INTERVENTION

This section will concentrate on therapeutic intervention in special care nurseries with high-risk infants whose evaluations make them candidates for programming, as opposed to later, postdischarge treatment of infants following dignosis of central nervous system dysfunction. Treatment of the older, diagnosed, infant or child is considered in other chapters of this volume.

As with evaluation, intervention with high-risk infants must be directed to those who should benefit most from it, timed so as to minimize adverse effects and maximize effectiveness, carefully selected as to scope and method, and well-integrated with the infant's total management program. Selection of infants in need of therapeutic intervention should be possible through application of the various evaluation principles just discussed and adverse effects minimized through the same measures suggested in the evaluation section. Selecting intervention methods, however, and integrating them into the infant's total program, is a more difficult task, as is evaluating the effectiveness of therapeutic intervention.

No studies of intervention with high-risk neonates designed specifically to improve motor control or conducted by physical therapists have been reported in the literature. In studies by members of other disciplines, information on the effects of various programs of stimulation on neurologic, neuromuscular, or motoric functioning is sparse. The typical intervention program reported has as its model the relatively healthy, preterm infant who is not typical of the critically ill, potentially neurologically damaged infant being followed by physical therapists in special care nurseries.[81,82] In addition, many evaluative studies of the effects of early intervention have a number of serious methodologic problems of commission or omission that limit the interpretation, understanding, and generalizability of their findings. A number of critical reviews have discussed the various methodologic differences and limitations of these intervention studies.[81,83–86]

Some theoretical background, rationale, and principles for effective intervention, however, can be construed from the work of others and will be discussed here, as will some possible areas of focus for intervention with high-risk neonates by physical therapists.

Support for the need of intervention with high-risk neonates stems from the numerous studies demonstrating that premature and other high-risk neonates are much more likely to have later developmental problems in almost every area of function than are full-term, low-risk neonates, especially if they are raised in environments with nonoptimal stimulation, such as may be the case in low socioeconomic situations.[87]

The theoretical bases for providing such intervention as early as possible in the life of the neonate are primarily derived from the theories of Hebb[88] and Piaget.[89] Hebb (as summarized by Wright[87]) proposes that the brain has two major types of tissue. Committed tissue is genetically programmed before birth to manage sensory input and motoric output (e.g., reflexive responses) in response to external activation. Associative (noncommitted) tissue functions are not predetermined at birth, but must be established by the wealth of sensorimotor experience occurring during the early years of life. Such functions can also be activated internally by "autonomous central processes." Associative tissue, therefore, is particularly vulnerable to early brain damage, which may destroy it directly or indirectly (by preventing normal early experiences from occurring).

Piaget's theory of development (as summarized by Wright[87]) emphasizes the importance of the first two years of life, termed the "sensorimotor" period, during which the infant builds from a rich sensorimotor experience base the abilities necessary for later higher level functions.

From these two theories came the corollary propositions that early deprivation of sensorimotor experience may result in developmental deficits, that early enrichment may enhance development,[84,87] and that infancy and the early years are sensitive periods or phases of heightened responsiveness, to sensorimotor stimulation.[90]

Many of the rationales used for research in early intervention can be seen to derive from these theories. The premature infant confined to an isolette in a special care nursery is considered sensorily deprived of the normal stimulation provided in the uterus and of that provided by parents in the home. In addition, the child and the parents are deprived of the normal opportunity to develop the reciprocal interaction considered necessary for normal attachment to each other.[82,84] Recently, some investigators have suggested that the special nursery environment may provide too much stimulation or an adequate amount, but inappropriate form of stimulation (e.g., monotonous, unpatterned, noncontingent).[83,86] Based on these differences in rationale, some programs are designed to make up for the lack of stimulation, others to provide extra stimulation to accelerate development, and others to provide improved quality of stimulation and experience.[86] In addition, some experiences are developed to simulate experiences within the uterus, others are aimed at simulating experiences available to a full-term neonate, while others are focused on manipulating the special care nursery experiences unique to the premature or high-risk neonate.[83,86]

The reports of research, primarily by psychologists and nurses, provide some hints for areas of focus for intervention with high-risk infants by physical therapists. Of particular interest would seem to be reports of the effects of intervention on activity level, effects of positioning, effects on motor development and muscle tone, and effects on oral motor functioning.

Effects on Activity Level

As Als and colleagues[61] have suggested, a number of very young premature and very stressed high-risk infants may demonstrate motoric imbalance in that they are unable to maintain motoric control while attending to other events or to inhibit motor activity once it is elicited by external or internal stimuli. A number of investigators have hypothesized that this uninhibited, continuous movement (especially of the limbs) poses a threat to survival in that it contributes to excessive burning of calories and weight loss.[91,92] The results of some studies with normal, full-term neonates suggest that continuous stimulation of almost any nature (e.g., auditory, visual, tactile, proprioceptive, thermal) has a quieting or "pacification" effect evidenced in a variety of systems. The effect is demonstrated by decreased and more regular heart rate and respiration, less crying, more sleep, and decreased motor activity.[92–94] In a more recent study, Chapman[91] attempted to assess the effects of patterned auditory stimulation on the motor activity of short-gestation infants (mean age at birth, 30 to 31 weeks of gestation). The infants received one of three types of auditory stimulation: (1) routine auditory stimulation in the isolette (control group); (2) taped maternal speech; or (3) taped music. Motor activity was measured by accelerometers[95] attached to the infants' wrists and ankles for 48 hours after discontinuation of the stimulation. No effects on motor activity were demonstrable in this study. Although this study produced no significant decrease in motor activity in short-gestation infants, the theoretical basis for such an effect appears sound. Perhaps, for the short-gestation infant, another sensory modality (e.g., tactile, kinesthetic, or proprioceptive) would be more appropriate or, perhaps assessment of motor activity should be done while the stimulus is being administered, and this compared with periods of no stimulation in the same infants, as well as with a separate control group receiving no stimulation.

Positioning has also been shown to affect activity level in normal, full-term infants. Brackbill and associates[96] demonstrated that two-day-old neonates placed in prone slept more, cried less, and moved less than when placed in supine. This effect has not been systematically evaluated in preterm and high-risk neonates. The prone position may be contraindicated when such things as umbilical artery catheters or chest tubes are required in very ill neonates but side-lying can be used during this time and the prone position used later when the medical condition permits.

Physiologic Effects of Positioning

The influence of body position on pulmonary function in healthy preterm infants has been investigated in several studies. Most report advantages of prone over supine in improved ventilation and patterns of breathing with only a negligible increase in the work of breathing.[97–99]

In addition, gastric emptying in term, preterm SGA, and respiratory distress syndrome infants was found to be more rapid in prone and right lateral positions than in supine and left lateral positions. Respiratory distress syndrome infants were found to have delayed gastric emptying and a high incidence of abdominal distention and pooling of feeds in the stomach in the supine and left lateral positions.[100]

One other study reports significantly increased blood pressure and decreased tcPo$_2$ in sick neonates when held in the knee-chest position[101] as when a lumbar puncture is obtained. Lucey[53] also lists lumbar puncture and diaper change as causes of hypoxemia in sick LBW infants, although the knee-chest position per se is not mentioned. Physical therapists must be careful when using a flexed position with sick neonates (as in attempting to decrease extensor muscle tone in the legs).

Effects on Motor Development, Maturation, and Muscle Tone

A number of studies, using a variety of sensory modalities, have demonstrated increased weight gain in infants receiving intervention, as compared with controls receiving only routine care.[102–106] Although not specifically a motor effect, such a short-term effect is certainly a worthwhile goal. Better nourished infants may be better able to cope with stressful neonatal events and better able to respond to developmental intervention and with their parents in social interactions.

Three investigators used the Graham/Rosenblith Scales to determine early developmental effects of intervention. Neal[107] reported a previous study of 28- to 32-week premature infants receiving vestibular stimulation imposed with a motorized rocking hammock. Katz[108] also studied 28- to 32-week infants but the intervention was in the form of taped recordings of the mother's voice. Both administered the Graham/Rosenblith Scales at 36 weeks conceptual age. Results favoring the experimental groups in both studies were found for the motor, auditory and visual scales. Neal also found better weight gain in her experimental group, while Katz also found better tactile-adaptive scores in her experimental group. Chapman[109] however, found no differences on the Graham/Rosenblith Scale between infants receiving auditory stimulation and controls.

In slightly older infants who received extra stroking, holding, and rocking as preterm neonates, Powell[110] found experimental group infants to have higher Bayley Mental and Motor Scale Scores at 4 months than did control infants, but these differences had disappeared at 6-month retesting. Following a program of stroking and rocking with preterm neonates, Rice[106] found more mature Landau and head righting reflexes and higher Bayley Mental scores at 4 months chronologic age (CA) in her experimental group as compared to a control group, but no differences in integration of primitive reflexes or in Bayley Motor scores. After using a multimodal program of enrichment (visual, auditory, tactile, and kinesthetic), Lieb and associates[111] found no differences between experimental and control preterm infants on the BNBAS, but significantly better Bayley Mental and Motor scores for the treated group at 6 months of age (measured from EDC). Few studies have followed infants beyond the age of six months following neonatal stimulation programs. In a preliminary report of her large-scale project, Chapman[109] reports no differences among auditory stimulation and control groups on Bayley Mental, Motor or Infant Behavioral Record scores at 9 and 18 months of age measured from the EDC.

Effects of Oral Motor Programs

In the neonate, the major goals of oral motor programs are associated with feeding. The therapist hopes the program will hasten the time when an infant can begin either bottle or breast feeding, will increase the amount of fluid that can be ingested at a feeding session (thereby reducing the need for supplementary gavage feeding), and will ultimately contribute to or facilitate normal weight gain.

A number of remedial programs for infants with oral motor problems are well described in the literature and serve as a basis for selecting oral stimulation techniques.[79,80,112,113]

A few controlled studies of the effects of oral stimulation programs with high-risk neonates have been reported. In three studies, the effects on nutrient intake were investigated. In a pilot study with 11 infants, Burpee[114] reported no significant differences between an experimental group receiving a program of oral stimulation and a control group receiving passive range of motion to the upper extremities, on measures of the quality of rooting and sucking, amount of formula consumed, number of sucks/2 minutes, or the time until sucking was initiated. The experimental group showed a trend to faster regaining of birth weight. Leonard and associates[115] found increased numbers of sucks per minute in five high-risk neonates during a feeding condition in which perioral stimulation was given as compared with two baseline measures the same day when no stimulation was given. The same treatment condition produced enhanced rates of sucking and increased volume of formula ingested in a larger group of high-risk neonates when compared with conditions of no stimulation and stimulation only before feeding.[116]

A number of interesting effects on high-risk neonates given nonnutritive sucking opportunities have also been reported. In the normal newborn, nonnutritive sucking tends to have a quieting effect in that it reduces crying and excessive movement, while enhancing the quiet, alert state during which the infant is most responsive to stimuli.[117] Anderson and Vidyasagar[118] provided nonnutritive sucking opportunities to 10 critically ill, very immature neonates and found their sucking ability to be unrelated to gestational age or weight at birth. Sucking scores were positively related to pH and negatively to P_{CO_2} and increased with closely time-related sucking opportunities. Although not observed in a controlled way, the authors believed that infant state and neuromuscular coordination were improved after very brief sucking activity. They suggest that such opportunities do not appear to have any adverse effects on the infant's medical condition and may, therefore, be safely used in efforts to enhance earlier oral feeding. Such sucking opportunities can be given even to infants who, for various medical reasons, cannot have nutritive sucking experience. Burroughs and associates[119] found that $tcPo_2$ levels in preterm infants increased during periods of nonnutritive sucking, and remained high or continued to increase during a contiguous period following the sucking session. Measel and Anderson[120] gave nonnutritive sucking opportunities to an experimental group of premature infants during and following tube feedings. Compared to a control group who did not suck, the experimental infants began bottle feeding earlier and, therefore, required fewer tube feedings, were discharged earlier, and tended toward more rapid weight gain.

In summary, the high-risk infant intervention research results suggest several goals compatible with those which physical therapists often state for older infants and young children with diagnosed central nervous system dysfunction and for acutely ill hospitalized patients: (1) effecting improvement in physiologic functions such as ventilation; (2) enhancing oral motor function for feeding; (3) normalizing muscle tone and activity level; and (4) facilitating general sensorimotor development.

FOLLOW-UP OF THE HIGH-RISK INFANT

After an infant has progressed to a medically stable state, whether transferred to an intermediate level nursery or discharged home, further developmental assessment and, perhaps, continuation or initiation of therapeutic intervention is in order. Diagnosis of definite central nervous system dysfunction is rarely possible during the period of critical illness. Following that period, however, early signs of dysfunction may provide a better indication of eventual prognosis and, as the infant matures, more subtle signs, previously masked by the initial perinatal problems or which are evident as more complex behaviors develop, may appear.

Just before the infant is discharged, the therapist may wish to repeat a "risk assessment" in order to select those infants most in need of continued developmental follow-up. A number of authors suggest that extremely important prognosticators for eventual outcome are both the speed and degree to which the infant responds to the management provided in the special care setting,[121] the persistence of deviant signs beyond the neonatal period,[122] and the cumulative effects of perinatal and later nonoptimal events.[55] The therapist, armed with the results of a series of assessments during the infant's nursery stay, should be able to identify infants who consistently demonstrated poor performance, responded poorly to intervention, and suffered a large number of nonoptimal perinatal insults. Arrangements for continued evaluation and treatment of these infants must be explored, if they are not to be followed within the same facility. Typically, most tertiary care facilities maintain follow-up clinics to which high-risk neonates are referred for specified lengths of time and which include developmental therapy personnel. A certain percentage of infants, however, who reside a great distance from the referral hospital, may receive pediatric care in their home communities. Such care may or may not include developmental assessment. Often, therefore, specific referral to a local developmental facility should be made from the discharging hospital.

A number of appropriate assessment tools for evaluation of the older infant are available (see Stengel et al., Chapter 2) and will not be reiterated here. A major question is likely to be: How soon can we be sure that physical therapy is indicated? This question stems from a limited amount of information about the normal course of development in infants who have sustained significant perinatal insults. The studies of their eventual outcome do not usually provide descriptions of the developmental behavior which occurred between the neonatal period and the age of outcome assessment. Do high-risk infants have delayed attainment of developmental milestones, delayed integration of primitive reflexes, or delayed appearance of postural reactions? Should results of developmental testing be interpreted for the chronologic or postconceptual age of premature infants and, if so, for how long is such adjustment necessary?

A longitudinal study of infants at very high risk for developing central nervous system dysfunction is being conducted at the University of North Carolina at Chapel Hill, which may provide some descriptive data related to these questions.[123] Preliminary analysis of the first group of high-risk infants to complete a 2-year evaluation indicated that unevenness in standardized motor test scores can be expected throughout the first year, but that 1- and 2-year motor outcome is predictable from assessments as early as 3 months (the correlation between the 3-month Bayley PDI and the 12-month PDI is 0.51; $p = 0.05$ and between the 6-month PDI and 24-month PDI is 0.68; $p = 0.02$).[124]

Niparko,[125] in a retrospective study of the records of 203 premature infants assessed with the Denver Developmental Screening test (DDST) during the first year of life, found that children born after 34 weeks gestation and known to be developmentally normal at 1 year usually performed normally on the DDST by 6 months, whether or not age was adjusted for prematurity. She suggested, however, that the difference between DDST results interpreted for chronologic age and adjusted age may improve the discrimination of the DDST.

The decision as to when to initiate intervention in the older high-risk infant must be made judiciously. The results of assessments may show tremendous variability in the first year of life in infants whose outcome will be normal; yet early deviations can also predict later poor motor performance.

Early motor deviations may also be predictive of later nonmotoric problems, such as the generalized developmental delay typical of the child with mental retardation. Early motor assessments, therefore, should not be used to label a child with a diagnosis of motoric dysfunction, but rather as warning signs requiring careful follow-up of the child's total development.

PARENT EDUCATION

In recent years, the NICU has been made increasingly more accessible to parents and close relatives of high-risk neonates, who are encouraged to visit early and frequently, to make contact with their infants, and to take part in their care when possible. If parents are encouraged to visit and participate in their high-risk neonate's programs, special care nursery personnel must be alert to their needs. Depending on their individual natures and the stage of adjustment to the birth of their sick neonate, some parents may want, and should be allowed, early and intensive contact, but others may prefer limited contact until their infant is healthier and more responsive. In one study, parents of the sickest infants had the highest levels of attachment.[126] Participation in a self-help group has been associated with increased frequency of visiting, increased satisfaction with medical care and information given, and improved quality of maternal-infant interaction.[127] Most important, however, is that parents be taught about their infant's *specific* capabilities so they will have some idea of what to expect and can avoid negative interactions.[128,129]

Although a sick or preterm infant may not provide the same social cues as does the healthy term infant, parents (and nursery staff) can be taught to read the cues given. Often these are physiologic, rather than social, cues and can indicate a desirable response to an event (e.g., the "pinking-up" of an infant calmed by maternal gentle stroking) or may signal the need to rest from stimulation (e.g., increased irregularity of heart or respiratory rates, or gaze aversion).

The BNBAS is frequently used in parent education to demonstrate to mothers (often high-risk mothers) their infants' unique capabilities, in hopes of encouraging appropriate mother-infant interactions. Widmayer and Field[130] found improved BNBAS interactive process scores at 1 month, better DDST fine motor adaptive abilities at 4 months and higher Bayley Mental scores at 12 months in healthy preterm infants whose mothers observed BNBAS assessments or completed the Mothers' Assessment of the Behavior of Her Infant Scale (MABI), an adaptation of the BNBAS, during the neonatal period. Bayley Motor scores for the experimental groups were also higher than for a control group, but the differences did not reach statistical significance.

Allowing parents to observe their infants' assessments may be a useful tool for teaching therapeutic intervention as well, although this has not been evaluated thoroughly with very high-risk infants.

Two studies have demonstrated increased visiting by mothers of infants involved in nursery-based intervention programs as compared with mothers of control infants.[131,132] Rosenfeld[132] suggests that the increased visiting might have resulted from the increased alertness and responsiveness also found in the stimulation group infants.

Desmond and associates[5,133] suggest that more attention needs to be paid to continuing parental support during the period following hospital discharge. Parents may feel their problems are largely over since the infant has survived, while at the same time they feel terribly afraid of assuming total responsibility for the child's care. The infant may have difficulty adjusting to family schedules and in establishing normal feeding and sleep-awake cycles. Recurring illness during early infancy is common and may require rehospitalization, reawakening parental fears about survival and long-term outcome. The early developmental course can be uneven or slow even in those children who eventually have normal outcomes, and in some a real disability begins to evolve. These and other common stresses (such as those associated with poverty, single and/or youthful parenthood) combine to make high-risk infants vulnerable to disorders of parenting such as child abuse, neglect, failure to thrive, and the Vulnerable Child Syndrome.[5,133]

During the period of posthospitalization follow-up, the physical therapist can contribute a great deal to education of parents and other family members. Since many preterm infants are discharged to their parents before or very close to their expected birth dates, families should be made aware of some of the basic differences in appearance and functioning between preterm infants reaching 40 weeks postconceptional age and infants born at term.

Healthy preterm, AGA infants usually reach normal size and weight by 40 to 42 weeks postconceptional age, but very immature, very ill preterm infants often have weight below the third percentile at term date with catch-up growth often occurring until the 6th through 9th month postterm. The SGA infant tends to remain small all through childhood.[5]

Positional disorders, though usually transient, may also be worrisome to parents. Positioning the hypotonic preterm infant in supine during the period of intensive care is often necessary for placement of umbilical catheters, chest tubes, and respiratory-support apparatus, but contributes to later persistence of the upper extremities in abduction and external rotation at the shoulders and may contribute to delay in bringing the hands together in the midline. Similarly, the lower extremities tend to be abducted and externally rotated at the hip, a poor position for later weight bearing. Desmond and associates[5] suggest that similar positional disorders can result from continuous prone placement.

Howard and associates[134] used a brief neurologic examination developed for full-term newborn infants to compare full-term neonates and preterm neonates at 40 weeks postconceptional age. They found a significant number of weak responses in the preterm group, particularly in head extension while seated, arm and leg traction, leg recoil, and the Moro reflex, despite a higher level of arousal. They also reported more asymmetric responses in the preterm group.

Behaviorally, the infant who, as a high-risk neonate was either extremely hypo- or hyperreactive, may continue to demonstrate some of these traits into the early months post term. The child may be difficult to arouse or difficult to console, or may show extremes of motoric imbalance. Caring parents may attempt to provide a stimulating environment for such infants, which may actually "overload" the infant causing withdrawal; conversely, they may feel the infant is responding aversively and tend to leave him or her alone.[58]

As the child matures, if a disability is diagnosed, parents must be helped to cope with this new problem and be guided to seek appropriate therapeutic help. Such support and follow-up should continue at least through the preschool years, as increasing evidence is being found that high-risk infants, even those with normal or near-normal cognitive and motoric functioning, frequently demonstrate marginal school readiness, disorders of attention, and learning disability when reaching school age.[133]

In summary, "the ultimate outcome for these infants will be greatly influenced by postnatal events, parental perceptions of the child, nurture provided by the home and quality of the health care environment after discharge from hospital care."[5]

STAFF EDUCATION

The contribution of the physical therapist to the care of the high-risk infant is not complete unless it includes a contribution to the ongoing education of his or her colleagues. Most levels II and III special care nurseries are located in facilities in which ongoing postgraduate education is an integral part of the institution's program, including both formal and informal training of resident physicians, special care nurses, medical social workers, nutritionists, and therapists. The physical therapist must participate in such educational programs both as a learner and a teacher.

This implies that the therapist must become an integral member of the nursery team, not just receive referrals for treatment of individual infants. Participation in nursery rounds, inservice education programs, on the job training programs, individual consultations, staff conferences, and ongoing research projects provides avenues for staff education to supplement the daily presence in the nursery for evaluation and intervention. Therapists may initially need to actively pursue referrals, while also continuing efforts to educate nursery staff as to which infants to refer for evaluation, and developing a formal protocol for referral.

Therapists tend to assume that special care nurses, since they are in constant attendance in the nursery, are available and eager to carry out daily therapy programs. This assumption should be critically evaluated, not taken for granted. The special care nursery is, as its name implies, a very special setting. Nurses in particular are subject to an almost impossible set of demands. The full-time routine nursing care of very sick neonates demands a huge proportion of their time and emotional energy. This is complicated by the constant need to be ready to respond to life-threatening crises, admissions at any time of the day or night, transport system coverage, the needs of the visiting parents, and other interruptions.[135] Small wonder that some may offer resistance to the suggestion that they must also be responsible for programs of developmental therapy.

Physical therapists must be practical, innovative, realistic, and available if they are to gain the support of nursing colleagues. They must evaluate carefully what care can reasonably be given by the nurses, innovative about demonstrating ways in which such procedures can be incorporated into the nursery routine, and be available to perform the therapy when nurses cannot.

Last, but definitely not least, to gain acceptance as valued special care nursery team members, physical therapists must be accountable for their programs. The fact that very little evidence of the effectiveness of physical therapy with high-risk neonates exists should be acknowledged and every effort made to remedy this situation. A number of suggestions for establishing accountability have been made by Campbell and Wilhelm.[136] For example, self-education before entering nursery practice to assure that services established are based on sound principles; development of protocols that include standardized methods of collecting patient data during treatment and long-term follow-up; establishing therapeutic goals that can be objectively measured; and contributing to the professional knowledge base through participation in planning and conducting clinical research at whatever level one's education permits, including publishing one's findings in the professional literature or presenting them at scientific meetings, whether these be well-documented case reports, single-subject experiments, or the results of more formal research.

REFERENCES

1. Parmelee AH, Haber A: Who is the "risk infant"? Clin Obstet Gynecol 16:376, 1973.
2. Schechner S: For the 1980s: How small is too small? Clin Perinatol 7:135, 1980.
3. Thompson JR, Reynolds J: The results of intensive care therapy for neonates: I. Overall neonatal mortality rates. II. Neonatal mortality rates and long-term prognosis for low birthweight neonates. J Perinat Med 5:59, 1977.
4. Baum D, MacFarlane A, Tizard P: The benefits and hazards of neonatology. In Chard T, Richards M (eds): Benefits and Hazards of the New Obstetrics. Clinics in Developmental Medicine, No. 64. Lippincott, Philadelphia, 1977.
5. Desmond MM, Wilson GS, Alt EJ, et al: The very low birth weight infant after discharge from intensive care: Anticipatory health care and developmental course. Curr Probl Pediatr 10:1, 1980.
6. Sostek AM, Quinn PO, Davitt MK: Behavior, development and neurologic status of premature and full-term infants with varying medical complications. In Field TM, Sostek AM, Goldberg S, et al (eds): Infants Born at Risk: Behavior and Development. SP Medical and Scientific Books, New York, 1979.
7. Hill A, Volpe JJ: Seizures, hypoxic-ischemic brain injury and intraventricular hemorrhage in the newborn. Ann Neurol 10:109, 1981.
8. Sarnat HB, Sarnat MS: Neonatal encephalopathy following fetal distress: A clinical and electroencephalographic study. Arch Neurol 33:696, 1976.
9. Finer NN, Robertson CM, Richards RT, et al: Hypoxic-ischemic encephalopathy in term neonates: Perinatal factors and outcome. J Pediatr 98:112, 1981.
10. DeSouza SW, Richards B: Neurological sequelae in newborn babies after perinatal asphyxia. Arch Dis Child 53:564, 1978.
11. Low JA, Galbraith RS, Muir D, et al: Intrapartum fetal asphyxia: A preliminary report in regard to long-term morbidity. Am J Obstet Gynecol 130:525, 1978.
12. MacDonald HM, Mulligan JC, Allen AC, et al: Neonatal asphyxia. I. Relationship of obstetric and neonatal complications to neonatal mortality in 38,405 consecutive deliveries. J Pediatr 96:898, 1980.
13. Mulligan JC, Painter MJ, O'Donoghue PA, et al: Neonatal asphyxia. II. Neonatal mortality and long-term sequelae. J Pediatr 96:903, 1980.
14. Scott H: Outcome of very severe birth asphyxia. Arch Dis Child 51:712, 1976.

15. Thomson AJ: Quality of survival after severe birth asphyxia. Arch Dis Child 52:620, 1977.
16. Yu VYH, Wood C: Perinatal asphyxia and outcome in very low birthweight infants. Med J Aust 2:278, 1978.
17. Hobel CJ, Oakes GK: Special considerations in the management of preterm labor. Clin Obstet Gynecol 23:147, 1980.
18. Lou HC: Perinatal hypoxic-ischemic brain damage and intraventricular hemorrhage: A pathogenetic model. Arch Neurol 37:585, 1980.
19. Wigglesworth JS: Pathophysiology of intracranial hemorrhage in the newborn. J Perinat Med, 9, Suppl 1: 90, 1981.
20. deCourten GM, Rabinowicz T: Intraventricular hemorrhage in premature infants: Reappraisal and new hypotheses. Dev Med Child Neurol 23:389, 1981.
21. Pasternak JF, Mantovani JF, Volpe JJ: Porencephaly from periventricular intracerebral hemorrhage in a premature infant. Am J Dis Child 134:673, 1980.
22. Pape KE: Intraventricular hemorrhage: Diagnosis and outcome. Birth Defects 17:143, 1981.
23. Fenichel GM: Neonatal Neurology. Churchill Livingstone, New York, 1980.
24. Ahmann PA, Lazzara A, Dykes FD, et al: Intraventricular hemorrhage in the high-risk preterm infant: Incidence and outcome. Ann Neurol 7:118, 1980.
25. Kosmetatos N, Dinter C, Williams ML, et al: Intracranial hemorrhage in the premature: Its predictive features and outcome. Am J Dis Child, 134:855, 1980.
26. Cooke RWI: Factors associated with periventricular hemorrhage in very low birthweight infants. Arch Dis Child 56:425, 1981.
27. Papile L-A, Burstein J, Burstein M, et al: Incidence and evolution of subependymal and intraventricular hemorrhage: A study of infants with birth weights less than 1,500 grams. J Pediatr 92:529, 1978.
28. Clark CE, Clyman RI, Roth RS, et al: Risk factor analysis of intraventricular hemorrhage in low-birth-weight infants. J Pediatr 99:625, 1981.
29. Dubowitz LMS, Levene MI, Morante A, et al: Neurologic signs in neonatal intraventricular hemorrhage: A correlation with real-time ultrasound. J Pediatr 99:127, 1981.
30. Levene MI, Wigglesworth JS, Dubowitz V: Cerebral structure and intraventricular hemorrhage in the neonate: A real-time ultrasound study. Arch Dis Child 56:416, 1981.
31. Krishnamoorthy KS, Shannon DC, DeLong GR, et al: Neurologic sequelae in the survivors of neonatal intraventricular hemorrhage. Pediatrics 64:233, 1979.
32. Rajani K, Goetzman BW, Kelso GF, et al: Prognosis of intracranial hemorrhage in neonates. Surg Neurol 13:433, 1980.
33. Robinson RO, Desai NS: Factors influencing mortality and morbidity after clinically apparent intraventricular hemorrhage. Arch Dis Child 56:478, 1981.
34. Siegel JD, McCracken GH Jr: Sepsis neonatorum. N Engl J Med 304:642, 1981.
35. Hill A, Shackelford GD, Volpe JJ: Ventriculitis with neonatal bacterial meningitis: Identification by real-time ultrasound. J Pediatr 99:133, 1981.
36. Sinclair JC, Torrance GW, Boyle MH, et al: Evaluation of neonatal-intensive-care programs. N Engl J Med 305:489, 1981.
37. McCormick MC: The regionalization of perinatal care. Am J Public Health 71:571, 1981.
38. Harris TR: Influence of newborn and maternal transport programs on neonatal mortality in the State of Arizona. In Sell EJ (ed): Follow-up of the High Risk Newborn—A Practical Approach. Charles C Thomas, Springfield, IL, 1980.

39. Hack M, Fanaroff AA, Merkatz IR: Current concepts: The low-birth-weight infant—Evolution of a changing outlook. N Engl J Med 301:1162, 1979.
40. Siegel E, Gillings D, Campbell S, et al: A controlled evaluation of regional perinatal care in North Carolina. Final Report, Grant MC-R-370424, Maternal and Child Health and Crippled Children's Services Research Grants Program, Bureau of Community Health Services, HSA, PHS, DHHS, 1982.
41. Shapiro S, McCormick MC, Starfield BH, et al: Relevance of correlates of infant deaths for significant morbidity at one year of age. Am J Obstet Gynecol 136:363, 1980.
42. Stavis RL, Krauss AN: Complications of neonatal intensive care. Clin Perinatol 7:107, 1980.
43. Lucey JF: Thoughts on double site TcPO₂ monitoring: Iatrogenic hypoxaemia and the patent ductus arteriosus epidemic. In Rolfe P (ed): Fetal and Neonatal Physiological Measurements. Pitman, London, 1980.
44. Gottfried AW, Wallace-Lande P, Sherman-Brown S, et al: Physical and social environment of newborn infants in special-care units. Science 214:673, 1981.
45. Lazzara A, Ahmann P, Dykes F, et al: Clinical predictability of intraventricular hemorrhage in preterm infants. Pediatrics 65:30, 1980.
46. Silverboard G, Lazarra A, Ahmann PA, et al: Comparison of lumbar puncture with computed tomography scan as an indicator of intracerebral hemorrhage in the preterm infant. Pediatrics 66:432, 1980.
47. Grant EG, Borts FT, Schellinger D, et al: Real-time ultrasonography of neonatal intraventricular hemorrhage and comparison with computed tomography. Radiology 139:687, 1981.
48. Sauerbrei EE, Digney M, Harrison PB, et al: Ultrasonic evaluation of neonatal intracranial hemorrhage and its complications. Radiology 139:677, 1981.
49. Thorburn RJ, Lipscomb AP, Stewart AL, et al: Prediction of death and major handicap in very preterm infants by brain ultrasound. Lancet 1(8230):1119, 1981.
50. Huch A, Huch R: Transcutaneous noninvasive monitoring of pO₂. Hosp Pract 11:43, 1976.
51. leSouef PN, Morgan AK, Soutter LP, et al: Comparison of transcutaneous oxygen tension with arterial oxygen tension in newborn infants with severe respiratory illnesses. Pediatrics 62:692, 1978.
52. Huch R, Lubbers DW, Huch A: Reliability of transcutaneous monitoring of arterial pO₂ in newborn infants. Arch Dis Child 49:213, 1974.
53. Lucey JF: Transcutaneous diagnosis in the high-risk neonate. Hosp Pract 16:108, 1981.
54. Hobel CJ, Hyvarinen MA, Okada DM, et al: Prenatal and intrapartum high-risk screening. I. Prediction of the high-risk neonate. Am J Obstet Gynecol 117:1, 1973.
55. Parmelee A, Kopp C, Sigman M: Selection of developmental assessment techniques for infants at risk. Merrill-Palmer Q 22:177, 1976.
56. Prechtl HFR, Beintema DJ: The neurological findings in newborn infants after pre and perinatal complications. In Jonxis JHP, Visser HKA, Troelska JA (eds): Nutricia Symposium: Aspects of Prematurity and Dysmaturity. Stenfert Kroese, Leiden, 1968.
57. Als H: II. Assessing an assessment: Conceptual considerations, methodological issues, and a perspective on the future of the Neonatal Behavioral Assessment Scale. Monogr Soc Res Child Dev 43:14, 1978.
58. Gorski PA, Davison MF, Brazelton TB: Stages of behavioral organization in the high-risk neonate: Theoretical and clinical considerations. Sem Perinatol 3:61, 1979.

59. Speidel BD: Adverse effects of routine procedures on preterm infants. Lancet 1(8069):864, 1978.
60. Long JG, Philips AGS, Lucey JF: Excessive handling as a cause of hypoxemia. Pediatrics 65:203, 1980.
61. Als H, Lester BM, Brazelton TB: Dynamics of the behavioral organization of the premature infant: A theoretical perspective. In Field T (ed): Infants Born at Risk. Spectrum, New York, 1979.
62. Brazelton TB, Parker WB, Zuckerman B: Importance of behavioral assessment of the neonate. Curr Probl Pediatr 7:1, 1976.
63. Andre-Thomas, Chesni Y, Saint-Anne Dargassies S: The Neurological Examination of the Infant. Little Club Clinics in Developmental Medicine, No. 1. National Spastics Society, London, 1960.
64. Paine RS: Neurologic examination of infants and children. Pediatr Clin North Am 7:471, 1960.
65. Paine RS: The immediate value of the neonatal neurological examination. In Child Neurology and Cerebral Palsy. Little Club Clinics in Developmental Medicine, No. 2. National Spastics Society, London, 1960.
66. Prechtl HFR, Beintema D: The Neurological Examination of the Full Term Newborn Infant. Clinics in Developmental Medicine, No. 12. Heinemann, London, 1964.
67. Prechtl HFR: The Neurological Examination of the Full Term Newborn Infant. 2nd Ed. Clinics in Developmental Medicine, No. 63. Lippincott, Philadelphia, 1977.
68. Graham FK: Behavioral differences between normal and traumatized newborns. I. The test procedures. Psychol Monogr 70(20):1–16, 1956.
69. Rosenblith JF, Anderson-Huntington R: Behavioral examination of the neonate. In Wilson JM (ed): Infants at Risk: Medical and Therapeutic Management. 2nd Ed. University of North Carolina at Chapel Hill, Chapel Hill, 1981.
70. Brazleton TB: Neonatal Behavioral Assessment Scale. Clinics in Developmental Medicine, No. 50. Lippincott, Philadelphia, 1973.
71. Saint-Anne Dargassies S: Neurological maturation of the premature infant of 28–41 weeks gestational age. In Falkner F (ed): Human Development. Saunders, Philadelphia, 1966.
72. Saint-Anne Dargassies S: Neurological Development in the Full-Term and Premature Neonate. Excerpta Medica, New York, 1977.
73. Prechtl HFR, Fargel JW, Weinmann HM, et al: Postures, motility and respiration of low-risk, pre-term infants. Dev Med Child Neurol 21:3, 1979.
74. Bosma JF: Examination of the mouth and pharynx of the infant. In Wilson JM (ed): Infants at Risk: Medical and Therapeutic Management. 2nd Ed. University of North Carolina at Chapel Hill, Chapel Hill, 1981.
75. Wolff PH: Abnormalities in the sequential organization of non-nutritive sucking. In Wilson JM (ed): Infants at Risk: Medical and Therapeutic Management. 2nd Ed. University of North Carolina at Chapel Hill, Chapel Hill, 1981.
76. Cowett RM, Lipsett LP, Vohr B, et al: Aberrations in sucking behavior of low-birthweight infants. Dev Med Child Neurol 20:701, 1979.
77. Bosma JF: Structure and function of infant oral and pharyngeal mechanisms. In Wilson JM (ed): Oral-Motor Function and Dysfunction in Children. University of North Carolina at Chapel Hill, Chapel Hill, 1978.
78. Carr J: Oral Function in Infancy. Cumberland College Reports, No. 15. South Wales, Australia, Cumberland College of Health Sciences, 1979.

79. Farber S: Neurohabilitation for the neonate. In Wilson JM (ed): Infants at Risk: Medical and Therapeutic Management. 2nd Ed. University of North Carolina at Chapel Hill, Chapel Hill, 1981.
80. Morris SE: Principles of oral-motor assessment. In Wilson JM (ed): Oral-Motor Function and Dysfunction in Children. University of North Carolina at Chapel Hill, Chapel Hill, 1978.
81. Campbell SK: Effects of developmental intervention in the special care nursery. In Wolraich ML, Routh D (eds): The Advances in Developmental and Behavioral Pediatrics, Greenwich CT, JAI Press 1983, pp 165–179.
82. Brown J, Hepler R: Stimulation—A corollary to physical care. Am J Nurs 76:578, 1976.
83. Field T: Supplemental stimulation of preterm neonates. Early Hum Dev 4:301, 1980.
84. Schaefer M, Hatcher RP, Barglow PD: Prematurity and infant stimulation: A review of research. Child Psychiatry Hum Dev 10:199, 1980.
85. Masi W: Supplemental stimulation of the preterm infant. In Field TM, Sostek AM, Goldberg H, Shuman HH (eds): Infants Born at Risk: Behavior and Development. SP Medical and Scientific Books, New York, 1979.
86. Cornell EH, Gottfried AW: Intervention with premature human infants. Child Dev 47:32, 1976.
87. Wright L: The theoretical research base for a program of early stimulation care, and training of premature infants. In Hellmuth J (ed): Exceptional Infant. Vol 2. Brunner/Mazel, New York, 1967.
88. Hebb DO: Organization of Behavior. Wiley, New York, 1949.
89. Piaget J: Origins of Intelligence in Children, trans. Cook M. International Universities Press, New York, 1952.
90. Rutter M: The long-term effects of early experience. Dev Med Child Neurol 22:800, 1980.
91. Chapman JS: The relationship between auditory stimulation and gross motor activity of short gestation infants. Res Nurs Health 1:29, 1978.
92. Brackbill Y: Cumulative effects of continuous stimulation on arousal levels in infants. Child Dev 42:17, 1971.
93. Brackbill Y: Continuous stimulation reduces arousal level: Stability of the effect over time. Child Dev 44:43, 1973.
94. Brackbill Y, Adams G, Crowell DH, et al: Arousal level in neonates and preschool children under continuous auditory stimulation. J Exp Child Psychol 4:178, 1966.
95. Schulman JL, Reisman JM: An objective measure of hyperactivity. Am J Ment Defic 64:455, 1959.
96. Brackbill Y, Douthitt TC, West H: Psychophysiologic effects in the neonate of prone versus supine placement. J Pediatr 82:82, 1973.
97. Schwartz FCM, Fenner A, Wolfsdorf J: The influence of body position on pulmonary function in low birthweight babies. S Afr Med J 49:79, 1975.
98. Hutchison AA, Ross KR, Russell G: The effect of posture on ventilation and lung mechanics in preterm and light-for-date infants. Pediatrics 64:429, 1979.
99. Martin RJ, Herrell N, Rubin D, et al: Effect of supine and prone positions on arterial oxygen tension in the preterm infant. Pediatrics 63:528, 1979.
100. Yu VYH: Effect of body position on gastric emptying in the neonate. Arch Dis Child 50:500, 1975.
101. Spahr JC, MacDonald HM, Mueller-Heubach E: Knee-chest position and neonatal oxygenation and blood pressure. Am J Dis Child 135:79, 1981.

102. Scarr-Salapatek S, Williams ML: The effects of early stimulation on low-birth-weight infants. Child Dev 44:94, 1973.
103. Karmer LI, Pierpont ME: Rocking waterbeds and auditory stimuli to enhance growth of preterm infants. J Pediatr 88:297, 1976.
104. White JL, Labarba RC: The effects of tactile and kinesthetic stimulation on neonatal development in the premature infant. Dev Psychobiol 9:569, 1976.
105. Field TM, Widmayer SM, Stringer S, et al: Teenage, lower-class, black mothers and their preterm infants: An intervention and developmental follow-up. Child Dev 51:426, 1980.
106. Rice RD: The effects of the Rice Sensorimotor Stimulation Treatment on the development of high-risk infants. Birth Defects 15:76, 1979.
107. Neal MV: Vestibular stimulation and development of the small premature infant. Commun Nurs Res 8:291, 1975.
108. Katz V: Auditory stimulation and developmental behavior of the small premature infant. Nurs Res 20:196, 1971.
109. Chapman JS: The effect of pre-term infants' decreasing mortality on their future morbidity: Preliminary examination of long-term outcomes of stimulation programs for preterm infants. Nurs Pap 10:31, 1978.
110. Powell LF: The effect of extra stimulation and maternal involvement on the development of low-birth-weight infants and on maternal behavior. Child Dev 45:106, 1974.
111. Lieb SA, Benfield DG, Guidubuldi J: Effects of early intervention and stimulation on the preterm infant. Pediatric 66:83, 1980.
112. Mueller HA: Facilitating feeding and prespeech. In Pearson PH, Williams CS (eds): Physical Therapy Services in the Developmental Disabilities. Charles C Thomas, Springfield IL, 1972.
113. Mueller HA: Feeding. In Finnie N (ed): Handling the Young Cerebral Palsied Child at Home. Dutton, New York, 1975.
114. Burpee B: Effects of oral stimulation in premature infants. In Wilson, JM (ed): Infants at Risk: Medical and Therapeutic Management. 2nd Ed. University of North Carolina at Chapel Hill, Chapel Hill, 1982.
115. Leonard EL, Trykowski LE, Kirkpatrick BV: Nutritive sucking in high-risk neonates after perioral stimulation. Phys Ther 60:299, 1980.
116. Trykowski LE, Kirkpatrick BV, Leonard EL: Enhancement of nutritive sucking in premature infants. Phys Occup Ther Pediatr 1:27, 1981.
117. Neeley CA: Effects of nonnutritive sucking upon the behavioral arousal of the newborn. Birth Defects 15:173, 1979.
118. Anderson GC, Vidyasagar D: Development of sucking in premature infants from 1 to 7 days post birth. Birth Defects 15:145, 1979.
119. Burroughs AK, Asonye UO, Anderson-Shanklin GC, et al: The effect of non-nutritive sucking on transcutaneous oxygen tension in noncrying, preterm neonates. Res Nurs Health 1:69, 1978.
120. Measel CP, Anderson GC: Nonnutritive sucking during tube feedings: Effect on clinical course in premature infants. JOGN Nurs 8:265, 1979.
121. Dubowitz LMS, Dubowitz V: The Neurological Assessment of the Preterm and Full-term Newborn Infant. Clinics in Developmental Medicine, No. 79. Lippincott, Philadelphia, 1981.
122. Prechtl HFR: Assessment methods for the newborn infants, a critical evaluation. In Stratton P (ed): Psychobiology of the Human Newborn. Wiley, Chichester, 1982.

123. Campbell SK, Wilhelm IJ: Developmental sequences in infants at high risk for central nervous system dysfunction: The recovery process in the first year of life. In Stack JM (ed): An Interdisciplinary Approach to the Optimal Development of Infants: The Special Infant. Human Sciences Press, New York, 1982.

124. Campbell SK, Wilhelm IJ, Attermeier SA, et al: Baby Research and Training Section progress report: Development of infants at risk for CNS dysfunction. In Slaton DS (ed): Caring for Special Babies. University of North Carolina at Chapel Hill, Chapel Hill, 1983, pp. 96–158.

125. Niparko N: The effect of prematurity on performance on the Denver Developmental Screening Test. Phys Occup Ther Pediatr 2:29, 1982.

126. Parmelee AH: Assessment of the infant at risk during the first year. In Sell EJ (ed): Follow-up of the High Risk Newborn—A Practical Approach. Charles C Thomas, Springfield IL, 1980.

127. Minde K, Shosenberg N, Marton P, et al: Self-help groups in a premature nursery—A controlled evaluation. J Pediatr 96:933, 1980.

128. Ross G: Parental responses to infants in intensive care: The separation issue reevaluated. Clin Perinatol 7:47, 1980.

129. Jeffcoate JA, Humphrey ME, Lloyd JK: Disturbance in parent-child relationship following preterm delivery. Dev Med Child Neurol 21:344, 1979.

130. Widmayer SM, Field TM: Effects of Brazelton demonstrations for mothers on the development of preterm infants. Pediatrics 67:711, 1981.

131. Brown JV, LaRossa MM, Aylward GP, et al: Nursery based intervention with prematurely born babies and their mothers: Are there effects? J Pediatr 97:487, 1980.

132. Rosenfeld AG: Visiting in the intensive care nursery. Child Dev 51:939, 1980.

133. Desmond MM, Vorderman AL, Salinas M: The family and premature infant after neonatal intensive care. Tex Med 76:60, 1980.

134. Howard J, Parmelee AH, Kopp CB, et al: A neurologic comparison of preterm and full-term infants at term conceptual age. J Pediatr 88:995, 1976.

135. Marshall RE, Kasman C: Burnout in the neonatal intensive care unit. Pediatrics 65:1161, 1980.

136. Campbell SK, Wilhelm IJ: Physical therapy in the special care nursery. In Pearson PH, Fieber N, (eds): Physical Therapy Services in the Developmental Disabilities. 2nd Ed. (in press).

5 | Brachial Plexus Injury

Roberta B. Shepherd

Although the occurrence of brachial plexus injury in the neonate has been reduced by improved obstetric techniques, as Eng[1] has pointed out, the current incidence is not negligible, and the resultant handicap can be very severe indeed. Unfortunately, it is the relatively small number of such infants seen by therapists that constitutes a problem, as there has been little investigation of new and more effective ways of ensuring maximum possible recovery of function.

Brachial plexus injuries are usually classified under three headings: *Erb or upper plexus type* (involving C5 and C6), *Klumpke or lower plexus type* (involving C8 and T1), and *Erb-Klumpke or whole arm type* (involving C5 to T1). Exact localization of the anatomic lesion is often difficult,[2,3] however, and many infants demonstrate a mixed upper and lower type. Considerable variation in the type of lesion occurs, ranging from a mild edema affecting one or two roots to total avulsion of the entire plexus. Involvement is usually unilateral and the results of the lesion are always immediately recognizable.

ETIOLOGY AND INCIDENCE

Injury to the brachial plexus in infants occurs most commonly as a result of a difficult birth.[4,5] The factors implicated include the following: high birth weight, a sedated, hypotonic, and therefore vulnerable infant, a heavily sedated mother, traction in a breech presentation or rotation of the head in a cephalic presentation, and a difficult cesarean extraction.

During the birth process, the trauma that injures the plexus may also injure the facial nerve, causing a mild facial paralysis.[1] Other complications include fractures of the clavicle or humerus, traction to the cervical cord with signs of upper motoneuron lesion, subluxation of the shoulder, and torticollis. The phrenic nerve (C4) may also be injured, causing an ipsilateral hemiparalysis of the diaphragm. Eng[1] reported an infant with a peripheral radial nerve lesion in addition to a bilateral Erb's paralysis.

Trauma to the shoulder region other than birth injury may also result in injury to the brachial plexus, although this is not common. Such trauma may include pressure from a body case,[6] falls involving traction and hyperabduction of the shoulder, and pressure from the neck-seal of a continuous positive airway pressure head box.[7]

The lower plexus may be injured as a result of pressure from congenital abnormalities such as cervical rib, abnormal thoracic vertebrae, or shortened scalenus anticus muscle. An unusual neuritis of the brachial plexus, called "paralytic brachial neuritis," which is of unknown etiology, has been described by Magee and DeJong.[8]

Incidence of brachial plexus injury has declined because of improved obstetric management of difficult labor.[1] According to the studies[3,9–11] available, actual incidence seems to vary. Adler and Patterson[3] reported that the incidence had declined from 1.56 to 0.38 per 1000 live births between the years of 1938 and 1962. However, Specht[10] in his 1975 review gave an incidence of 0.57 per 1000 and Davis and associates[11] reported in 1978 that the current incidence was approximately 0.6 per 1000 live births.

PATHOLOGY

In order to understand the mechanism of injury, it is necessary to study the anatomy of the brachial plexus and its relationship to its surrounding structures. The reader is referred to the many anatomy texts available. Figure 5-1 illustrates diagrammatically the three main trunks of the plexus.

In theory, any force that alters the anatomic relationship between neck, shoulder, and arm may result in injury to the plexus. The plexus is attached by fascia to the first rib medially and to the coracoid process of the scapula laterally. Lateral movement of the head with depression of the shoulder girdle will stretch the nerves and compress them against the first ribs. Forced abduction (hyperabduction) of the shoulder with traction on the arm will stretch the nerves and compress them under the coracoid process. The former will cause injury to the upper plexus, the latter to the lower plexus. Where the trauma is severe and stretch reaches a certain force, complete avulsion of the nerves will result.

Stretching of the nerve roots or trunk of the plexus may result in injuries ranging from swelling of the neural sheath with blocking of nerve impulses, to hemorrhage and scar formation, to axonal rupture with wide separation of fragments.[12] The nerve roots may be completely avulsed from the cord. A combination of these lesions is common and this will be reflected in the electromyographic (EMG) findings.[12] If avulsion occurs, there will be some hemorrhage in the subarachnoid space, and the presence of blood in the cerebrospinal fluid will therefore suggest this more serious injury. Some authors[13,14] recommend the use of somatosensory cerebral evoked potentials for specific

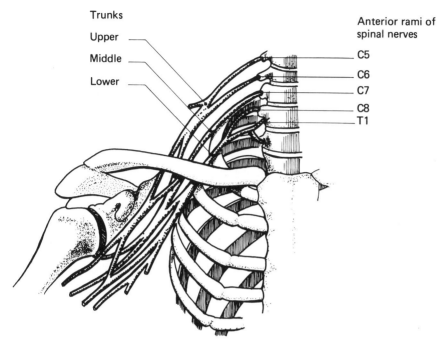

Fig. 5-1. The three main trunks of the brachial plexus.

diagnosis of dorsal root avulsion. Presence of Horner's syndrome* indicates an intraspinal avulsion of the root of T1 with involvement of the sympathetic fibers.

Regeneration of nerves is unlikely following complete axonal rupture. However, most brachial plexus lesions are less severe, and in these cases recovery occurs due to resolution of edema and hemorrhage, or to regrowth of nerve fibers down the sheath. In the latter case, recovery will be slow due to the distance over which regenerating axons must grow. Regrowth, if it occurs, proceeds at approximately 1 mm/day. In the upper arm type, this regeneration is usually complete by 4 to 5 months, in the whole arm type, by 7 to 9 months.[12]

Eng[1] describes serial electromyographic studies that depict the evolution of the disorder. The lesion is indicated by decreased voluntary motor unit activity and the presence of denervation potentials in the form of fibrillation and sharp wave potentials. Regeneration is signified by the appearance of small polyphasic motor units. As recovery progresses, there is an increase in the number of motor units recorded, a decrease in denervation potentials, and eventually a return of excitability of the nerves to electrical stimuli. Degen-

---

* Horner's syndrome: deficient sweating, recession of eyeball into the orbit, abnormal pupillary contraction, and ptosis.

erative changes in muscles are indicated by absent motor unit activity and paucity of denervation potentials plus nonconduction.

In adults, denervation of a muscle is followed by changes in the contractile properties of that muscle. A denervated muscle atrophies with shrinkage of individual muscle cells and thickening of endomysium, perimysium, and epimysium. Studies by Stefanova-Uzunova and colleagues[15] suggest that if denervation occurs at birth, there is also impairment of the normal developmental changes in the contractile properties of muscle that should occur postnatally.

DIFFERENTIAL DIAGNOSIS AND PROGNOSIS

The principle other causes of upper limb paralysis in infancy that need to be excluded are upper motoneuron lesions (lesions of the cervical cord or brain) and lower motoneuron lesions (lesions of the anterior horn cell) such as occur in poliomyelitis. Although the clinical appearance of the upper limb in hemiplegia and brachial plexus paralysis may be similar in terms of the arm's posture and absence of movement in either the whole arm or in certain muscle groups, hemiplegia can usually be easily differentiated by careful analysis of lower limb function and by the testing of reflexes. In upper motoneuron lesions, tendon reflexes are present and hyperactive in both limbs on the affected side or in all four limbs. In addition, there is sustained ankle clonus and a persistent Babinski sign. A spinal cord lesion is also characterized by sensory abnormalities over the trunk and involvement of the bladder.

Poliomyelitis may be confused with the whole arm type of brachial plexus lesion, but can usually be differentiated by the typical clinical picture and by the presence of intact sensation.

Most cases of brachial nerve injury have a favorable prognosis.[10,16] It is not the extensiveness of the involvement but the severity of the involvement, that is, the degree of neural damage, which gives the clue to prognosis. Eng[1] reported that electromyographic findings on the extent of the involvement did not correlate with the rate of recovery. For example, an extensive paralysis that is merely a neurapraxic lesion may recover completely, while a lesion of only C5 and C6, if complete axonal rupture is involved, may not recover at all.

PHYSICAL THERAPY EVALUATION

Evaluation is necessary as an aid to diagnosis, as a record of progress, and, by providing a detailed analysis of function, as an important stage in the problem-solving process. An important part of the physical therapy evaluation is the analysis of motor function, the objective of which is to gain the most complete picture possible of the infant's current status, the reasons for dysfunction, and the problems that may arise in the future. For analysis of motor function to be sufficiently thorough, the therapist must understand the muscle function required for the performance of everyday movements. In the case of infants, the therapist must also understand the development of motor control that occurs as the infant's brain matures and it becomes possible to practice increasingly complex motor tasks.

Analysis of motor function is made by observation of muscle contraction and movement in comparison with normal function at that age, and by passive movement to gauge the length of muscles and to gain a subjective impression of the muscle contraction that occurs in response to these movements. Motor function may be recorded on videotape, cine film, or still photograph. Muscle activity may be documented by an electromyographic recording or on a muscle chart.

Sensory loss may not correspond to the extent of motor loss. Sensory testing is not possible with any degree of accuracy in young infants, and the problem is compounded by the muscle paralysis. Response to pin prick can be tested, using the infant's appearance of discomfort as a guide, and the result can be recorded on a body chart. O'Riain[17] describes a "wrinkle" test that may be helpful. The fingers are immersed in water at 40°C for 30 minutes. Normal skin wrinkles, but denervated skin does not. Wrinkling returns as the skin is reinnervated. In older children, two-point discrimination can be tested using an esthesiometer; however, the functional significance of such testing is doubtful.

Analysis of Motor Function

Presence of movement is assessed by *observation* of the following:

1. Spontaneous movement and posture as the infant lies in the suspine and prone positions and is moved around, cuddled, and talked to
2. Motor behavior during testing of reflexes and reactions, particularly of the Moro reflex, the placing reaction of the hands, the Galant (trunk incurvation) reflex, the neck righting reaction, the parachute reaction

Observation will give some indication of muscle activity, and this can be graded and recorded on a chart as, for example,

0 = Absent
1 = Present, but lacking full range of movement
2 = Present throughout a full range of movement

This chart is upgraded at subsequent visits, the therapist always searching actively for the presence of muscle contraction in different parts of range and different relationships to gravity.

Although it is usual in the literature to see a list of the typically denervated muscles in the various types of lesion, the therapist should take care not to assume weakness and paralysis in certain muscles and normal function in others. Careful analysis of motor function will frequently reveal a mixed lesion.

Several authors describe the use of *electromyographic assessment*.[12,18-20] Eng[1] suggests that electromyography is useful in topographically delineating the extent and severity of the injury, and in giving information about expected recovery. Electromyography would also provide the therapist with the information needed in planning treatment, as electromyographic signs of return usually precede clinical evidence of function by several weeks. Serial electromyographs are commenced within the first 2 weeks after birth and are repeated at 6- to 8-week intervals for as long as is indicated.

The appearance of decreased denervation potentials and the appearance of reinnervation potentials may predate subjective clinical evidence by several weeks. The appearance of these electromyographic findings should therefore be followed immediately by intensified therapy to stimulate activity in these muscles. Electromyographic information would therefore enable the therapist and parents to concentrate on the eliciting of motor activity and training of motor control in particular muscles at a time when the therapist may not be able to recognize the first signs of motor activity. Although excessive fatigue should be avoided, specific motor stimulation at this point in recovery may be crucial to the infant's ability to make the most of neural recovery, and it is probable that electromyography should be used more extensively than at present in order to guide the motor training program.

Patterns of Muscle Dysfunction

In the *upper arm type*, the dysfunction may involve the following muscles: rhomboids, levator scapulae, serratus anterior, deltoid, supraspinatus, infraspinatus, biceps brachii, brachioradialis, brachialis, supinator and long extensors of the wrist, fingers, and thumb (Fig. 5-2).

In the *lower arm type*, dysfunction involves the intrinsic muscles of the hand and the extensors and flexors of the wrist and fingers. Many infants demonstrate some mixture of upper and lower type dysfunction.

In the *upper and lower arm types*, problems arise as a result of the paralysis or weakness of certain muscles, the unopposed activity of other muscles, and the resultant muscle imbalance. These problems include persistent and abnormal movement habits, abnormal posturing of the arm (Fig. 5-3), soft tissue contracture, glenohumeral subluxation or dislocation (Fig. 5-4), posterior displacement of the humeral epiphysis and posterior radial dislocation, and, eventually, skeletal deformity and poor bone growth.

The resting position of the arm after brachial plexus injury is at the side. This factor, plus the paralysis or weakness of the shoulder abductors and flexors and the scapular retractors and protractors, together with overactivity of the unopposed shoulder adductors and medial rotators results eventually in soft tissue contracture.

Paralysis of the rhomboideus muscle together with the unopposed activity and eventual contracture of the muscles that link the humerus to the scapula (muscles subscapularis, teres minor, latissimus dorsi) cause the scapula to adhere to the humerus, and any flexion or abduction movement of 'he arm will

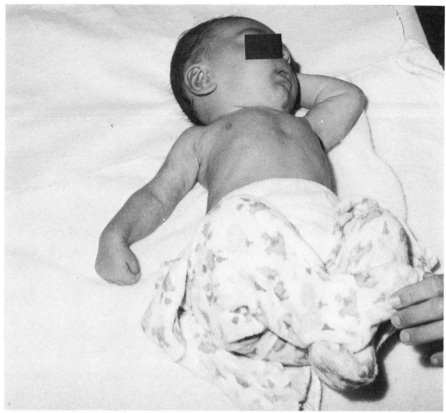

Fig. 5-2. Infant of 4 weeks with partial paralysis of the right arm.

be accomplished in a 1:1 ratio instead of the normal 6:1 humeroscapular relationship in the first 30 degrees of movement.

Abnormal posturing of the arm reflects the muscle imbalance but also the
substitution of habitual incorrect motor activity. The typical posturing of the
neonate with the upper arm type of paralysis (adducted, medially rotated shoulder, extended and pronated forearm, flexed wrist) gives way to an elevated,
slightly abducted, medially rotated and pronated arm as some muscle activity
returns and as the infant makes compensatory (and abnormal) movements in
attempts to use the arm.

It is common to see abnormal combinations of movement components, for
example, the combination of wrist flexion and forearm pronation with finger
extension for grasp. This is similar to the abnormal synergic activity seen as
part of the motor dysfunction resulting from central nervous system (CNS)
lesions. In the case of brachial plexus lesions, it may be that these abnormal
combinations of activity result from the child's attempts at using a poorly
aligned arm with as yet inadequate return of muscular function. The consequent

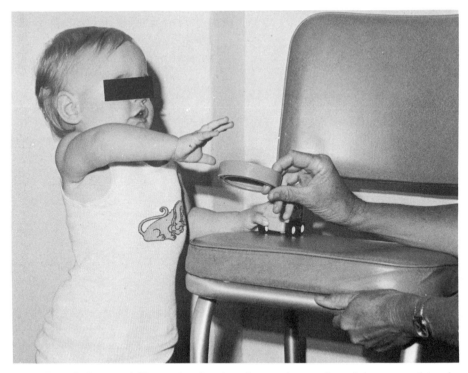

Fig. 5-3. Infant aged 13 months showing abnormal posturing of the arm and trunk.

lack of motor "skill" is seen therefore as an inability to eliminate muscle activity that is unnecessary for the function being attempted.

Other authors refer to these movements as "synkinetic movements" or "associated movements." Contractions of the biceps brachii and deltoid muscles have been noted to occur in conjunction with inspiratory movement.[16,21] Esslen[22] found synchronous motor unit potentials in different muscles supplied by the same nerve. De Grandis and colleagues[23] described a 13-year-old girl who was incapable of extending her fingers without flexing the forearm and wrist, and a 15-year-old girl whose strong finger flexion was associated with flexion of the forearm and wrist. The authors concluded that there is simultaneous innervation by the same motoneurons of one or more "motor subunits" in different muscles. They suggested also that inability to perform some movements may be due to simultaneous contraction of antagonistic muscles and not due to lack of muscle strength. Tada and associates,[24] in their study of rats, discussed disordered recovery and suggested that functionally different neurons as well as the correct neurons participate in the regeneration of the disrupted nerves.

In the *whole arm type*, there may be no apparent muscle activity anywhere in the limb. In whole arm paralysis, major problems are caused by the depen-

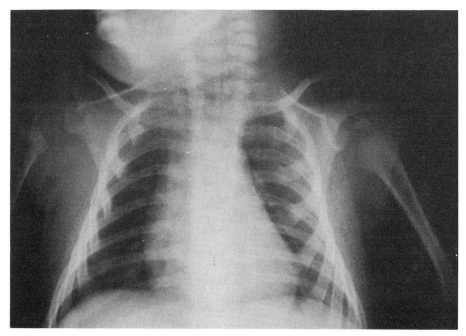

Fig. 5-4. Radiograph of infant showing dislocation of the right glenohumeral joint.

dent position of the arm with resultant stretch of soft tissues, together with a lack of muscle activity with which to preserve the integrity of the glenohumeral joint. This results in subluxation and dislocation of the glenohumeral joint.

Other problems that result from muscle paralysis are "learned nonuse," delay in achieving certain motor milestones such as balanced sitting, and inability to perform two-handed functions.

Analysis of Respiratory Function

Phrenic nerve paralysis, resulting in decreased movement of the ipsilateral thorax with respiratory distress and cyanosis, may mimic diaphragmatic hernia.[25]

Hemiparalysis of the diaphragm should be suspected whenever there are persistent physical and x-ray findings of atelectasis and unilateral diaphragmatic elevation. However, examination of diaphragmatic function using electromyography and fluoroscopy should be carried out on all infants with the upper or whole arm type of paralysis. Where electromyography is unavailable, assessment will involve observation of thoracic and abdominal movement in order to detect motor asymmetry.

PHYSICAL THERAPY

The infant should rest for the first few days to allow hemorrhage and edema to resolve. Physical treatment then commences, with the major objectives being to ensure the optimal conditions for recovery of motor function, to provide the stimulation necessary to enable muscles to resume function as soon as sufficient neural regeneration has taken place, and to train motor control.

In order to ensure the optimal conditions for recovery, the problems of soft tissue contracture, disorganization of movements at the shoulder and shoulder girdle joints, neglect of the limb, and incorrect movement habits must be prevented. In order to ensure that maximal functional recovery will follow neural regeneration, therapy must include specific careful training of functional movement once the affected muscles are reinnervated and capable of contraction. If recovery does not occur, the objectives of physical therapy will change to provide for the specific training which will be necessary following surgery to transplant muscles or arthrodese joints.

The role of physical therapy must be seen, therefore, to extend beyond the maintenance of joint range and stimulation of movement, and must take into account the need to develop ways of preventing or minimizing disorganized movement in the limb, of training motor control, and preventing neglect of the arm. In addition, the therapist must train the parents to carry out treatment at home. Treatment must follow on from a detailed analysis of each problem, both existing and potential. The effects of each step in therapy should be subject to reevaluation to ensure that unproductive methods are discarded, new methods are introduced, and analysis has been correct.

In order to appreciate the effects of muscle dysfunction and to determine the objectives of treatment, it is necessary to understand the normal functions of the involved muscles and the way in which an infant normally acquires motor control of the upper limb.

Motor Training

A program of specific motor training should commence within the first 2 weeks of the infant's life. Although there can be no activity in muscles that are not innervated, this early motor training probably serves several purposes: to stimulate activity in muscles whose nerve supply is only temporarily disconnected; to enable muscles to be activated as soon as nerve regeneration has taken place; and to prevent, or minimize, soft tissue contracture, the syndrome of neglect, and habituation of incorrect (abnormal) movements.

Motor training should be specific and carefully monitored, the therapist using manual guidance and verbal feedback to ensure that the infant moves correctly, that is, activates the correct muscles for the movement. In selecting the muscles upon which to focus attention, it may be helpful to consider that certain of the involved muscles are particularly essential for function, for example, the abductors, flexors, and lateral rotators of the shoulder, together with the scapular rotators, retractors and protractors, the supinators of the

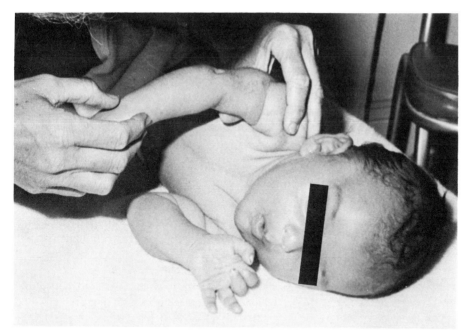

Fig. 5-5. Infant aged 4 weeks. Attempting to elicit activity in the deltoid muscle by encouraging the infant to take his hand to his face. This would require the muscle to work both concentrically and as a fixator.

forearm, the wrist extensors and radial deviators, and the palmar abductor of the thumb. Of course, this is not to suggest that these are the only muscles to be trained, but only to point out that there is an urgent need to train these muscles as early as recovery will allow, before habitual overactivity of the nonparalyzed muscles and contracture of soft tissues make it impossible for the recovering muscles to demonstrate their optimal activity.

Training should commence under the best possible conditions for each muscle, taking into account leverage, the relationship of the limb to gravity (Figs. 5-5, 5-6), the fact that an eccentric contraction can often be elicited before a concentric contraction (Fig. 5-7), and the need for proper alignment in order to encourage the correct muscle action (Fig. 5-8). Hence with every muscle to be trained, the therapist must search actively for the presence of muscle contraction, checking different sectors of the movement range, different relationships to gravity, and trying to elicit eccentric activity if concentric activity is not present.

Unless the therapist initiates these activities, the earliest manifestations of recovery of motor activity in particular muscles may pass unnoticed. In the earliest stage of recovery a muscle may not be able to contract under certain conditions of leverage. For example, the deltoid may not be strong enough to raise the arm from the side but may be able to hold the arm and let it down a few degrees from a horizontal position in sitting (Fig. 5-7) or in a vertical

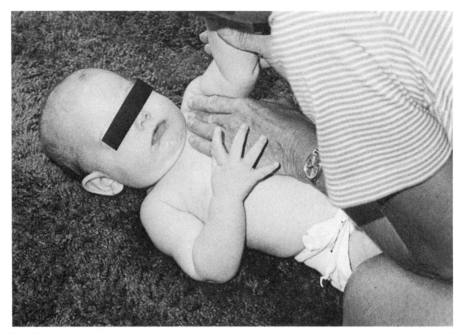

Fig. 5-6. Infant aged 4½ months. Encouraging activity in the deltoid muscle to hold the arm in flexion as he reaches up to touch the therapist's face.

position in lying (Fig. 5-6). Similarly, the wrist extensors may not be able to contract strongly enough to lift the hand from a position of total wrist flexion, but they may be able to contract eccentrically from a shortened position, or the radial extensor may be able to contract to radially deviate or lift the wrist from the table.

Motor training should continue for as long as recovery is still occurring. It may be that nerves have the potential for recovery for a relatively long period of time. Gatcheva[26] reports electromyographic evidence of reinnervation and the return of nerve conduction for 6 to 8 years after brachial plexus injury and suggests that it is essential to continue rehabilitation for many years. Gatcheva's observation is contrary to the usual opinion that recovery takes place within the first two years. However, the therapist should continue with periods of intensive motor training, using electromyography to provide guidance as to recovery.

Manual Guidance. Manual guidance to each movement is essential (Figs. 5-9, 5-10) in order that the desired muscle activity can be encouraged and incorrect movements prevented. For example, if the therapist attempts to elicit motor activity by encouraging reaching and other movements without appropriate guidance and control (Fig. 5-3), the infant, who will tend to use the stronger muscles or those that have the greatest advantage, will practice incorrect movements, and these substitution movements will quickly become

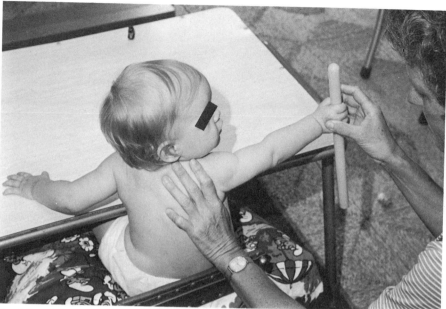

Fig. 5-7. Infant aged 13 months. Attempting to elicit eccentric deltoid activity in the inner range. Therapist guides correct scapula movement with her left hand.

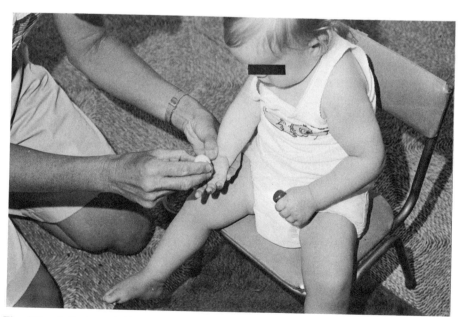

Fig. 5-8. Infant aged 13 months. Encouraging grasp and release with the forearm in supination. She will only spontaneously grasp and release in pronation.

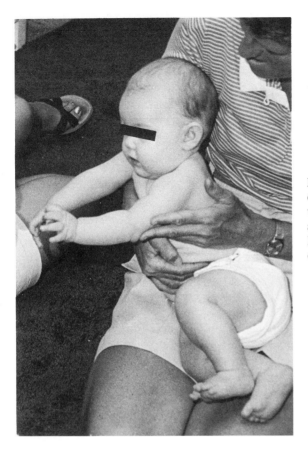

Fig. 5-9. Manual guidance to ensure the infant reaches forward with shoulder in correct alignment. Without guidance he would hold it in some abduction.

learned. This point must be kept in mind even with the young infant, as it will be difficult for the abnormal substitution movements to be "unlearned" once they have become well established, at least not until the infant is old enough to concentrate for longer periods on motor training and practice. In certain cases, muscles with the potential to recover fail to develop maximal function because of the establishment of poor movement habits. For this reason, a simple and accurate method of discovering the earliest manifestations of muscle activity by electromyography must be developed and utilized so that the therapist and parents can have advance notice of muscle reinnervation and concentrate their attention on stimulating recovering muscles to ensure their best possible recovery of function. Of course, where there has been severe disruption of nerve supply, there may be no recovery of function, no matter how skilled the therapist.

Fitts[27] and Fitts and Posner[28] have pointed out that the first stage in motor learning is *cognitive*, that is, the beginner tries to "understand" the overall idea of the task and what it demands; the second stage is *associative*, a period of continuous adjustment and reorganization of motor behavior in which com-

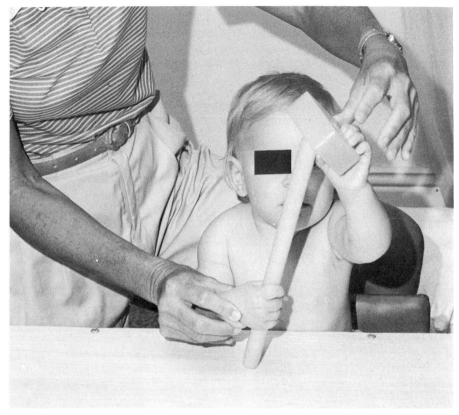

Fig. 5-10. Manual guidance to encourage supination of the right forearm, and to ensure the correct forearm alignment for grasping.

ponents are tried out and put together; and the third stage, the *autonomous* or automatic stage, is characterized by coordinated execution of the task, requiring little cognitive control and suffering less from distractions. Although there is an increasing lack of conscious awareness during this stage, learning does not cease. It is generally assumed that movement in infants can only be stimulated at an automatic level by play or by "facilitation" of movement. However, it is my experience that even small babies are able to "learn" movement at a cognitive level, that is, by "thinking" about the movement and by reacting to feedback from the therapists and parents about the success or otherwise of their performance. The therapist should not keep the infants practicing any movement for more than a few moments as they have little ability to concentrate and will resent being held in one position for too long. It may be that motor training of infants would be more effective if it concentrated on stimulating the infant's cognitive awareness of what he or she must do, rather than solely on eliciting an automatic response. One problem with stimulating movement at an automatic level is that it is so often done with insufficient

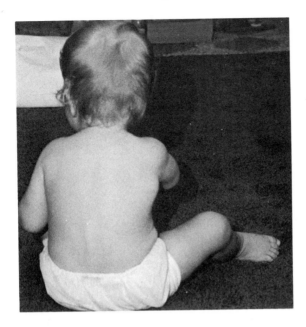

Fig. 5-11. Note the abnormal relationship between the scapula and the humerus on the right side. The scapula is protracted and moves with the humerus instead of adhering to the thoracic wall.

guidance. This results in the infant practicing what, in a sense, he or she can already do, which, without guidance, will frequently be an incorrect movement.

Verbal Feedback and Reinforcement. The infant's correct attempts at using the arm should be rewarded, so that he or she receives feedback as an aid to learning. *Verbal feedback* of successful performance, with reinforcement from tone of voice, smile, and a general attitude of pleasure, seems to have meaning even for small infants, who will usually strive to repeat the performance. Manual guidance, which ensures that the infant is as successful as possible, together with verbal feedback, will mean that therapy sessions are fun and motivating for the infant.

Behavior therapy is also a helpful method of ensuring maximal learning of the desired motor behavior. Behavior therapy involves positive reinforcement by smiling and saying "good boy" or by giving actual rewards, and shaping, which means reinforcing successive approximations of the desired behavior. For example, if the child will not concentrate on practice of a particular activity, he or she is rewarded for practicing for 2 minutes, then for 3 minutes, and so on.

Treatment of Movement Disorganization. Disorganization of scapulohumeral movement is frequently a serious problem (Fig. 5-11). Not only should therapy aim to prevent contracture of muscles such as subscapularis, which link the scapula and the humerus, it must also aim to stimulate the rhomboids and serratus anterior muscles to contract. Passive movement that ensures the normal range of shoulder abduction and flexion will have no real effect if the muscles that retract, protract, and rotate the scapula are inactive or weak. Figures 5-12 and 5-13 show two ways of ensuring that the scapular retractors

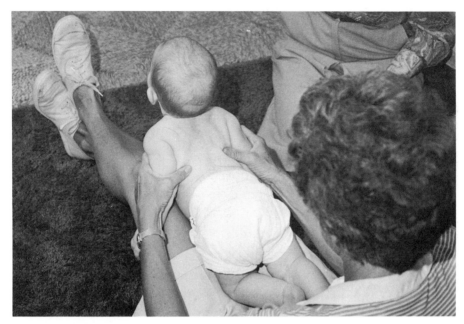

Fig. 5-12. Infant aged 4½ months. One method of encouraging the scapular retractors to contract.

have the maximal opportunity to contract, but once contraction with the arm by the side is possible, they should be encouraged to contract with the arm progressively more and more abducted. Training the serratus anterior muscle is more difficult, but the therapist should stabilize the scapula against the thoracic wall while the infant takes weight through the hand. Therapy should aim to train a more normal relationship both between the protractors and retractors themselves and between these muscles and the muscles for which they act as stabilizers and synergists.

Attempts should be made to elicit activity in the supinators of the forearm, where these are weak or paralyzed, as early as possible in infancy. Unfortunately, an infant in the early months can accomplish much of what he or she wants to do with the forearm in a pronated position (Fig. 5-14), so specific ways of training active supination must be instituted by the therapist (Figs. 5-15 and 5-16). It is worth noting that active supination is easier to elicit if the elbow and arm are stabilized to prevent other movements (Fig. 5-15). The elbow-flexed position also favors the contraction of biceps brachii, which is the most efficient supinating muscle in this position. Supination is not only more difficult to localize with the elbow extended, it is also less likely to be elicited, as the supinator muscle needs to be of good strength to act in this position. The therapist should be aware that forced passive supination of the forearm when the pronators are contracted may reinforce the tendency toward dislocation of the radius.[12] Passive movements are in any case of no value, as

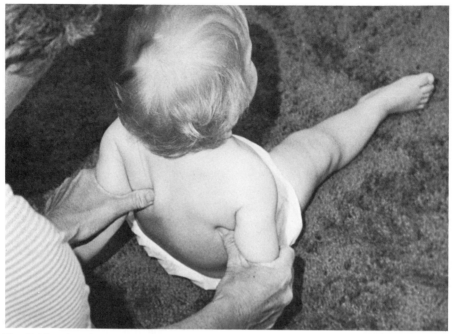

Fig. 5-13. Another method of encouraging the scapular retractors to contract (see Fig. 5-12). The infant's weight is shifted backward onto her hands.

the infant will persist in using the hand in the pronated position, and passive movement will not stimulate active contraction of the supinators. Some other ways to stimulate specific motor activity are illustrated in Figures 5-17 to 5-19.

Biofeedback. Biofeedback or sensory feedback therapy is potentially a means of reinforcing the required motor behavior in infants and children. The development of biofeedback devices may eventually progress to the stage where they are simple and accurate enough to give an irresistible signal to an infant, which will be motivation for further correct practice.

Orthoses. If during training sessions the infant's movements are not guided and controlled by the therapist or parent, it is possible that potential improvement in recovering muscles will not take place. Potential improvement may also be inhibited if abnormal alignment of a joint (or joints) is maintained during the day, encouraging the infant to practice only the incorrect muscle activity.

The correct use of splinting will prevent excessive use of unopposed or relatively unopposed muscles until the child can be trained to contract only those muscles necessary for a movement and to eliminate activity in others not required for the movement. In this way, the further development of abnormal movement combinations may be prevented, and the child may have a better chance of regaining functional use of the limb.

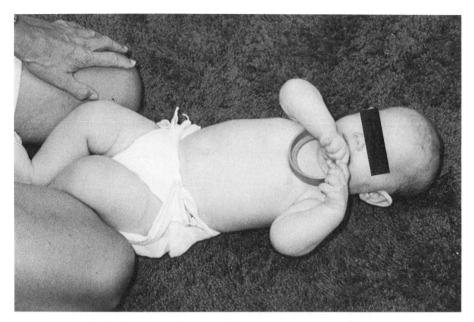

Fig. 5-14. Note the incorrect alignment of the wrist and forearm. If the infant continues practicing without control of his wrist and forearm position, this posturing may become habitual even though recovery of the affected muscle takes place.

To make it possible for the correct muscle activity to be practiced, a small, light splint may be worn for a significant part of the day. For example, an infant with paralysis of the palmar abductor of the thumb may need a small molded-plastic splint to hold the thumb in palmar abduction, but this should only be worn for periods of the day to help in using the hand effectively and must not interfere with what normal movement he or she has. Similarly, a small wrist splint may be worn for part of the day to encourage activity in the wrist extensors with the hand in the correct alignment. Dynamic splinting may be useful to reinforce wrist extension in infants with a C7 paralysis.[1]

Similarly, with increasing age and assertiveness, the infant will practice what he or she likes, whether the movement is correct or not, and at this stage the provision of an orthotic device may be effective in preventing incorrect practicing and in encouraging correct movement. If a splint is used it must be designed so it does not discourage or impede the movement wanted. Therapy to stimulate activity in particular muscles in the older infant can be combined with the use of a biofeedback training device, which will also make therapy sessions enjoyable and enable appropriate home practice.

Electrotherapy. The use of electrotherapy is controversial. Its efficacy is difficult to assess. Eng and colleagues[1,12] suggested that the use of galvanic current of sufficient intensity to cause a maximum muscle contraction under isometric conditions may prevent wasting of denervated muscle and loss of

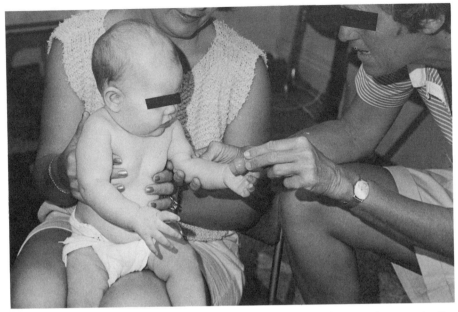

Fig. 5-15. Holding the elbow in flexion probably makes it easier to activate supination of the forearm.

awareness of the affected limb. Electrotherapy should be discontinued as soon as muscle function returns.

Soft Tissue Contracture

Passive Movements. Many authors[1,29] stress the importance of passive movements in preventing soft tissue contracture, particularly scapulohumeral adhesion. Passive movements must, however, be done gently to avoid damage to the unprotected shoulder joint. Zancolli[30] comments that forceful manipulation is one of the factors that contributes to an alteration in the anatomy of the glenohumeral joint. Although it is important to prevent contracture of the muscles that link scapula to humerus, the normal relationship between scapula and humerus, and the necessity for controlled scapular movement as the glenohumeral joint is abducted or flexed,[31] must be taken into account. The scapula should not be manually restrained once the humerus is moved beyond 30 degrees of range. Elevation of the arm without rotation of the scapula and without lateral rotation at the glenohumeral joint will damage the glenohumeral joint by causing the humerus to impinge upon the immobile acromion process. Abduction or flexion of the arm should therefore not take place without associated and appropriate scapular movement, which should be assisted if necessary. It must be noted that full range at the shoulder can only be maintained if good function recovers in the deltoid, supraspinatus, infraspinatus, and rhomboid muscles.

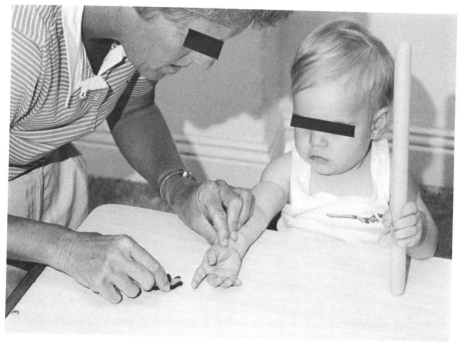

Fig. 5-16. Once the infant has some active supination, this movement should also be encouraged with the elbow extended.

Particular care must also be taken in teaching the infant's parents how to do passive movements. Parents should receive instruction in the anatomy of the shoulder so that they understand the movements they must do and the importance of keeping within the normal range. They should understand the anatomic reasons why they must be careful not to overmobilize and why they must be gentle. They should be warned not to proceed with any movement that causes the infant to cry. Unfortunately, without this knowledge, a parent may severely injure the infant's arm.

Soft tissue contracture will ultimately be prevented only if activity recovers in the affected muscles. Passive movements will not lead to the restoration of active function. Therapy must therefore concentrate not only on ensuring the optimal position and alignment of joints, but most particularly on the stimulation of active movement.

Splinting. Splinting, particularly where it involves the shoulder, remains a controversial issue.[4] Although some authors have recommended it, evidence exists that several of the problems that arise in these infants may be directly related to the type of splinting used.

In the upper arm type, some authors have suggested that the arm be held in abduction and lateral rotation by pinning the sleeve to the pillow or by a "statue of liberty" splint, or held in abduction and midrotation by an ab-

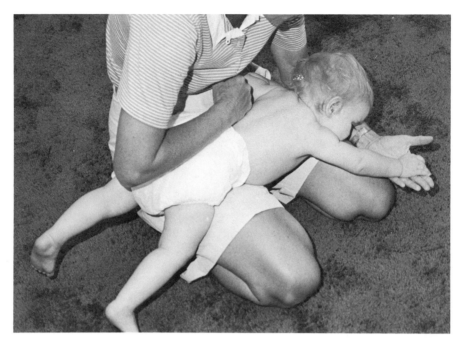

Fig. 5-17. Training the deltoid muscle and the scapular retractors. The therapist is eliciting eccentric contractions by encouraging the infant to lower her hand toward the therapist's hand.

duction splint. Some of these authors in subsequent articles and other authors[1,2,4,25,32–34] have pointed out, however, that splinting the arm in this position may lead to "overmobility" of the glenohumeral joint, and that this positioning may be a factor that contributes to pathology in the glenohumeral joint, even to anterior dislocation.[12] Although there seems to be sufficient evidence to discontinue the use of the types of shoulder splinting listed above, it should be possible for therapists and bioengineers to design a means of supporting the humerus in the glenohumeral cavity that will not discourage use of the limb and will not predispose to joint dysfunction. This type of splint would not be necessary for the majority of infants with brachial plexus injury, but may be helpful for the infant with extensive paralysis around the shoulder.

Neglect of the Arm, or "Learned Nonuse"

Neglect of a paralyzed arm is relatively common in hemiplegic infants and children and in adults following stroke.[35] It appears also to occur in some infants with brachial plexus lesions and may be an important contributing factor to the failure to develop motor control. The infant's initial attempts to use his arm result in failure and he may cease trying. Neglect may also be a factor in preventing recovery of muscle function that could potentially have occurred

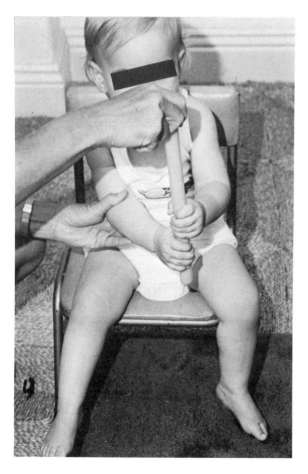

Fig. 5-18. Practicing grasp and release and shoulder flexion by placing hand over hand. Therapist ensures correct alignment.

as a result of nerve regeneration. Several reports in the literature mention infants with good return of muscle function, who nevertheless ignored the arm and refused to use it.[1,25] Wickstrom[2] attributed this neglect to the lack of development of "functional cerebral motor patterns of coordination." Zalis and colleagues[36] suggested that transitory interruption of peripheral nerve pathways at birth prevented the establishment of normal patterns of movement and the organization of body image. Taub[37] has described what he calls "learned nonuse," which is demonstrated by monkeys after either deafferentation or brain lesion, and which is primarily due, according to Taub, to a learning phenomenon. The animals learn *not* to use the affected limb because they can perform in a satisfactory manner with the remaining limbs and no motivating factor exists to encourage them to use the affected limb. This habitual nonuse persists so that even when the limb becomes potentially useful, the animal does not seem aware of this possibility. Other authors[38] have described similar findings. Consequently, motor training procedures for infants with brachial plexus lesions should probably be carried out in conjunction with short periods of re-

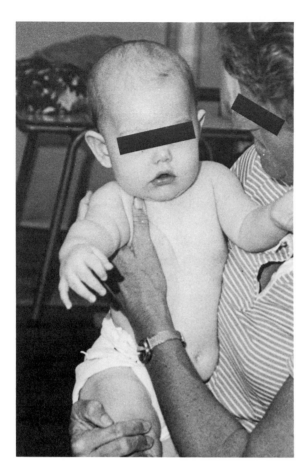

Fig. 5-19. If the parents hold the infant like this, the tendency to abduct instead of flex the shoulder is controlled and the movement of flexion is encouraged.

straint of the unaffected arm (Fig. 5-20). One study with two hemiplegic infants[39] involved restraint of the intact arm during the early training sessions for short periods during the day. After 6 months of training, both children were able to use successfully the previously paretic arm and hand.

Sensory Unawareness

Specific attempts should be made in treatment to stimulate sensory awareness, but it is probable that active movement of the arm is itself the major source of sensory input. When the infant is old enough sensory "games" can be played, such as locating certain objects in sand, localizing touch stimuli, and recognizing and naming common objects while blindfolded.

Abnormal Respiratory Function

Where diaphragmatic paralysis exists, respiration can be aided by oxygen with continuous positive airway pressure or continuous negative pressure.[40,41] If the nerve lesion is a neurapraxia, there will be eventual recovery of dia-

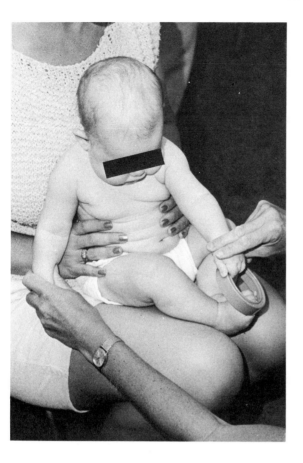

Fig. 5-20. Restraint of the unaffected limb is also carried out during training sessions. The arm can be restrained within a vest instead of manually.

phragmatic function, but during the period of paralysis, it is important to prevent respiratory problems such as atelectasis. Positioning with the paralyzed side underneath should be avoided. Postural drainage in the prone position at a 45° angle should be carried out at home for short periods during the day with the objective of preventing retention of secretions in the relatively immobile parts of the lung.

SURGICAL TREATMENT

Surgery is not usually performed in infancy, although some authors suggest that, with certain lesions, surgical intervention may help in removal of hematomas or neurolysis of adhesions,[6] and others[42] suggest early surgical exploration and repair by nerve graft. In the older child, surgery to stabilize joints, tendon transplantation, and soft tissue elongation are performed with the objective of gaining some improvement in function.[43,44] Zancolli[30] describes surgical techniques aimed at improving function and cosmesis of the shoulder.

CONCLUSION

Brachial plexus injury at birth may be followed by considerable disability involving muscle paralysis and weakness, soft tissue contracture, loss of sensation and sympathetic changes. The major loss of function is the infant's inability to use the hand effectively, and the therapist, sensitive to the child's needs, must set about the task of analyzing treatment approaches to this problem with as much knowledge as can be gathered. Therapists should question whether existing treatment procedures are logical in terms of a biomechanical and anatomic understanding of the dysfunction, and develop more effective ways of training motor control and of preventing habitual substitution movements and "learned nonuse" of the limb. It is probable that most infants could regain better motor function if put on a more specific motor training program that at present appears to exist.

REFERENCES

1. Eng GD: Brachial plexus palsy in newborn infants. Pediatrics 48:18, 1971.
2. Wickstrom J: Birth injuries of the brachial plexus: Treatment of defects of the shoulder. Clin Orthop 23:187, 1962.
3. Adler JB, Patterson RL: Erb's palsy: Long-term results of treatment in eighty-eight cases. J Bone Joint Surg [Am] 49:1052, 1967.
4. Johnson EW, Alexander MA, Koenig WC: Infantile Erb's palsy (Smellie's palsy). Arch Phys Med Rehabil 58:175, 1977.
5. Czurda R, Meznik F: Zur Therapie und Prognose der Plexuslähmung beim Neugeborenen. Paediatr Paedol 12:137, 1977.
6. Swaiman KF, Wright FS: Neuromuscular Diseases of Infancy and Childhood. Charles C Thomas, Springfield IL 1970.
7. Turner T, Evans J, Brown JK: Monoparesis. Complication of constant positive airways pressure. Arch Dis Child 50:128, 1975.
8. Magee KR, DeJong RN: Paralytic brachial neuritis. JAMA 174:1258, 1960.
9. Tan KL: Brachial palsy. J Obstet Gynaecol Br Commonw 80:60, 1960.
10. Specht EE: Brachial plexus palsy in the newborn. Clin Orthop 75, 110:32, 1975.
11. Davis DH, Onofrio BM, MacCarty CS: Brachial plexus injuries. Mayo Clin Proc 53, 12:799, 1978.
12. Eng GD, Koch B, Smokvina MD: Brachial plexus palsy in neonates and children. Arch Phys Med Rehabil 59:458, 1978.
13. Zverina E, Kredba J: Somatosensory cerebral evoked potentials in diagnosing brachial plexus injuries. Scand J Rehabil Med 19:47, 1977.
14. Landi A, Copeland SA, Wynn Parry CB, et al: The role of somatosensory evoked potentials and nerve conduction studies in the surgical management of brachial plexus injuries. J Bone Joint Surg 62B 4:492, 1980.
15. Stefanova-Uzunova M, Stamatova L, Gatev V: Dynamic properties of partially denervated muscle in children with brachial plexus birth palsy. J Neurol Neurosurg Psychiatry 44:497, 1981.
16. Gjorup L: Obstetrical lesion of the brachial plexus. Acta Neurol Scand, suppl K42 18:9, 1966.

17. O'Riain S: New and simple test of nerve function in the hand. Br Med J 3:615, 1973.
18. Bufalini C, Pescatori G: Posterior cervical electromyography in the diagnosis and prognosis of brachial plexus injuries. J Bone Joint Surg 51B:627, 1969.
19. Leffert RD: Brachial plexus injuries. N Engl J Med 291, 20:1059, 1974.
20. Stanwood JE, Kraft GH: Diagnosis and management of brachial plexus injuries. Arch Phys Med Rehabil 52:52, 1971.
21. Robinson PK: Associated movements between limb and respiratory muscles as a sequel to brachial plexus birth injury. Johns Hopkins Med J 89:21, 1951.
22. Esslen E: Electromyographic findings on two types of misdirection of regenerating axons. Electroencephalogr Clin Neurophysiol 12:738, 1960.
23. De Grandis D, Fiaschi A, Michieli G, et al: Anomalous reinnervation as a sequel to obstetric brachial plexus palsy. J Neurol Sci 1(43):127, 1979.
24. Tada K, Ohshita S, Yonenobu K, et al: Experimental study of spinal nerve repair after plexus brachialis injury in newborn rats: A horseradish peroxidase study. Exp Neurol 2(65):301, 1979.
25. Rose FC: Paediatric Neurology. Blackwell, Oxford, 1979.
26. Gatcheva J: Early diagnosis and long term management of obstetric paralysis. Int Rehabil Med 3(1):126, 1979.
27. Fitts PM: Perceptual motor skill learning. In Melton AE (ed): Categories of Human Learning. Academic Press, New York, 1964.
28. Fitts PM, Posner MI: Human Performance. Prentice-Hall, London, 1973.
29. Shepherd RB: Physiotherapy in Paediatrics. 2nd Ed. Heinemann, London, 1980.
30. Zancolli EA: Classification and management of the shoulder in birth palsy. Orthop Clin North Am 12:433, 1981.
31. Cailliet R: The Shoulder in Hemiplegia. Davis, Philadelphia, 1980.
32. Carter S, Gold AP: Neurology of Infancy and Childhood. Appleton-Century-Crofts, New York, 1974.
33. Schut L: Nerve injuries in children. Surg Clin North Am 52:1307, 1972.
34. Aitken J: Deformity of elbow joint as sequel to Erb's obstetrical paralysis. J Bone Joint Surg [Br], 34:352, 1952.
35. Carr JH, Shepherd RB: A Motor Relearning Programme for Stroke. Heinemann, London, 1983.
36. Zalis OS, Zalis AW, Barron KD, et al: Motor patterning following transitory sensory-motor deprivation. Arch Neurol 13:487, 1965.
37. Taub E: Somato-sensory deafferentation research with monkeys: Implications for rehabilitation medicine. In Ince LP (ed): Behavioral Psychology in Rehabilitation Medicine: Clinical Applications. Williams and Wilkins, Baltimore, 1980.
38. Yu J: Functional recovery with and without training following brain damage in experimental animals: A review. Arch Phys Med Rehabil 57:38, 1976.
39. Schwartzman RJ: Rehabilitation of infantile hemiplegia. Am J Phys Med 53:75, 1974.
40. Bucci G, et al: Phrenic nerve palsy treated by continuous positive pressure breathing by nasal cannula. Arch Dis Child 49:230, 1974.
41. Weisman L, Woodall J, Merenstein G: Constant negative pressure in the treatment of diaphragmatic paralysis secondary to birth injury. Birth Defects 12, 6:297, 1976.
42. Gilbert A, Khouri N, Cartioz H: Exploration chirurgicale du plexus brachial dans la paralysic obstétricale. Rev Chir Orthop 66:33, 1980.

43. Hoffer MM, Wickenden R, Roper B: Brachial plexus birth palsies: Results of tendon transfers to the rotator cuff. J Bone Joint Surg 60A:691, 1978.
44. Manske PR, McCarroll HR, Hale R: Biceps tendon rerouting and percutaneous osteoclasis in the treatment of supination deformity in obstetrical palsy. J Hand Surg 5:153, 1980.

6 | Down Syndrome

Susan R. Harris

Physical therapy for children with Down syndrome received relatively little attention prior to the early 1970s. Whereas children with more obvious physical handicaps, such as those with cerebral palsy or meningomyelocele, have received services from pediatric therapists for many years, children with Down syndrome have been less apt to be the focus of evaluation and treatment. Clinical research during the past decade has demonstrated that there are many aspects of this syndrome that warrant attention from pediatric therapists, such as significant developmental motor delay during infancy and early childhood,[1-3] perceptual-motor deficits,[4] and a variety of orthopedic disorders.[5] This chapter focuses primarily on the physical therapist's evaluation and treatment of children with Down syndrome. Other issues addressed are the incidence, etiology, and pathology of this disorder as well as medical, educational, and family involvement for children with Down syndrome.

ETIOLOGY

Down syndrome has long been recognized as one of the most common causes of mental retardation.[6,7] The overall incidence of this disorder is one in every 660 live births with an increased incidence occurring with advanced maternal age.[8] Advanced paternal age has also been implicated as a factor contributing to increased risk for giving birth to a child with Down syndrome.[9,10] Individuals with Down syndrome comprise at least 10 percent of the moderately to severely retarded population.[8]

The etiology of this disorder was first described by Lejeune and colleagues in 1959 based on chromosome analysis of affected individuals.[11] In 91 percent of cases of Down syndrome, there is an extra small chromosome present on the twenty-first pair of chromosomes. This chromosome abnormality is labeled more specifically as trisomy-21[6] and develops as a result of nondisjunction of

169

two homologous chromosomes during either the first or second meiotic division.[12] Approximately 3 to 4 percent of individuals with Down syndrome have a chromosomal abnormality known as translocation in which there is breakage of two nonhomologous chromosomes with subsequent reattachment of the broken pieces to other intact chromosome pairs. Risk of recurrence of a second child with Down syndrome to parents who are translocation carriers varies from 2 to 10 percent, making the risk of recurrence much greater than with the nondisjunction type of trisomy-21.[12] The remaining 4 percent of cases of Down syndrome represent mosaic disorders in which some cells within the individual are normal and some are trisomy-21.

PATHOLOGY

Neuropathology

The neuropathology associated with Down syndrome has been explored by a number of researchers. The overall brain weight of individuals with Down syndrome averages 76 percent of the brain weight of normal individuals with the combined weight of the cerebellum and brainstem being proportionately even smaller, an average of 66 percent of the weight of the cerebellum and brainstem in normal individuals.[13] The reduction in size of the cerebral hemispheres is especially apparent at the frontal poles causing Cowie[14] to speculate that this particular aspect of neuropathology may have some bearing on the persistence of the palmar grasp reflex in infants with Down syndrome, since a lesion in the frontal lobe of an adult may result in a forced grasp.

Other gross neuropathologic findings include the more rounded shape of the brains of children with Down syndrome, which may be secondary to the brachycephaly associated with this syndrome.[15] The brains of infants with Down syndrome show smaller convolutions than those of normal infants of comparable age, indicating their relative neurologic immaturity.[16]

In addition to these gross neurologic differences, there are a number of cytologic distinctions that characterize the brains of individuals with Down syndrome. Marin-Padilla[17] studied the neuronal organization of the motor cortex of a 19-month-old child with Down syndrome and found various structural abnormalities in the dendritic spines of the pyramidal neurons of the motor cortex. He suggested that these structural differences may underlie the motor incoordination and mental retardation characteristic of individuals with Down syndrome. Loesch-Mdzewska,[18] in his neuropathologic study of 123 brains of individuals with Down syndrome aged 3 to 62, also frequently found neurologic abnormalities of the pyramidal system in addition to the reduced brain weight noted by the other researchers cited above.

Benda noted a lack of myelinization of the nerve fibers in the precentral areas and frontal lobes of the cerebral cortex and in the cerebella of infants with Down syndrome, suggesting a lack of central nervous system maturity.[16] As Lipton[19] has pointed out, the laying down of myelin sheaths contributes to the rapid increase in the size of the brain between the ages of 2 and 6 in normal children.

Another neuropathologic study conducted on the brains of five adults with Down syndrome who had died at ages ranging from 21 to 62 showed a significant decrease in the number of pyramidal neurons in the hippocampus when compared to brains of normal individuals of comparable ages.[20] This finding combined with a significant increase in Alzheimer neurofibrillary tangles demonstrated a quantitative similarity of types of neurons between the brains of adults with Down syndrome and the brains of adults with Alzheimer's dementia.[21] Such similarities suggest that individuals with Down syndrome are at risk for demonstrating clinical characteristics of premature senility.

In addition to the neuropathologic findings associated with Down syndrome, there are a number of other pathologic characteristics, many of which warrant medical intervention. The following sections will discuss a number of these associated deficits and medical management.

Cardiovascular Anomalies

Congenital heart defects are very common in individuals with Down syndrome. Cardiac anomalies were present in 60 percent of individuals with Down syndrome for whom autopsies were performed in one report.[6] The two most common cardiac anomalies reported are atrioventricular canal defects and ventriculoseptal defects.[6] Many congenital heart defects can be repaired surgically. It is extremely important that the child's therapist be aware of the presence and extent of any cardiac defects, particularly those severe enough to influence the course of evaluation and treatment. Children with heart defects need not be excluded from receiving therapy, but close consultation with the child's physician and careful monitoring of response to treatment is strongly advised.

Sensory Deficits

Another common medical problem that may indirectly influence the child's response to physical therapy is hearing loss. In a recent study of 107 individuals with Down syndrome, binaural hearing loss was noted in 64 percent of the subjects tested.[22] Otitis media is a frequently recurring medical problem that contributes to hearing deficiencies in individuals with Down syndrome.[6] Visual defects are also much more common in individuals with Down syndrome than in the general population. Strabismus (usually esotropia) was noted in 41.3 percent of a sample of 75 institutionalized individuals with Down syndrome.[23] Nystagmus, cataracts, and myopia were frequently found.[23] Other ocular findings of less clinical significance were the presence of Brushfield spots in the iris and the characteristic upward and outward slanting of the palpebral fissures. Interestingly, the presence of epicanthal folds—a classic clinical diagnostic feature of Down syndrome—was noted in only 17.3 percent of this institutionalized sample.[23]

With regard to visual perception, a frequent area of deficit in all handicapped populations, a recent study examining the ability of school-age children with Down syndrome to replicate and match block structures concluded that the inability to replicate the structures was due to a perceptual-motor deficit rather than to a defect in visual perception, since the subjects were able to correctly match like structures. The author concluded that visual perception was intact in this sample of children.[4]

Orthopedic Problems

Of particular interest to physical therapists are the number and types of orthopedic problems associated with Down syndrome, due in part to the generalized hypotonia and ligamentous laxity characteristic of this disorder. Diamond and colleagues[5] evaluated the prevalence of orthopedic deformities among a sample of 265 persons with Down syndrome, 107 of whom were institutionalized patients, with the remainder being outpatients. A much greater prevalence of major orthopedic problems existed among the institutionalized sample. The two major foot deformities noted were metatarsus primus varus and pes planus (secondary to severe ligamentous laxity). Both of these disorders frequently required the prescription of special shoes and occasionally surgical intervention. Patellar instability resulting in subluxation or dislocation was present in 23 percent of the subjects and usually was managed surgically. Hip subluxation or dislocation occurred in 10 percent and also required surgical intervention.[5]

While thoracolumbar scoliosis was present in 52 percent of individuals in this sample, most of the curves were defined as "mild to moderate," and only one case required surgery.[5] Physical therapists who work with children with Down syndrome should be aware of their propensity for developing such orthopedic deformities and should provide periodic musculoskeletal evaluation such as posture screening and range-of-motion evaluation of hips and knees.

One of the most serious orthopedic problems associated with Down syndrome is the propensity for atlantoaxial dislocation. Because of the laxity of the transverse odontoid ligament,[24] there may be "excessive motion of C1 on C2,"[25] which can result in subluxation or dislocation of the atlantoaxial joint. Andrews[26] reported in 1981 that 33 cases of atlantoaxial dislocation in individuals with Down syndrome had been cited in the medical literature. Radiologic examination of various samples of persons with Down syndrome has demonstrated atlantoaxial dislocation in 12 to 20 percent of the subjects.[27] Although the majority of cases with dislocation have been clinically asymptomatic, a small number of individuals have shown myelopathy, including spastic quadriplegia.

Early symptoms associated with atlantoaxial dislocation include gait changes (ankle instability and increased difficulty in walking),[25] urinary retention,[25] torticollis,[4,24] reluctance in moving the neck, and increased deep tendon reflexes.[27] Posterior arthrodesis of C1 to C2 is recommended in cases of atlantoaxial dislocation without neurologic symptomatology, whereas posterior stabilization and fusion of C1 to C2 are recommended for cases with early neurologic involvement.[25] Whaley and Gray[27] advise a radiologic examination for any child with Down syndrome who has limited neck movement or a gait disturbance.

Physical therapists who work with children with Down syndrome should be acutely aware of the increased risk for atlantoaxial dislocation. While every effort should be made to mainstream the handicapped child into recreational activities engaged in by their nonhandicapped peers, particular caution should be exercised in involving the child with Down syndrome in strenuous gymnastics and tumbling or contact sports, such as football and wrestling, since the ligamentous laxity of the atlantoaxial joint makes it "less resistant to superimposed flexion trauma."[25]

Hypotonia

In addition to the foregoing complications associated with Down syndrome that frequently warrant medical or surgical management, there are several other characteristic features of this disorder that indicate the need for evaluation and treatment by qualified developmental therapists. One of the hallmarks of Down syndrome and, in fact, one of the most characteristic diagnostic features at birth is generalized hypotonia.[28] Particularly evident during the early years,[1,29] the hypotonia is probably a major contributing factor to the significant motor delay characterizing the period of infancy and early childhood in children with Down syndrome. These characteristics are discussed in more detail in the following sections which address the physical therapist's role in the evaluation and treatment of children with this disorder.

Finally, other medical problems appearing with greater frequency among individuals with Down syndrome than among those in the normal population include seizure disorders (5 to 6 percent), duodenal stenosis, leukemia, and senile dementia.

PHYSICAL THERAPY EVALUATION

The physical therapist who participates in the evaluation of a child with Down syndrome should be cognizant of the medical problems associated with this disorder as well as being aware of recent research reports which have explored the degree of motor delay, the interrelationship of mental and motor delay, and the effects of the generalized hypotonia on other aspects of development. The first part of this section will provide a review of recent literature examining these concerns, with the latter part of the section directed at specific evaluation strategies based on these research findings.

Review of Motor Deficits Associated with Down Syndrome

The most common motor deficit associated with Down syndrome is hypotonia or low muscle tone.[7,15,30] Estimates vary as to the percentage of infants with Down syndrome who display hypotonia,[31–34] but a 1970 study by Cowie[29] of the neurologic development of 79 infants with Down syndrome indicated that marked hypotonia was universally present in the infants tested. In their study of 86 children with Down syndrome at the Nebraska Psychiatric Institute, McIntire and coworkers[35] described hypotonia as the most frequently observed characteristic and also indicated that it was found in all major muscle groups including neck, trunk, and extremities for 98 percent of the population tested.

A number of researchers have demonstrated a relationship between low muscle tone and delayed motor development. Crome and colleagues,[36] in their neuropathologic study of the brains of individuals with Down syndrome, speculated that the lower weight of the cerebellum and brainstem characteristic of this population may account for the muscular hypotonia, which in turn is probably a major influence on early motor development. In their descriptive retrospective report on the developmental data of 612 noninstitutionalized children with Down syndrome ranging in age from birth to 16 years, Melyn and White[37] found a wide range of development in every attribute they tested, including motor and speech milestones derived from the norms of Gesell and Amatruda.[38] These researchers suggest that one of the most influential characteristics affecting early motor development is degree of hypotonia. They further implicate hypotonia of the speech musculature as a contributing factor in the delayed speech development that characterizes children with Down syndrome.[36]

LaVeck and LaVeck,[2] in their administration of the mental and motor scales of the Bayley Scales of Infant Development[39] to 20 female and 20 male infants with Down syndrome ranging in age from 12 to 36 months, found that the mean mental quotients were significantly higher than the mean motor quotients and that the average motor age lagged 2.86 months behind the average mental age. The authors suggested that this significantly greater delay in motor development may be related to the hypotonia associated with Down syndrome and not solely to the mental retardation, since a comparison group of developmentally delayed non-Down-syndrome infants, many of them with known or suspected neurologic deficits, were not as severely delayed in psychomotor functioning as were the infants with Down syndrome. In replicating this study with younger infants with Down syndrome (2.7 to 21.5 months), Harris[3] reported similar findings in that significantly greater delays were noted in motor development than in mental development as measured on the Bayley scales.

Not only has hypotonia been implicated as a contributing factor in delayed motor development and delayed speech acquisition in infants and young children with Down syndrome, but it has also been shown to be correlated with lags in affective and cognitive development. Cicchetti and Sroufe,[40] in their longitudinal study of 14 infants with Down syndrome ranging in age from 4 to 24 months, demonstrated that the four most hypotonic infants were not only the most delayed in affective expression, but also scored the lowest on measures of cognitive development as shown by the mental scale of the Bayley[39] and the Uzgiris-Hunt scales of cognitive development.[41] Cowie, in her neurologic study of 79 infants with Down syndrome from birth to 10 months, also noted a correlation between extreme hypotonia and poor performance on the Bayley Scales.[29]

The lowered muscle tone characteristic of Down syndrome has also been shown to contribute to slower reaction time and depressed kinesthetic feedback. O'Connor and Hermelin[42] compared reaction time on a task between a group of children with Down syndrome and a comparable group of non-Down-syndrome retarded children. They theorized that the slower reaction time which characterized the group of children with Down syndrome was due, in part, to the marked hypotonia. They also hypothesized that the hypotonia contributed to a lessened degree of kinesthetic feedback, another sensory deficit characteristic of individuals with Down syndrome.[42]

In a more recent study, the relationship of muscle tone (as evaluated during the first year of life in 89 infants with Down syndrome) with later outcome variables was assessed.[43] The authors reported that muscle tone ''was a powerful predictor of all the outcome variables including language acquisition, motor and social development, and mental functioning.''[43] While hypotonia is most pronounced during infancy and tends to diminish with increasing age, individuals with Down syndrome remain hypotonic throughout life.

Although hypotonia is the most frequently mentioned neuromotor deficit mentioned in describing the characteristics of infants and young children with Down syndrome, a number of additional problems also have been noted. In her longitudinal study of 79 infants with Down syndrome from birth to 10 months, Cowie[29] administered comprehensive neurologic examinations during the neonatal period, at 6 months, and at 10 months. In addition to the universal finding of marked hypotonia, Cowie also noted a persistence of primitive reflexes past the time when they should normally disappear. These reflexes included the palmar and plantar grasp reflexes, the stepping reflex, and the Moro reflex.[29] My own clinical observations of infants with Down syndrome suggest that primitive reflexes are present in a diminished state (hyporeflexia) and do not persist past the time when they would normally be integrated, with the possible exception of the plantar grasp reflex. Cowie's third major neurologic finding was a delay in the development of normal postural tone as indicated by the severe headlag evident during elicitation of the traction response and the lack of full antigravity extension noted when testing for the Landau response.[29]

Cowie speculates that the possible neurologic causes for these clinical findings are delayed cerebellar maturation, the relatively small size of the brainstem and cerebellum, and maturational delay of descending pathways from the motor cortex.[36]

Because of the multiplicity of medical, cognitive, and motor problems associated with Down syndrome, evaluation by the physical therapist must be comprehensive and must reflect information from members of the interdisciplinary assessment team. In light of the frequency of major medical problems associated with this disorder, the therapist should work in close consultation with the child's physician. Prior to performing an evaluation, the therapist should obtain current medical information about the child's cardiac status, risk for atlantoaxial dislocation, any history of seizures, and results of visual and auditory examinations. Information from the child's teacher concerning IQ, any behavioral problems, and known reinforcers for positive behavior should also be gleaned. The parents' goals and expectations about the evaluation process should also be derived. Reports from psychologists, speech therapists, nurses, and nutritionists may also be available and should be examined prior to conducting the evaluation.

Qualitative Evaluation

The physical therapist's evaluation should be directed at a qualitative assessment of the child's movement patterns as well as a developmental assessment of the child's gross motor and fine motor functional skills. For example, it has been my experience that a number of young infants with Down syndrome may roll from prone to supine as early as 1 to 2 months of age, a developmental motor milestone that is first performed by normal infants at approximately 4 months of age. A qualitative evaluation of this "precocious" motor skill in infants with Down syndrome reveals that their ability to move out of prone into supine is accomplished because of a lack of cocontraction of muscles in the trunk and an inability to grade movement so that any initiation of rolling results in a marked "flip over" into supine rather than a graded ability to smoothly execute the transition. Delayed righting reactions in the head and trunk also appear to contribute to this early ability to flip over from prone to supine (Fig. 6-1).

Another motor milestone that frequently appears in developmental assessment tools is the ability to rise to sitting independently from a prone-lying or supine-lying position.[39] Lydic and Steele[44] have noted an important qualitative difference in the manner in which infants with Down syndrome accomplish this motor skill as compared to the manner in which normal infants rise to sitting: "Advancing from a prone to a sitting posture, the child with Down's syndrome who has received no therapeutic intervention characteristically spreads his legs until he is in full-split position with his legs 180 degrees from each other and then uses his hands (or his head) to push up into the sitting position with the legs still in partial- to full-split position or tailor style." (Fig. 6-2). These authors suggest that this qualitative difference may be due in part to the hypermobility of the hip joints as well as lack of active trunk rotation.[44]

While a number of qualitative differences in movement patterns may be observed during administration of a developmental assessment tool, it is optimal to conduct a separate qualitative assessment as well. The Movement Assessment of Infants (MAI)[45] is a suggested evaluation instrument for examining qualitative aspects of movement in infants with Down syndrome, since it assesses four different components of movement: postural tone, primitive reflexes, automatic reactions, and volitional movement (see Chapter 2 for a review of this test). Since research has suggested that the generalized hypotonia, delayed integration of primitive reflexes, and delayed development of automatic reactions characteristic of infants with Down syndrome[29] may all contribute to the documented delays in achieving motor milestones, it is im-

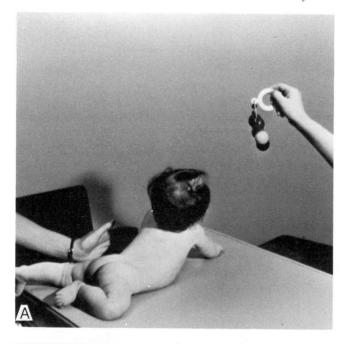

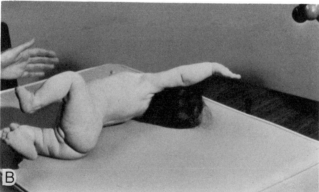

Fig. 6-1. Rolling prone to supine (4 months of age).

portant for physical therapists to evaluate these qualitative aspects of movement as well as assessing the child's developmental motor level (Fig. 6-3).

Qualitative evaluation of older children with Down syndrome should include analysis of the manner in which they perform functional activities such as gait[46] and task analysis of fine motor activities, such as shoe-tying or prevocational skills. In light of the frequency of associated orthopedic problems,[5] posture screening and range-of-motion evaluation of hips and knees should also be included as part of the global physical therapy assessment.

Assessment of developmental motor level is also an integral part of the physical therapist's evaluation of the child with Down syndrome. Whenever

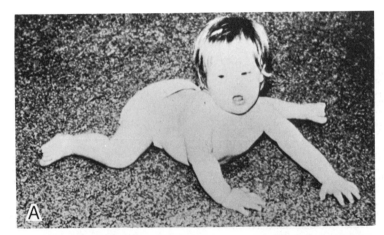

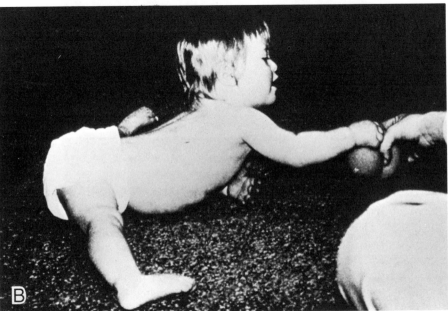

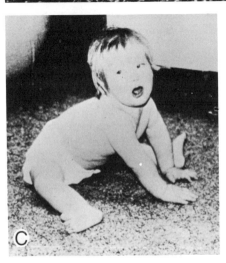

Fig. 6-2. Advancing from prone to sitting posture without trunk rotation. (Reprinted from Physical Therapy 59:1489–1494, 1979 with the permission of the American Physical Therapy Association.)

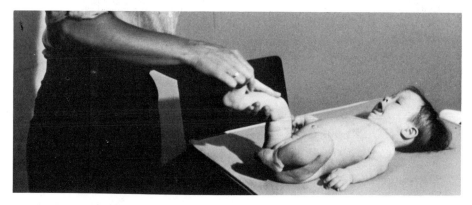

Fig. 6-3. Administering the MAI to a 4-month-old infant. (Item 2 in Muscle Tone: extensibility of heelcords).

possible, a standardized norm-referenced motor assessment tool should be used. Documentation of degree of developmental motor delay is important for several reasons: (1) to qualify the child for placement in a special education or developmental disabilities program, (2) to justify the receipt of physical therapy services, and (3) to serve as a baseline measure in documenting change as a result of intervention.

Developmental Evaluation

Physical therapists are limited in their choice of developmental motor assessment tools which are both standardized and norm-referenced. A standardized tool uses consistent or standardized assessment procedures and frequently utilizes standardized equipment in the form of a test kit. In order for an assessment instrument to reflect the degree of motor delay of the child with Down syndrome as compared to normal chronologic age mates (a norm-referenced tool), normative data must have been collected on samples of children from a cross section of ethnic and socioeconomic strata for each age level represented on the test. The availability of acceptable reliability and validity data also contributes to the utility of a particular test.

In evaluating developmental motor levels of infants with Down syndrome, the therapist may choose either the Bayley Scales of Infant Development[39] or the Gesell and Amatruda Developmental Examination.[47] Both Mental and Motor Scales are available as part of the Bayley, but there is no differentiation of gross motor and fine motor skills. The Motor Scale consists primarily of gross motor items but also includes some fine motor items, particularly at the younger age levels. A number of items on the Mental Scale also require fine motor abilities.

The Bayley Scales have been used repeatedly in assessing developmental motor levels of infants with Down syndrome in a number of research studies.[1–3,48,49] Although the upper limit of the age range for the Bayley is 30 months,

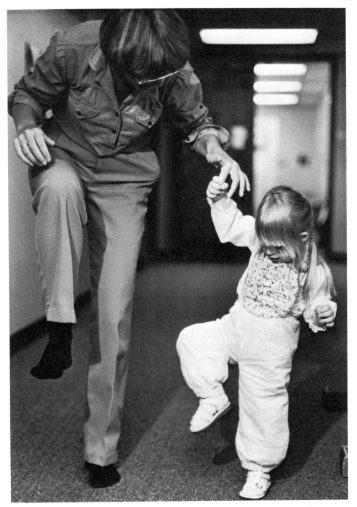

Fig. 6-4. Administering the Bayley Motor Scale to a 3-year-old. (Item 52: Stands on left foot with help).

many preschoolers with Down syndrome are functioning at or below this level. Since it is possible to derive an age-equivalent score for both the Mental and Motor Scales, it is frequently possible to continue to use the Bayley for assessing developmental levels in 3-, 4-, and even some 5-year-old children with Down syndrome. Fig. 6-4 shows the Bayley Motor Scale being administered to a 3-year-old child with Down syndrome.

The Gesell, also a standardized assessment instrument, was renormed between 1975 and 1977 on a sample of 1053 children ranging in age from 4 weeks to 36 months.[47] There are five fields of behavior evaluated on the Gesell: adaptive, gross motor, fine motor, language, and personal-social. In each field of behavior, the child's "maturity level" can be derived, although it is impossible to determine a specific age level if a wide scatter of items is passed and failed. A developmental quotient is derived by using the following formula:

$$DQ = \frac{\text{maturity age}}{\text{chronologic age}} \times 100$$

In assessing young children with Down syndrome, the Gesell has an advantage over the Bayley in that both a gross motor and a fine motor quotient can be derived. Eipper and Azen,[50] in a comparison of the Gesell based on earlier norms (1940s) and the current version of the Bayley administered to a sample of children with Down syndrome, concluded that the Gesell is more appropriate for clinical use because of its ease and speed of administration, and the Bayley is more applicable for research purposes because it more reliably estimates developmental age.

For assessing motor development in older children with Down syndrome, there are two available instruments which are both standardized and norm-referenced: the Bruininks-Oseretsky Tests of Motor Proficiency[51] and the Test of Motor Impairment by Stott and colleagues.[52] Normed in 1973, the Bruininks-Oseretsky consists of 46 items that examine running speed and agility, balance, bilateral coordination, strength, upper limb coordination, response speed, visual motor control, and upper limb speed and dexterity.[53] This test is appropriate for children with motor ages between 4.5 and 14.5 years. The complete battery can be administered in 45 to 60 minutes with the additional option of using a 15 to 20-minute short form; both gross motor and fine motor ages can be derived. A limitation in using the Bruininks-Oseretsky with children with Down syndrome is the complexity of the verbal directions for administering each item. Since young children of normal intellect frequently have difficulty interpreting the directions on the Bruininks-Oseretsky, any child with a mental age of less than 5 years would also have difficulty trying to comply with the complex instructions.

The Test of Motor Impairment, although normed and standardized for ages 5 to 13 years, is oriented toward assessing children with more subtle forms of neural dysfunction such as the child with "minimal brain damage."[52] For this reason, this test is probably inappropriate for assessing motor development of the child with Down syndrome.

Two other new motor assessment tools may be appropriate for use with children with Down syndrome: the Miller Assessment for Preschoolers[54] and the Peabody Developmental Motor Scales.[55] The Miller Assessment for Preschoolers (MAP) is a standardized tool that was normed on 1200 preschoolers in the late 1970s. Both a screening test and a more comprehensive clinical evaluation are available as part of the MAP. The clinical evaluation examines such areas as ocular abilities, quality of movement, and sensory integration.[54]

The Peabody Developmental Motor Scales (PDMS) were first published in 1974.[56] Norms are currently being collected on a standardized version of the PDMS; the revised tool is scheduled to be available as a kit in October 1982.[55] The age range on which the PDMS is being normed is birth to 6 years 11 months.

The tool consists of both gross motor and fine motor scales, thus enabling the derivation of developmental quotients in both areas. The earlier version of the PDMS[56] has been used in research studies on infants with Down syndrome.[49]

Self-Care Evaluation

In addition to evaluating the general developmental motor level of the child with Down syndrome, the physical therapist may also be called upon to assess the child's abilities in the areas of self-help or daily living skills. Campbell[57] has suggested a problem-oriented approach to the evaluation of self-care skills in which the therapist assesses the child's abilities in a particular self-care area and then hypothesizes about the possible factors which may be interfering with the achievement of age-appropriate skills. Possible interfering problems may include neuromotor deficits or inappropriate behaviors. One goal of programming, then, is to minimize the effects of the interfering behaviors by developing alternative strategies for treatment.[57] For example, in the child with Down syndrome who is having difficulty drinking from a cup, two hypothesized causes of interfering problems might be the generalized hypotonia affecting the oral musculature resulting in inadequate lip closure (neuromotor deficit) or the existence of inappropriate behaviors such as throwing or dropping the cup. By observing the child during feeding time, the therapist can hypothesize about which type of behavior is interfering with the achievement of independent drinking and then develop appropriate alternative strategies. If the failure to drink successfully is due to poor lip closure, a program designed to increase tone in the oral muscles through such activities as vibration or chin tapping might be recommended. Hypotonia of the jaw muscles probably contributes to the inability to close the lips.

If inappropriate behaviors, such as dropping or throwing the cup, are interfering with the achievement of independent drinking, rather than a true neuromotor deficit, a behavioral program of systematically ignoring the inappropriate behavior or of modeling appropriate cup drinking with an empty cup might be preferred alternative strategies.

Feeding is, in fact, one of the most important self-care areas to be evaluated by the physical therapist who works with infants and children with Down syndrome. Neuromotor deficits such as hypotonia of the oral muscles and delayed appearance of oral reflexes are frequent concerns in working with this population.[58] Of particular concern is the hypoactive gag reflex which may contribute to aspiration or choking during feeding. Palmer has identified five specific feeding problems commonly seen in children with Down syndrome: (1) poor suck and swallow in early infancy, (2) drooling secondary to poor tongue and lip control from hypotonia, (3) presence of the protrusion reflex of the tongue, (4) chewing difficulties, and (5) xerostomia or dry mouth leading to swallowing difficulties.[58] The underdeveloped bones of the facial skeleton contribute to a smaller oral cavity[59] and create the illusion that the tongue is abnormally large.

Specific eating problems identified by mothers of children with Down syndrome include difficulty in using utensils; difficulty in chewing foods, particularly meat; difficulty in drinking from a cup; and regurgitation of food.[60] Pipes and Holm,[61] in a review of medical charts of 49 children with Down syndrome seen at an interdisciplinary diagnostic center, reported feeding practices that were developmentally inappropriate for more than half of the children in the sample. These included failure to offer table food when appropriate, failure to encourage self-feeding, and persistence of bottle feeding.[61] Part of the evaluation role of the physical therapist is to determine the child's developmental readiness for certain foods and feeding practices and to encourage parents and teachers to provide foods that are developmentally appropriate.

Avoidance of foods that are particularly difficult to chew, swallow, and digest should also be advised. Pomeranz[62] has cautioned that celery, carrots, popcorn, and peanuts should not be given to any child under the age of six. Since many older children with Down syndrome continue to exhibit developmentally delayed oral motor patterns, caution should be exercised in allowing them to eat such difficult-to-handle foods.

While eating difficulties are particularly prevalent among younger children with Down syndrome, excessive caloric intake and resultant obesity were found to be problems in 50 percent of the children over the age of 5 years in the study of Pipes and Holm.[61] Cronk[63] reported excessive weight as compared to length in 30 percent of a sample of children with Down syndrome ranging in age from birth to 3 years. The physical therapist who works with children with Down syndrome should be cognizant of this risk for obesity and should encourage exercise programs that will facilitate caloric expenditure as well as being developmentally appropriate.

In assessing the feeding and oral motor development of the child with Down syndrome, the physical therapist should work closely with other members of the interdisciplinary team, particularly the nutritionist, speech therapist, and pediatrician. Pipes and Holm[61] suggest the use of a developmental feeding table, modified from Gesell and Ilg,[64] for the evaluation of feeding skills in children with Down syndrome (Table 6-1). Palmer[58] advises using the prespeech evaluation schedule developed by Mueller[65] to assess feeding problems in children with Down syndrome that may result from neuromotor dysfunction.

Summary

Three general strategies have been suggested when conducting physical therapy evaluation of a child with Down syndrome: qualitative evaluation of movement patterns, developmental evaluation of gross and fine motor skills, and evaluation of self-care skills, particularly feeding. One of the primary goals in conducting a physical therapy evaluation is to establish programming objectives that will serve as the framework for the plan of treatment. The following section will address an objective-oriented approach to developing an appropriate treatment plan for the child with Down syndrome. A review of treatment strategies previously reported in the literature will also be provided.

Table 6-1. Progression of Feeding Behavior in Normal Children

Developmental Stage	Approximate Age (Months)	Food Introduced	Observed Behavior
Sucking or suckling (reflexive at birth)		Bottle	Nipple grasped with slight tongue curling and lip seal
Head erect in supported sitting	4	Strained fruit	Tongue protrudes before swallowing; food ejected; mouth poises to receive spoon
Looks at objects in hands; beginning bilateral reaching	5	Crackers; piece of cheese	Food grasped in a squeeze and brought to mouth; munching movements; lips close on swallowing
Bites (nipple, fingers); grasps large objects with palmar grasp; hands to mouth	6		
Pincer grasp (inferior); pokes with index finger	9–10	Peas and carrots	Interested in feel of food; finger-feeds
Uses spoon to scoop (e.g., sand); empties spoon to mouth upside down or sideways	15	Custard; macaroni and cheese	Fills spoon by pushing into food; tongue licks food on lips
Turns pages in books; builds two-block tower	18	Hamburger in gravy; ice cream	Begins to inhibit spoon turning; skilled finger-feeding

Copyright The American Dietetic Association. Adapted by permission from Journal of the American Dietetic Association, 77:277, 1980.

PHYSICAL THERAPY

The goals of this section on treatment are (1) to provide an overview of therapy programs for infants and children with Down syndrome that have been described in the recent literature, and (2) to outline an objective-oriented approach to treatment based on information gleaned from typical evaluation strategies described in the foregoing section. A case study of an infant with Down syndrome will be used to exemplify the objective-oriented approach to treatment. A case study of an older child with Down syndrome will be used to highlight the physical therapist's role as a consultant.

Review of Therapy Programs in the Literature

In spite of the well-documented motor problems associated with Down syndrome, relatively few intervention programs reported in the medical and educational literature are specifically aimed at remediating these problems. Two well-known early intervention programs for Down syndrome, the Down's Syndrome Infant Learning Program at the University of Washington[66,67] and the University of Minnesota's Project EDGE,[68] make no specific mention of the use or importance of physical therapy services in their curricula.

A search of the Down syndrome literature from the past 15 years reveals only a handful of articles specifically pertaining to physical therapy for children with Down syndrome. Each of these programs will be discussed briefly with regard to their strengths and limitations for use with children with Down syndrome.

Kugel[69] reported on an 18-month pilot study of seven institutionalized infants with Down syndrome aged 4 to 17 months at the initiation of the study. This research was conducted at the University of Nebraska Mental Retardation Clinical Research Center. One of the goals of this program was the encouragement of motor skills through individualized management plans for physical and occupational therapy. General guidelines for developing motor skills for all the infants included activities designed to improve head and neck control and to facilitate developmentally appropriate sitting, creeping, standing, and walking.

While the goals of this program are congruent with those that have been recommended in more recently reported studies,[49] the treatment techniques specified do not seem appropriate and in some cases would be contraindicated. One example cited is the use of techniques to improve head and neck control.[69] The author reports that nurses and aides were encouraged, by the instruction of the physical therapist, to conduct activities aimed at increasing mobility of the head such as pull-to-sit without head support. Since research has demonstrated that children with Down syndrome are already hypermobile due to the decreased muscle tone and joint laxity[70] and also exhibit a persistent and severe head lag during pull-to-sit,[29] it would appear that such activities as described here would be entirely inappropriate and possibly contraindicated. A preferred method for facilitating head righting into flexion in the infant with Down syndrome would be to partially eliminate the effects of gravity by starting the pull-to-sit at a 45- to 60-degree angle with the child sitting in the therapist's or parent's lap and by giving support at the shoulders rather than pulling on the hands (Fig. 6-5).

Although Kugel[69] reports that, at the conclusion of the study, the infants in the program were functioning "up to age in gross motor activities," he fails to report what measurement instruments were used and what scores were achieved. The absence of a control or comparison group in this study also minimizes the value of its reported effects.

Another physical therapy program for infants with Down syndrome cited in the literature was that carried out at Cheltenham Group Hospitals in England and reported by Hughes.[71] Hughes's article is purely descriptive of her 10 years experience in working with infants with Down syndrome. The author espouses a developmental approach to treatment with emphasis on proprioceptive and other sensory stimulation. The only specific treatment strategies mentioned are the suggested use of three basic postures: early prone-lying, side-sitting, and early weight bearing in standing. While the first two postures are certainly developmentally appropriate, the encouragement of early weight bearing in standing before adequate trunk and hip control have been achieved may actually promote hyperextension of the hips and knees and contribute to greater joint laxity. Aside from the three static postures suggested, the author fails to describe any other therapeutic strategies. Since it has been my experience that

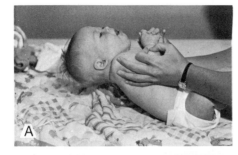

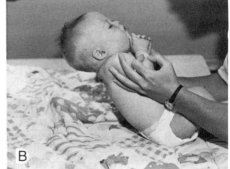

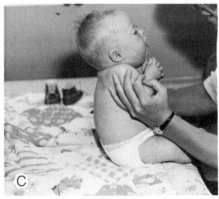

Fig. 6-5. Pull-to-sit with support at the shoulders (4-month-old infant).

infants with Down syndrome tend to get "stuck" in static postures, it would be preferable to recommend strategies for facilitating movement into and out of appropriate postures and emphasizing functional activities.

A second article from the British physical therapy literature presents a descriptive approach to the treatment of children with Down syndrome which is similar to that described by Hughes. York-Moore[72] also recommends early prone positioning to encourage head raising as well as advocating more finely graded pull-to-sit activities from supine. Early weight bearing is encouraged, but specific graded activities for first strengthening lower extremities are provided toward the achievement of this goal. While York-Moore stresses the importance of good balance in sitting, she does not provide any treatment strategies for facilitating balance or protective reactions.[72] Both York-Moore[72] and Hughes[71] have presented treatment approaches based largely on the use of static postures with little discussion of how to facilitate movement into and out of these postures.

Another early intervention program for children with Down syndrome has been described by Connolly and Russell.[73] Their article describes an interdisciplinary program at the University of Tennessee Child Development Center in which 40 children with Down syndrome, from birth to 3 years of age, were included. Physical therapy consisted of gross motor activities including "muscle strengthening, range of motion, sensory and gross motor stimulation."[73] The use of vibrators for the stimulation of weak extensor muscles as well as for oral facilitation and sensory stimulation was also included as part of the intervention. Equipment included beach balls, which were used for facilitation of righting reflexes and neck and back extension.

In an effort to measure the success of their intervention strategies, Connolly and Russell[73] compared the achievement of gross motor milestones for their group of infants with those achieved by the infants with Down syndrome in a descriptive study of untreated infants by Fishler and colleagues[74] using the Gesell Developmental Scales.[75] The authors reported that all gross motor milestones were achieved at an earlier age by the children in the study group. In a follow-up study with 20 of these same children,[76] the authors show that there was earlier acquisition of both motor and self-help skills among the children who received early intervention as well as statistically significant differences in terms of intelligence and social quotients in favor of the group of treated children as compared to a similar group of noninstitutionalized children with Down syndrome who had not received early intervention.

One of the first reported studies on the effects of physical therapy on the improvement of motor performance in infants with Down syndrome was reported by Kantner and associates.[77] The intervention technique used was vestibular stimulation of the horizontal and vertical canals for a period of 10 days. Infants were placed in the laps of volunteers who were seated in a hand-operated rotary chair. Two infants with Down syndrome received treatment and two others were utilized as controls. Motor performance as measured by an assessment scale developed for use in the study was one of the two dependent variables examined. Since one of the treatment group subjects failed to cooperate during posttesting, the reported results are based solely on the posttest measurements of the one treatment subject remaining and of the two control subjects. Since the experimental group subject gained 16 points on the motor scale and the mean gain for the control group subjects was 0.75 point, the authors concluded that the treatment was responsible for the 15.25-point difference in mean gain. The extremely small number of subjects used in the study as well as the lack of mention of random assignment to groups makes the authors' strong concluding statement that the treatment was effective highly questionable.

Harris[78] suggested a transdisciplinary developmental therapy model for the infant with Down syndrome that utilizes treatment goals based on the neurodevelopmental treatment approach[79] and sensory integrative therapy.[80] Oral treatment techniques developed by Mueller[81] were also suggested as part of this model. It was suggested that specific, individualized therapy objectives, based on these more generic treatment goals, should be developed for each infant as part of this model program.

In 1980, Piper and Pless[82] published the results of a study which evaluated the effects of a biweekly developmental therapy program on the improvement of mental development in a sample of infants with Down syndrome. Infants in the experimental group received two hours of developmental programming each week for a period of six months, while infants in the control group received no intervention services during this same period. No significant between-group differences were found on any of the change scores on the Griffiths Mental Developmental scales. A number of limitations such as the relatively short duration and limited intensity of the intervention program were discussed in analyzing the differences in the results of this study to those of several earlier studies.

In a controlled experimental study designed to assess the effects of neurodevelopmental therapy on improving motor performance in a group of infants with Down syndrome, Harris[49] reported that, although there were no significant differences between groups on either the Bayley Scales of Infant Development[39] or the Peabody Developmental Motor Scales,[56] there was a significant difference in favor of the treatment group in the achievement of specific individualized therapy objectives, such as: "S. will correct her head to vertical and display a C-curve in trunk when tipped laterally to left and to right 3 out of 4 times in each direction" (Fig. 6-6). This finding lends support to the importance of early motor intervention for infants with Down syndrome. However, as the author points out, there is certainly an urgent need for further studies designed to examine the efficacy of various treatment approaches on improving motor abilities in children with Down syndrome. While experimental research with large numbers of children is beyond the scope of most clinical settings, it is incumbent upon the clinicians in our profession to develop at least strategies for the systematic documentation of individual changes as a result of their therapeutic intervention. Through an objective-oriented approach to treatment, such changes can be monitored and those facets of the treatment package that are most successful can be maximized.[83]

Treatment by Objectives

One of the primary goals of conducting a comprehensive evaluation for a child with Down syndrome is to develop a treatment plan which includes objectives aimed at improving the child's motor abilities. Through the qualitative assessment of the child's movement patterns, postural tone, primitive reflexes, and automatic reactions, the therapist can ascertain which aspects of movement may be interfering with the achievement of age-appropriate motor milestones. The results of a standardized developmental assessment will provide the therapist with additional information about which specific milestones the child is lacking. In addition to evaluating the general levels of gross and fine motor development, specific evaluation of self-care areas, such as feeding, will provide further information for developing a comprehensive treatment plan. Finally, the therapist should collect observational data of the child in the educational or home environment to determine if there are any interfering problems, such as specific neuromotor deficits or attentional deficits, which are preventing the acquisition of functional skills.[51] All information gleaned from such a comprehensive evaluation is then utilized by the therapist in developing treatment objectives that are both functional and developmentally appropriate for the particular child.

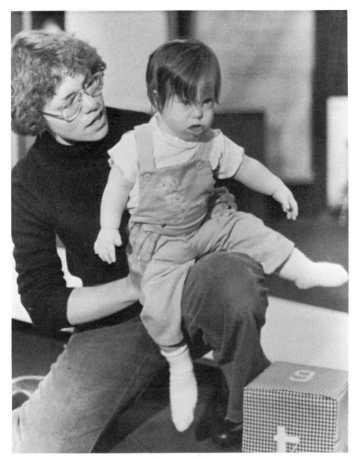

Fig. 6-6. Individualized therapy objective. S. will correct her head to vertical and display a C-curve in trunk when tipped laterally to left and to right (13-month-old infant).

Input from other professionals on the interdisciplinary team and from the child's parents should also be used in developing objectives that are relevant to their overall goals for the child. In developing a treatment plan for older children with Down syndrome, input from the child herself as to what aspects of her own motor performance she would like to improve should also be sought. Perhaps learning to tie her shoes independently is a very important goal for a school-age girl with Down syndrome, in which case this goal should become a part of the overall treatment plan.

The following case studies illustrate the development of a treatment plan based on specific evaluation data. One study is of an infant with Down syndrome for whom direct treatment is indicated, and the other is a 12-year-old girl with Down syndrome for whom specific consultation and outside referral is warranted. Both of these case summaries demonstrate that children with

Down syndrome have very special needs that frequently require consultation, evaluation, and treatment by a physical therapist. While portions of these case summaries are fictitious, they both represent examples of children with Down syndrome with whom the author has been involved in both evaluation and treatment. The breadth of associated physical, medical, and nutritional problems that frequently accompany a diagnosis of Down syndrome should not be overlooked by physical therapists concerned with evaluation and treatment of the "whole child."

Case Study: Patrick

Patrick is a 17-month-old infant with Down syndrome who lives at home with his parents and is enrolled in a developmental infant intervention program. Chromosome analysis shortly after birth revealed that Patrick has the standard trisomy-21 nondisjunction type of Down syndrome. In addition, he has a severe congenital heart defect for which the risks of surgical intervention are so great that surgery is inadvisable. Patrick exhibits bilateral esotropia which has been conservatively treated by alternate eye patching with no observable improvement. Patrick's pediatrician, after consultation with his cardiologist, has recommended evaluation and treatment by a physical therapist with the advice that excessive fatigue should be avoided.

Patrick's initial physical therapy evaluation was conducted on two separate occasions to minimize the chance of fatiguing him. During the first phase of the evaluation, the Movement Assessment of Infants (MAI) and Bayley Motor Scales were administered, since there is some overlap of items on these two tools. Administration of the postural tone section of the MAI revealed that Patrick was severely hypotonic as measured by items evaluating extensibility of joints, consistency of muscles, passivity of hands and feet (amplitude and duration of flapping of a distal extremity when it is shaken by the examiner), and ability to assume antigravity postures in prone, supine, and prone suspension. Evaluation of primitive reflexes indicated there was no retention of early reflexes that would interfere with motor progress. Assessment of automatic reactions revealed immaturities in lateral head righting and head righting into flexion during pull-to-sit. Although head righting into extension could be accomplished when Patrick was in prone position, it was observed that he needed to hyperextend his neck and rest his head back on his upper trunk in order to maintain this posture. Prone equilibrium reactions were absent, although beginning truncal equilibrium reactions were elicited in ventral suspension and supported sitting. Forward and sideways protective extension reactions in the arms were present inconsistently.

The volitional movement section of the MAI was administered concurrently with the Bayley Motor Scale. Patrick was able to sit independently when placed and was able to free his hands to play with toys although he frequently propped forward on extended arms as probable compensation for his low trunk tone. He was unable to get into or out of sitting independently, nor was he able to pull to standing. Patrick could progress forward on his abdomen and could rock in the quadruped position; he was unable to creep in quadruped. Fine motor skills included the ability to grasp cubes using a radial digital grasp, to scoop or rake the pellet, and to combine two cubes. On the Bayley Motor Scale, Patrick achieved a raw score of 35, which converted to an age equivalent of 7 to 8 months at chronologic age (CA) 17 months.

During the second evaluation session, the Bayley Mental Scale was administered to Patrick and an oral motor evaluation and feeding inventory were conducted. Patrick achieved a basal level of 6 months on the Bayley Mental Scale with his highest pass at 12 months (turns pages of book). He received a raw score of 83, which converted to an age equivalent of 7 to 8 months, identical to his age equivalent on the Bayley Motor Scale. The oral motor evaluation revealed no interfering influence of primitive oral reflexes; however, the gag reflex was hypoactive. In spite of the severe generalized hypotonia, Patrick maintained his tongue in his mouth and his mouth closed more than 50 percent of the evaluation time. Delayed dental development was apparent because of the absence of canine teeth. Patrick chewed using an up-and-down munching pattern. Patrick's mother was questioned about his feeding habits, and it was learned that he was eating some table foods as well as finger-feeding crackers and cookies but not yet using a spoon. He was beginning to drink from a cup with assistance.

A summary of the physical therapy evaluation results for Patrick (CA = 17 months) is as follows:

Test	Developmental Level/Findings
Movement Assessment of Infants	Severe hypotonia, appropriate absence of primitive reflexes, delayed development of automatic reactions (6-month level)
Bayley Motor Scale	7–8 months
Bayley Mental Scale	7–8 months
Feeding Inventory	6–10 months

Patrick's greatest area of delay appears to be in the development of age-appropriate automatic reactions. According to Fiorentino,[84] prone equilibrium reactions and forward protective extension should appear between 6 and 8 months in the normal infant. Patrick's absence of prone equilibrium reactions and the inconsistent appearance of forward protective responses would suggest that automatic reactions are significantly delayed. It could also be hypothesized that the severe truncal hypotonia might contribute to the failure to elicit age-appropriate equilibrium responses. The results of Patrick's oral motor assessment (see Table 6-1 for reference) indicate that his skills in this self-care area are certainly in line with his general mental and motor development as measured by the Bayley.

In developing a comprehensive treatment plan for Patrick, it is suggested that the problem-oriented approach described by Campbell[57] be utilized. Based on the foregoing evaluation, it could be hypothesized that Patrick's severe hypotonia is interfering with his attainment of age-appropriate motor skills. This hypothesis is based, in part, on two observations: (1) there were no obvious inappropriate behaviors such as throwing, refusal to comply, or self-stimulatory mannerisms that appeared to interfere with Patrick's achievement of various items, and (2) recent studies examining the relationship of hypotonia in Down syndrome to delays in affective, cognitive,[40] motor,[2] and feeding development[85] show a high level of consistency between the degree of hypotonia and the degree of delay in these other domains. Severe congenital heart disease in young children with Down syndrome has also been shown to contribute to greater delays in feeding and social development.[85]

Based on these observations, it would appear that Patrick's severe hypotonia is interfering with his achievement of more age-appropriate developmental milestones. Using Campbell's problem-oriented approach,[57] the first goal of treatment, therefore, would be to increase muscle tone. Since muscle tone is difficult to quantify clinically,[49] specific objectives written to reflect underlying improvements in tone must be devised as subsets of this more generic goal. In Patrick's case, some specific developmental motor objectives based on deficits revealed in his evaluation would include (1) Patrick will rise to sitting independently using trunk rotation, and (2) Patrick will get out of sitting independently using trunk rotation. Each of these objectives should then be further task-analyzed, and an instructional sequence should be developed (Table 6-2). Objectives should always be written in terms of child-achievement,[83] such as "*Patrick* will get into sitting independently using trunk rotation." In addition, the therapist's activities directed at the achievement of the objective may also be specified as part of the treatment plan for each goal and objective (Table 6-2).

Based on the results of Patrick's evaluation, another important goal would be to improve automatic reactions. An example of an objective that would work toward this goal would be as follows: "When placed in prone on the therapy ball, Patrick will display a C-curve in the trunk when tipped laterally to left and to right, 2 out of 3 times to each side." Examination of the evaluation data in the areas of feeding and fine motor skills shows that Patrick is beginning to finger-feed crackers and cookies and is able to scoop or rake the pellet used in Bayley testing. A combined feeding/fine motor objective that is both developmentally and functionally appropriate is as follows: "Patrick will pick up 2 out of 3 Cheerios presented to him at the table using an inferior pincer grasp."

In developing an objective-oriented treatment plan for Patrick, the therapist should include ideas from his parents, teachers, and any other professionals who are working with him. Certain objectives may be more appropriate than others based on environmental factors in the home or classroom, parental desires for the achievement of specific skills, nutritional needs, and so on. Treatment planning should be interdisciplinary and treatment delivery, particularly when working with young infants, should be transdisciplinary with the parent serving as the primary caregiver. Harris[78] has suggested that, in light of the severe motor problems that characterize infants with Down, the physical

Table 6-2. Developing an Instructional Sequence

NAME: *Patrick*   CHRONOLOGICAL AGE: *17 months*

Goal: To improve muscle tone in trunk.

Objective 1:   Patrick will get into sitting independently using trunk rotation by January 1, 1984.

Instructional Sequence:

1.1   P. will roll from supine to sidelying with therapist assist at hips, to right and to left, 3 out of 4 times, for 3 consecutive therapy sessions.

1.2   P. will roll from supine to sidelying with therapist prompt at hip, to right and to left, 3 out of 4 times, for 3 consecutive therapy sessions.

1.3   P. will roll from supine to sidelying independently, to right and to left, 3 out of 4 times, for 3 consecutive therapy sessions.

1.4   P. will push up from sidelying to position halfway between sidelying and sitting using both hands, with therapist assist at hips, to right and to left, 3 out of 4 times, for 3 consecutive therapy sessions.

1.5   P. will push up from sidelying to position halfway between sidelying and sitting using both hands, with therapist prompt at hip, to right and to left, 3 out of 4 times, for 3 consecutive therapy sessions.

1.6   P. will push up from sidelying to position halfway between sidelying and sitting using both hands, independently to right and to left, 3 out of 4 times, for 3 consecutive therapy sessions.

1.7   P. will push up from sidelying into sitting position with therapist assist at hips, to right and to left, 3 out of 4 times, for 3 consecutive therapy sessions.

1.8   P. will push up from sidelying into sitting position with therapist prompt at hip, to right and to left, 3 out of 4 times, for 3 consecutive therapy sessions.

1.9   P. will push up from sidelying to sitting position independently, to right and to left, 3 out of 4 times, for 3 consecutive therapy sessions.

Therapist Activities Directed Toward Goal:

1.   Joint approximation down through shoulders in sitting.
2.   Joint approximation upward through buttocks while bouncing on therapy ball.
3.   Joint approximation through shoulders and hips while in quadruped.
4.   Facilitation of trunk righting while sitting on ball in 6 planes of motion: forward, backward, right, left, right diagonal, and left diagonal.
5.   Manual resistance to shoulders and hips during rolling: supine to prone and prone to supine.
6.   Manual facilitation at hip of supine → sitting: to right and to left.

or occupational therapist may be the most appropriate coordinator of the intervention services.

Case Study: Carole

Carole is a 12-year-old girl with Down syndrome who was referred to the physical therapist by her special education teacher for posture screening. Her teacher had noted an increasing propensity by Carole to tilt her head toward the right while sitting at her desk and during recess activities. Carole is in a classroom for trainable mentally retarded youngsters in a junior high school. She was recently evaluated on the Peabody Developmental Motor Scales by her adaptive physical education teacher; her gross motor age equivalent was 4 years 9 months. Both her classroom and physical education teacher are also concerned about a recent weight gain causing her to become moderately obese.

In this instance, the physical therapist has been called upon to serve as a consultant in evaluating two specific concerns: (1) the head tilt to the right, and (2) the recent weight gain. Since Carole has recently had a developmental motor examination and is participating in a developmentally oriented physical education program, there is no need to further evaluate her level of gross motor skills. In Carole's case, the physical therapy evaluation consisted of range-of-motion assessment of the neck and posture screening. Range-of-motion evaluation of the neck revealed range within normal limits but Carole complained of pain in her neck during lateral flexion to the left. The therapist also questioned Carole about any numbness or tingling in her arms and legs, neither of which she reported. Posture screening demonstrated a mild thoracic scoliosis with convexity toward the left in standing, which disappeared during forward trunk flexion. There was no obliquity noted in the posterior rib cage.

With the assistance of the school nurse, Carole's height and weight measurements were also taken and plotted on a growth grid. While her height was below the 5th percentile for her age and sex, her weight was in the 30th percentile. On the basis of these evaluation findings, the therapist then called Carole's parents to share these results and to suggest that their pediatrician be contacted. At the parents' request, the therapist called Carole's pediatrician directly to discuss the postural and weight gain concerns. Cognizant of the risk for atlantoaxial dislocation, particularly in light of the clinical symptoms of neck pain and torticollis, the therapist suggested to the pediatrician that Carole be referred to an orthopedist to evaluate the possible presence of subluxation or dislocation and to take baseline x-rays of the scoliosis. Then it was suggested to the pediatrician that Carole's diet should be further evaluated by a nutritionist in light of the recent weight gain and the discrepant growth measurements.

In this instance, the physical therapist served primarily as a consultant in evaluating two specific areas of concern. Because of the grave risks associated with a possible atlantoaxial dislocation, referral to the appropriate specialist was the important first course of action. Establishing an exercise program for weight reduction or for correction of the scoliosis were inappropriate goals until the more immediate concerns were further evaluated. The therapist also advised Carole's classroom and physical education teachers to limit her involvement in strenuous physical activities until receiving the evaluation results from the orthopedist.

Measuring Change as a Result of Treatment

One of the purposes of the objective-oriented approach to treatment is to provide a system for measuring progress or change as a result of therapy. By utilizing measurable therapy objectives in treating the child with Down syndrome, the therapist can establish a baseline for each objective and then systematically monitor the child's progress toward the achievement of that objective by collecting data during each treatment session. O'Neill and Harris[83] have outlined procedures for developing goals and objectives for handicapped children and have emphasized the importance of measuring the child's ongoing

Table 6-3. Daily Data Sheet

Student's Name   Patrick

Objec- Patrick will get into sitting independently using trunk rotation by January 1, 1984.
tive #1

Steps 1 P. will roll from supine to sidelying with assist at hips.   Criterion 75% for 3 sessions
       2 P. will roll from supine to sidelying with prompt at hips.   Criterion 75% for 3 sessions
       3 P. will roll from supine to sidelying independently.   Criterion 75% for 3 sessions

Date	Data Taker	1	2	Trials 3	4	5	Crit. reach *	Step #	Comments
11/15/83	SH	+	−	+	+		*	1	
11/16/83	SH	+	+	+	+		*	1	
11/17/83	SH	+	+	+	+		*	1	Proceed to Step 2 at next PT session.

performance in meeting those objectives. Table 6-3 shows a typical data sheet that could be used for measuring Patrick's progress toward the achievement of the objective presented in his case study summary.

By utilizing measurable objectives in the treatment of the child with Down syndrome, the therapist can also establish the methodology for incorporating a single-subject research design into the clinical setting. Martin and Epstein[86] have described procedures for utilizing single-subject research in the treatment of the child with cerebral palsy. Such procedures are also applicable for conducting clinical research on children with Down syndrome. Wolery and Harris[87] have presented strategies for the interpretation of single-subject research designs that include visual analysis of graphed data, which is the simplest and most appropriate method for use in the typical clinical setting.

Summary

The foregoing section has presented a review of the recent literature describing physical therapy for the child with Down syndrome as well as an objective-oriented approach to treatment. Case studies of an infant and an older child with Down syndrome were used to exemplify the therapist's role in evaluation, treatment, and consultation. The importance of utilizing a data system to monitor the child's progress toward the achievement of therapy objectives was also discussed.

The role of the physical therapist in working with the child with Down syndrome should not be limited solely to evaluation and treatment. As was emphasized in this section previously, the therapist must also be concerned with the involvement of the child's family as well as with other professionals on the interdisciplinary team in the evaluation and treatment of the child. The following section will discuss the therapist's role in interacting with family members and other professionals with the goal of ensuring the best services for the "whole child."

PARENT/CLIENT EDUCATION

Because infants with Down syndrome are usually diagnosed at birth, based on typical clinical signs and symptoms,[28] and because this diagnosis is usually confirmed within a few weeks through chromosome analysis, their parents are confronted very early on with the realization that their child may be seriously handicapped. Mourning the loss of the expected normal infant has been described as being parallel to the stages of grief associated with the permanent loss of a loved one.[88] In addition, parents of retarded children are confronted with "chronic sorrow"[89] based on the realization that their child may never be able to live totally independent of them and will remain their responsibility throughout their lives.

Because of the availability of early diagnosis, intervention for the infant with Down syndrome may begin as early as 2 to 3 weeks of age. A transdisciplinary approach, in which the parent is the primary interventionist and the therapist is the team facilitator, has been espoused[78] and is described in greater detail in the previous section. In such a model, the therapist, who may serve as the primary professional contact for the family during the early months of the infant's life, must be cognizant of the mourning process described by Solnit and Stark.[88] By relating positively toward the infant, but within realistic developmental goals, the therapist can promote attachment and adjustment by the parents toward their child with Down syndrome.[90]

In addition, support groups made up of parents of infants with Down syndrome and other handicapping conditions may provide a valuable adjunct to early treatment and may help promote early acceptance of the handicapped child through the realization that they are not the only ones dealing with this dilemma.[90] Two excellent references for parents of children with Down syndrome of which the physical therapist should be aware are *To Give an Edge* by Horrobin and Rynders[91] and *Teaching your Down's Syndrome Infant: A Guide for Parents* by Hanson.[92] Suggested periodicals for parents are: *Down's Syndrome News*, a newsletter written by parents and professionals (P.O. Box 1527, Bronwood, Texas) and *Sharing our Caring*, a newsletter written by parents with practical advice on raising the child with Down syndrome (P.O. Box 196, Milton, Washington 98354).

Education of parents and other family members of individuals with Down syndrome should include genetic counseling about the nature of the occurrence of the chromosome abnormality as well as risks of recurrence. Based on the infant's karyotype and the age of the parents, the risks of giving birth to another child with Down syndrome can be estimated. Parents should be counseled that, although Down syndrome is a genetic disorder, it does not tend to "run in families," except for the translocation type in which the risk of recurrence is between 2 and 10 percent.[12] Physical therapists should be aware of the location and availability of genetic counseling services within their geographic area.

While a transdisciplinary approach has been suggested for treatment of the infant with Down syndrome in an effort to limit the number of different interventionists or "handlers,"[78,93] intervention for the preschool or school-age child should be interdisciplinary, utilizing the talents of the special education teacher, the speech therapist, the physical or occupational therapist, and the adaptive physical education specialist. Consultation as needed should be available from other specialists, including the physician, psychologist, nurse, and audiologist. It is important to recognize that intelligence quotients of individuals with Down syndrome vary widely, with some individuals performing in the mildly retarded ranges, whereas others may function at the severely and profoundly retarded levels. School placement options may range from an integrated classroom or resource room for the child with mild mental retardation to a self-contained classroom for the more severely handicapped child. Every effort should be made to place the child in the "least restrictive environment" as mandated by Public Law 94-142.[94]

Educational and family concerns surrounding the adolescent with Down syndrome may include the need for prevocational and vocational training as well as eventual placement in a setting which will maximize opportunities for independent or semiindependent living, such as a group home or supervised apartment setting. The therapist who works in a job setting where there are teenagers with Down syndrome may become involved in the evaluation and training of independent living skills for the purpose of enhancing their clients' opportunities for placement in semi-independent living situations.

RECENT TRENDS IN MANAGEMENT

In addition to the medical and therapy management strategies discussed earlier in this chapter, several other management strategies directed at improving the well-being of children with Down syndrome have been reported in the recent research literature.

Drug and Nutrition Therapy

The effects of the administration of 5-hydroxytryptophan and pyridoxine on the motor, social, intellectual, and language development of young children with Down syndrome was recently examined in a double-blind study by a group of investigators who had encountered mixed results in previous studies that had evaluated these forms of therapy.[95] Administration of 5-hydroxytryptophan is directed at raising the blood levels of serotonin, a neurotransmitter which has been found to be present in decreased levels in children with Down syndrome. Pyridoxine has been reported to act in a similar fashion.[96] The primary goal of these modes of therapy is to increase muscle tone with secondary aims of enhancing motor, mental, and social skills.

Shortly after birth 89 children with Down syndrome were randomly assigned to one of four treatment groups and were evaluated in this study during their first 3 years of life.[95] One group received 5-hydroxytryptophan, the second group received pyridoxine, the third group received a combination of 5-hydroxytryptophan and pyridoxine, and the fourth group received a placebo. There were no significant differences among the groups on muscle tone ratings, Bayley Mental or Motor Scales, or on the REEL language scale.[97] The authors concluded that their generally negative findings were in agreement with several previously published studies.[96,98,99]

Another recent study examined the effects of vitamins and nutritional supplements on improving IQ in a group of 16 retarded children, 5 of whom were children with Down syndrome.[100] Statistically significant IQ gains were noted in the group of children who received the vitamins and nutritional supplements as compared to a comparable group who received placebos during the first 4 months of the study. The first portion of this study was double-blind; during the second 4-month phase of the study, all subjects received the vitamins and nutritional supplements. Other changes reported during the first phase of the study in children who received the supplements were improvements in visual acuity and a decrease in hyperactive behavior. The authors were cautious in supporting their conclusions and suggested that replications of this study be done in an attempt to confirm or disconfirm their findings. One such replication, exclusively involving school-age children with Down syndrome, is currently being conducted at the University of Washington's Child Development and Mental Retardation Center.

Patterning Therapy

Another controversial type of therapy that has been advocated for children with Down syndrome as well as for more severely brain-damaged children is the Doman-Delacato approach to treatment, otherwise known as "patterning therapy."[101] Based on the assumption that passive manipulation of the limbs and head can affect brain development,[102] the goal of this approach to therapy is to achieve neurologic organization or "the process whereby the organism, subject to environmental forces, achieves the potential inherent in its genetic endowments."[102] In a recent study conducted by investigators at Yale University, 45 seriously retarded youngsters were assigned to one of three treatment groups: a group which received a modified sensorimotor patterning treatment, a second group which received additional individualized attention from foster grandparents, and a third no-treatment control group.[103] The authors employed 22 different dependent measures in analyzing the effects of treatment, including scores on the neurologic profile developed by the Institute for the Achievement of Human Potential where the patterning method is taught. No significant differences were noted between the two treatment groups on any of the measures following the one-year interventions. The authors concluded that "No evidence was found that treatment resulted in an improvement of the children's performance over what would be expected on the basis of attention (as assessed by the performance of the motivational group) and maturation."[103] Physical therapists who work with children with Down syndrome should be familiar with such studies, since their opinions of alternative forms of therapy may be sought out by the parents of the children with whom they work.

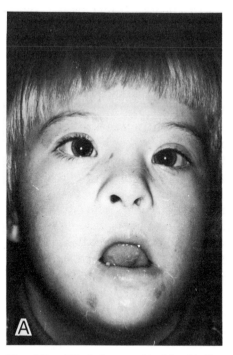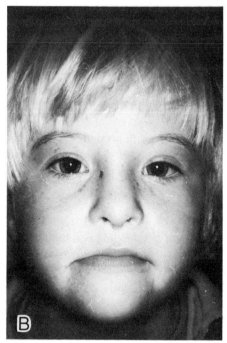

Fig. 6-7. (A) A 6-year-old girl with Down syndrome. (B) The same girl after nasal augmentation and tongue reduction. (Lemperle G, Radu G: Facial plastic surgery in children with Down's syndrome. Plast Reconstr Surg 66:337, 1980.)

Surgery

A new type of surgical management for individuals with Down syndrome is the use of facial reconstructive surgery to "normalize" their facial characteristics (Fig. 6-7).[104] In Frankfurt, Germany 67 children with Down syndrome, ranging in age from 2 to 22 years, underwent surgery. The plastic surgery was aimed at correcting six features: (1) the epicanthal folds, (2) the oblique eyelid axes, (3) the saddle nose, (4) the macroglossia (large tongue), (5) hypotonia of the lower lip, and (6) the receding chin (micrognathia). Such intervention is highly controversial. A leading medical researcher in Down syndrome, in reviewing this paper, has commented that several of these features tend to improve with age (the epicanthal folds and macroglossia) and that such treatment should be highly individualized depending upon the needs and feelings of the child, the family, and the school or community in which the child is involved.[105] As Hunt has suggested,[59] the tongue is *not* really abnormally large but only gives this appearance because of the underdeveloped bones of the jaw and face.

CONCLUSION

The goal of this chapter has been to describe the role of physical therapy in the management of children with Down syndrome. A review of the recent literature has demonstrated increasing involvement by physical therapists in providing descriptive approaches to therapy for this population as well as in providing controlled research studies to examine the effects of therapy on improving various aspects of development. An urgent need exists for continued involvement by physical therapists in both the treatment of individuals with Down syndrome as well as involvement in clinical research studies, including the documenting of individual gains made in the typical clinical setting through systematic monitoring of objective-oriented progress. My own involvement in the management of infants with Down syndrome and in interaction with their families has been an extremely rewarding and positive experience and it is my personal wish that this chapter will stimulate similar interest and involvement on the part of other pediatric therapists.

DEDICATION

This chapter is dedicated to the memory of Joshua Doe and to all the other children with Down syndrome who have helped me to grow and learn.

REFERENCES

1. Carr J: Mental and motor development in young mongol children. J Ment Defic Res 14:205, 1970.
2. LaVeck B, LaVeck GD: Sex differences in development among young children with Down syndrome. J Pediatr 91:767, 1977.
3. Harris SR: Relationship of mental and motor development in Down's syndrome infants. Phys Occup Ther Pediatr 1:13, 1981.
4. Stratford B: Perception and perceptual-motor processes in children with Down's syndrome. J Psychol 104:139, 1980.
5. Diamond LS, Lynne D, Sigman B: Orthopedic disorders in patients with Down's syndrome. Orthop Clin North Am 12:57, 1981.
6. Coleman M: Down's syndrome. Pediatr Ann 7:90, 1978.
7. Kirman BH: Genetic errors: Chromosome anomalies. In Kirman BH, Bicknell J (eds): Mental Handicap, Churchill Livingstone, Edinburgh, 1975.
8. Robinson NM, Robinson HB: The Mentally Retarded Child: A Psychological Approach. McGraw-Hill, New York, 1976.
9. Sasaki M: Paternal origin of the extra chromosome in Down's syndrome. Lancet 2:1257, 1973.
10. Uchida IA: Paternal origin of the extra chromosome in Down's syndrome. Lancet 2:1258, 1973.
11. Lejeune J, Gauthier M, Turpin R: Les chromosomes humain en culture de tissus. C R Acad Sci [D] (Paris), 248:602, 1959.
12. Novitski E: Human Genetics. Macmillan, New York, 1977.
13. Crome L: Pathology of Down's disease. In Hilliard LT, Kirman BH (eds): Mental Deficiency. 2nd Ed. Little, Brown, Boston, 1965.
14. Cowie VA: Neurological aspects of early development of mongols. Clin Proc Child Hosp DC 23:64, 1967.
15. Penrose LS, Smith GF: Down's Anomaly. Churchill Livingstone London, 1966.

16. Benda CE: The Child with Mongolism (Congenital Acromicria). Grune & Stratton, New York, 1960.
17. Marin-Padilla M: Pyramidal cell abnormalities in the motor cortex of a child with Down's syndrome: A Golgi study. J Comp Neurol 167:63, 1976.
18. Loesch-Mdzewska D: Some aspects of the neurology of Down's syndrome. J Ment Defic Res 12:237, 1968.
19. Lipton MA: Early experience and plasticity in the central nervous system. In Tjossem TD (ed): Intervention Strategies for High Risk Infants and Young Children. University Park Press, Baltimore, 1976.
20. Gath A: Cerebral degeneration in Down's syndrome. Dev Med Child Neurol 23:814, 1981.
21. Ball MJ, Nuttall K: Neurofibrillary tangles, granulovacuolar degeneration, and neuron loss in Down syndrome: Quantitative comparison with Alzheimer dementia. Ann Neurol 7:462, 1980.
22. Balkany TJ, Downs MP, Balkany DJ, et al: Hearing problems in children with Down's syndrome. Down Syndr Pap Abstr Profess 2:5, 1979.
23. Jaeger EA: Ocular findings in Down's syndrome. Trans Am Ophthalmol Soc 78:808, 1980.
24. Curtis BH, Blank S, Fisher RL: Atlantoaxial dslocation in Down's syndrome: Report of two patients requiring surgical correction. JAMA 205:464, 1968.
25. Giblin PE, Micheli LJ: The management of atlanto-axial subluxation with neurologic involvement in Down's syndrome: A report of two cases and review of the literature. Clin Orthop 140:66, 1979.
26. Andrews LG: Myelopathy due to atlanto-axial dislocation in a patient with Down's syndrome and rheumatoid arthritis. Dev Med Child Neurol 23:356, 1981.
27. Whaley WJ, Gray WD: Atlantoaxial dislocation and Down's syndrome. Can Med Assoc J 123:35, 1980.
28. Hall B: Mongolism in newborns: A clinical and cytogenetic study. Acta Paedri Scand, suppl 154, 1964.
29. Cowie VA: A Study of the Early Development of Mongols. Pergamon, Oxford, 1970.
30. Benda CE: Mongolism: A comprehensive review. Arch Pediatr 73:391, 1956.
31. Cummins H, Talley C, Platou RV: Palmar dermatoglyphics in mongolism. Pediatrics 5:241, 1950.
32. Levinson A, Friedman A, Stamps F: Variability of mongolism. Pediatrics 16:43, 1955.
33. McIntire MS, Dutch SJ: Mongolism and generalized hypotonia. Am J Ment Defic 68:669, 1964.
34. Wagner HR: Mongolism in orientals. Am J Dis Child 103:706, 1962.
35. McIntire MS, Menolascino FJ, Wiley JH: Mongolism—Some clinical aspects. Am J Ment Defic 69:794, 1965.
36. Crome L, Cowie V, Slater E: A statistical note on cerebellar and brainstem weight in mongolism. J Ment Defic Res 10:69, 1966.
37. Melyn MA, White DT: Mental and developmental milestones of noninstitutionalized Down's syndrome children. Pediatrics 52:542, 1973.
38. Gesell A, Amatruda C: Developmental Diagnosis: Normal and Abnormal Child Development. 2nd Ed. Hoeber, New York, 1947.
39. Bayley N: Bayley Scales of Infant Development. Psychological Corporation, New York, 1969.
40. Cicchetti D, Sroufe LA: The relationship between affective and cognitive development in Down's syndrome infants. Child Dev 47:920, 1976.

41. Uzgiris IC, Hunt JM: Assessment in infancy: Ordinal scales of psychological development. University of Illinois, Urbana, 1975.
42. O'Connor N, Hermelin B: Speech and Thought in Severe Subnormality. Pergamon, Oxford, 1963.
43. Reed RB, Pueschel SM, Schnell RR, et al: Interrelationships of biological, environmental and competency variables in young children with Down syndrome. Appl Res Ment Retard 1:161, 1980.
44. Lydic JS, Steele C: Assessment of the quality of sitting and gait patterns in children with Down's syndrome. Phys Ther 59:1489, 1979.
45. Chandler LS, Andrews MS, Swanson MW: Movement Assessment of Infants: A Manual. Movement Assessment of Infants, Rolling Bay, WA, 1980.
46. Parker AW, Bronks R: Gait of children with Down syndrome. Arch Phys Med Rehabil 61:345, 1980.
47. Knobloch H, Stevens F, Malone AF: Manual of Developmental Diagnosis: The Administration and Interpretation of the Revised Gesell and Amatruda Developmental and Neurologic Examination. Harper & Row, Hagerstown, MD, 1980.
48. Dameron LE: Development of intelligence of infants with mongolism. Child Dev 34:733, 1963.
49. Harris SR: Effects of neurodevelopmental therapy on motor performance of infants with Down's syndrome. Dev Med Child Neurol 23:477, 1981.
50. Eipper DS, Azen SP: A comparison of two developmental instruments in evaluating children with Down's syndrome. Phys Ther 58:1066, 1978.
51. Bruininks RH: Bruininks-Oseretsky Test of Motor Proficiency. American Guidance Service, Circle Pines, MN, 1978.
52. Stott DH, Moyes FA, Henderson SE: Test of Motor Impairment. Brook Educational Publishing, Guelph, Ontario, 1972.
53. Connolly B: Bruininks-Oseretsky tests of motor proficiency. Totline 8(1):21, 1982.
54. Miller LJ: Get yourself on the MAP. Totline 8(1):17, 1982.
55. Fewell R: Personal communication. April 20, 1982.
56. Folio R, DuBose RF: Peabody Developmental Motor Scales, IMRID Behavioral Science Monograph No. 25. George Peabody College, Nashville, TN, 1974.
57. Campbell P: Daily living skills. In Haring NG (ed): Developing Effective Individualized Education Programs for Severely Handicapped Children and Youth. Bureau of Education for the Handicapped, Washington, DC, 1977.
58. Palmer S: Down's syndrome. In Palmer S, Ekvall S (eds): Pediatric Nutrition in Developmental Disorders. Charles C Thomas, Springfield, IL, 1978.
59. Hunt PJ: Oral motor dysfunction in Down's syndrome: Contributing factors and interventions. Phys Occup Ther Pediatr 1(4):69, 1981.
60. Calvert SD, Vivian VM, Calvert GP: Dietary adequacy, feeding practices and eating behavior of children with Down's syndrome. J Am Diet Assoc 69:152, 1976.
61. Pipes PL, Holm VA: Feeding children with Down's syndrome. J Am Diet Assoc 77:277, 1980.
62. Pomeranz VE: Choking: The best cure is prevention. Parents 57:76, 1982.
63. Cronk CE: Growth of children with Down's syndrome: Birth to age 3 years. Pediatrics 61:564, 1978.
64. Gesell A, Ilg FL: Feeding Behavior of Infants: A Pediatric Approach to the Mental Hygiene of Early Life. Lippincott, Philadelphia, 1937.
65. Mueller H: Pre-speech Evaluation and Therapy. Paper presented at the Bobath Course at Sussex Rehabilitation Center, Long Island, NY, 1973. Cited in Palmer S, Horn S: Feeding Problems in Children. In Palmer S, Ekvall S (eds): Pediatric Nutrition in Developmental Disorders. Charles C Thomas, Springfield, IL, 1978.

66. Hayden AH, Dmitriev V: The multidisciplinary preschool program for Down's syndrome children at the University of Washington model preschool center. In Friedlander BZ, Sterritt GM, Kirk GE (eds): Exceptional Infant. Vol 3. Brunner/Mazel, New York, 1975.

67. Hayden AH, Haring NG: Early intervention for high risk infants and young children: Programs for Down's syndrome children. In Tjossem TD (ed): Intervention Strategies for High Risk Infants and Young Children. University Park Press, Baltimore, 1976.

68. Rynders JE, Horrobin JM: Project EDGE: The University of Minnesota's communication stimulation program for Down's syndrome infants. In Friedlander BZ, Sterritt GM, Kirk GE (eds): Exceptional Infant. Vol 3. Brunner/Mazel, New York, 1975.

69. Kugel RB: Combatting retardation in infants with Down's syndrome. Child Today 17:188, 1970.

70. Zellweger H, Simpson J: Chromosomes of Man. Heinemann, London, 1977.

71. Hughes NAS: Developmental physiotherapy for developmentally handicapped babies. Physiotherapy 57:399, 1971.

72. York-Moore R: Physiotherapy management of Down's syndrome. Physiotherapy 62:16, 1976.

73. Connolly B, Russell F: Interdisciplinary early intervention program. Phys Ther 56:155, 1976.

74. Fishler K, Share J, Koch R: Adaptation of Gesell developmental scales for evaluation of development in children with Down's syndrome (mongolism). Am J Ment Defic 68:642, 1964.

75. Gesell A, Amatruda C: Developmental Diagnosis. Hoeber, New York, 1941.

76. Connolly B, Morgan S, Russell FF, et al: Early intervention with Down syndrome children: Follow-up report. Phys Ther 60:1405, 1980.

77. Kantner RM, Clark DL, Allen LC, et al: Effects of vestibular stimulation on nystagmus response and motor performance in the developmentally delayed infant. Phys Ther 56:414, 1976.

78. Harris SR: Transdisciplinary therapy model for the infant with Down's syndrome. Phys Ther 60:420, 1980.

79. Bobath K, Bobath B: Cerebral palsy. In Pearson PH, Williams CE (eds): Physical Therapy Services in the Developmental Disabilities. Charles C Thomas, Springfield, IL, 1972.

80. Ayres AJ: Sensory Integration and Learning Disorders. Western Psychological Services, Los Angeles, 1972.

81. Mueller HA: Facilitating feeding and prespeech. In Pearson PH, Williams CE (eds): Physical Therapy Services in the Developmental Disabilities. Charles C Thomas, Springfield, IL, 1972.

82. Piper MC, Pless IB: Early intervention for infants with Down syndrome: A controlled trial. Pediatrics 65:463, 1980.

83. O'Neill DL, Harris SR: Developing goals and objectives for handicapped children. Phys Ther 62:295, 1982.

84. Fiorentino MR: Reflex Testing Methods for Evaluating C.N.S. Development. 2nd Ed. Charles C Thomas, Springfield, IL, 1973.

85. Cullen SM, Cronk CE, Pueschel SM, et al: Social development and feeding milestones of young Down syndrome children. Am J Ment Defic 85:410, 1981.

86. Martin JE, Epstein LH: Evaluating treatment effectiveness in cerebral palsy: Single-subject designs. Phys Ther 56:285, 1976.

87. Wolery M, Harris SR: Interpreting results of single-subject research designs. Phys Ther 62:445, 1982.

88. Solnit A, Stark M: Mourning and the birth of a defective child. Psychoanal Study Child 16:523, 1961.

89. Olshansky S: Chronic sorrow: A response to having a mentally defective child. Soc Casework 43:190, 1962.

90. Irvin NA, Kennell JH, Klaus MH: Caring for parents of an infant with a congenital malformation. In Klaus MH, Kennell JH (eds): Maternal-Infant Bonding. Mosby, St. Louis, 1976.

91. Horrobin JM, Rynders JE: To Give an Edge. Minneapolis, MN, Colwell Press, 1974.

92. Hanson M: Teaching Your Down's Syndrome Infant: A Guide for Parents. University Park Press, Baltimore, 1977.

93. Haynes UB: The national collaborative infant project. In Tjossem TD (ed): Intervention Strategies for High-Risk Infants and Young Children. University Park Press, Baltimore, 1976.

94. Public Law 94-142. Education For All Handicapped Children Act of 1975 (S.6). 94th Congress, 1st Session, 1975.

95. Pueschel SM, Reed RB, Cronk CE, et al: 5-Hydroxytryptophan and pyridoxine. Am J Dis Child 134:838, 1980.

96. Coleman M, Steinberg L: A double blind trial of 5-hydroxytryptophan in trisomy-21 patients. In Coleman M (ed): Serotonin in Down's Syndrome. American Elsevier, New York, 1973.

97. Bzoch KR, League R: The Receptive-Expressive Emergent Language Scale for the Measurement of Language Skills in Infancy. The Tree of Life Press, Gainesville, FL, 1970.

98. Partington MW, MacDonald MRA, Tu JB: 5-hydroxytryptophan (5-HTP) in Down's syndrome. Dev Med Child Neurol 13:362, 1971.

99. Weise P, Koch R, Shaw KNF, Rosenfeld MJ: The use of 5-HTP in the treatment of Down's syndrome. Pediatrics 54:165, 1974.

100. Harrell RF, Capp RH, Davis DR, Peerless J, Ravitz LR: Can nutritional supplements help mentally retarded children? An exploratory study. Proc Natl Acad Sci USA 78:574, 1981.

101. Chapanis NP: The patterning method of therapy: A critique. In Black P (ed): Brain Dysfunction in Children. Raven Press, New York, 1981.

102. LeWinn EB: Human Neurological Organization. Charles C Thomas, Springfield, IL, 1969.

103. Sparrow S, Zigler E: Evaluation of a patterning treatment for retarded children. Pediatrics 62:137, 1978.

104. Lemperle G, Radu D: Facial plastic surgery in children with Down's syndrome. Plast Reconstr Surg 66:337, 1980.

105. Coleman M: Current papers of special interest. Down Syndr Pap Abstr Profess 4(4):2, 1981.

7 | Myelodysplasia

June E. Bridgford

Myelodysplasia is one of the most complex congenital anomalies compatible with life. Commonly accompanied by hydrocephalus, the anatomic complexity of the primary nervous and skeletal system defects belies the conventional thinking that simply equates myelodysplasia with traumatic paraplegia. In addition to the medical and surgical procedures needed to treat the anomalies present at birth effectively, the secondary problems that occur and recur present a significant challenge to all the health care professions.

ETIOLOGY AND PATHOLOGY

Terminology

Considering the multifaceted nature of neural tube defects, it is not surprising to find a vast and varied nomenclature associated with them. The term spina bifida is defined here as a congenital vertebral defect characterized by lack of dorsal arch fusion. The term myelodysplasia refers to the wide variety of congenital spinal cord and nerve root abnormalities generally associated with spina bifida and characterized by varying degrees of spinal cord function.[1]

Open myelomeningocele is a general label used by Sharrard[2] to describe the spinal cord and vertebral defects associated with approximately 85 percent of surviving spina bifida births. The deficiency in lower extremity sensation and motor control characteristic of this group have been specifically delineated into different patterns by several authors.[2-4] Based on the extent of intact spinal cord reflex activity, Stark and Baker[4] have developed one of the more frequently used methods of labeling these patterns. They define four types (I to IV) with two subtypes (a,b).

From 65 to 100 percent of infants born with open myelomeningoceles are reported to have varying degrees of central nervous system abnormalities that lead to hydrocephalus.[5-7] The primary abnormality responsible for the hydrocephalic condition is commonly called an Arnold-Chiari malformation. The levels of severity of the malformation have been classified into types I to III (or IV).[3] This classification system is unrelated to that of spinal cord function described in the previous paragraph.

Pathogenesis and Epidemiology

Although investigated for over 300 years, the pathogenesis and etiology of spina bifida, myelodysplasia, and Arnold-Chiari malformation are still not clearly understood. Divergent theories of failed caudal neuropore closure and ruptured spinal cord central canal continue to be explored.[5,8–11] The etiology of this complex of defects is believed to be multifactorial. Numerous environmental factors[12–15] and genetic patterns[16–21] have been investigated, but the specific factors causing the condition remain unknown. Also unexplained, is the reduced incidence of spina bifida births, across the United States, to an overall rate of 0.50:1000 births in 1979.[22,23]

DIAGNOSIS AND MANAGEMENT

Prenatal Diagnosis

One of the major developments in myelodysplasia research during the past ten years has been the discovery of a means of prenatal diagnosis of open defects. Elevated levels of alpha-fetoprotein within the amniotic fluid as well as maternal serum, between 16 and 18 weeks of pregnancy, have been found predictive of open neural tube defects.[24–27] Prenatal screening projects have been conducted in the United Kingdom, as well as the United States, resulting in an 80 to 85 percent detection rate.[28] Since these projects have not been without their problems, debate continues regarding the feasibility of implementing a nationwide screening program in the United States.

Advances in Medical and Surgical Management

During the past decade, significant progress has been made in the medical and surgical management of myelodysplastic and hydrocephalic children. Although long-term follow-up information is not yet available, the techniques for neonatal closure of myelodysplasic defects have improved. The surgical microscope has paved the way for development of microneurosurgical methods that facilitate anatomic reconstruction of the open spinal cord as well as improved preservation of functional neural tissue.[29] Increased understanding of the dynamics of shunt obstruction and infection has resulted from the development of radiologic methods such as computed tomography and radioisotope ventriculography. Children with nonfunctioning shunts in place who were thought, because of absence of clinical symptoms, to have arrested hydrocephalus, have been found to have significantly dilated ventricles or compensating hydromyelia. This insidious level of brain damage has been proposed as the cause of gradual loss of upper and/or lower extremity function, an increase in scoliosis and/or decrease in cognitive function.[30] Although limited to a small population of patients, promising results from the use of acetazolamide and furosemide to influence the production of cerebrospinal fluid have been reported.[31] Use of clean intermittent catheterization techniques appear to be providing more effective management of urinary incontinence than surgical diversion methods.[32–35]

Advances in the orthopedic management of myelodysplasia patients reflect an increased understanding of criteria which identify those most likely to benefit from various procedures. Several follow-up studies now support the use of iliopsoas transfers and acetabuloplasties with only those children demonstrating essentially normal quadriceps function and high potential for adult ambulation.[36–38] For the individual who is potentially with bilateral long leg braces or dependent upon a wheelchair for mobility, soft tissue release, femoral osteotomy, and tendon division or excision of the iliopsoas and adductor muscle groups are recommended to manage hip flexion deformities. Thus the recent changes made in orthopedic management of the hips of myelodysplasia patients reflect a consensus that fewer and less complex procedures need to be done rather than the development of additional procedures.

The recent changes in orthopedic management of spinal deformities, however, do reflect the development and refinement of new surgical techniques. A frequently used method for stabilization of many myelodysplastic scoliosis and lordoscoliosis deformities is now a two-stage combination of anterior and posterior spinal fusion. The anterior fusion, stabilized by Dwyer instrumentation, precedes by two weeks the posterior fusion stabilized by Harrington rod instrumentation.[39,40] In an effort to eliminate the need for postoperative cast immobilization, Allen and Ferguson[39] have reported short-term success with a method of posterior stabilization called segmental spinal instrumentation. The kyphotic deformities of myelodysplasia patients still present a major management problem. In an effort to provide increased spinal stabilization, while eliminating the need for body jacket casting, a procedure called anterior-posterior plating has been implemented to a limited extent.[41]

Delineation of Associated Problems

Progress has been made in understanding the multiple complex problems associated with myelodysplasia and hydrocephalus. The extent to which the upper extremities of these children can be effected by central nervous system dysfunction is more clearly appreciated.[42–48] Numerous authors have reported studies that delineate the variety of ways in which the perceptual motor dysfunction of myelomeningocele hydrocephalic patients can be manifested.[49–52] Understanding of the relationship between cognitive skills, language development, and Cocktail Party Syndrome in this population has increased.[53–55] Awareness of the effects of myelodysplasia and the multiple hospitalization periods required for its management on psychosocial development, as well as family interaction patterns, has increased.[56-59] While these associated problem require further investigation to be thoroughly understood, the studies that hav been reported focus attention on aspects of the function and development « myelodysplasia children that warrant consideration during physical therap evaluation and habilitation.

PHYSICAL THERAPY EVALUATION

Since the primary and secondary problems resulting from myelodysplas defects are so numerous and interrelated, it is obviously important that th physical therapist focus upon a primary purpose of that evaluation. The lengthy detailed evaluation of clinical symptoms that either have little to do with actu. treatment planning or duplicate the evaluations of other health care provide are pitfalls to be avoided. In general terms, the primary purpose of physic therapy evaluation, for this population, is to define each individual's currer and potential secondary neuromusculoskeletal problems that are amenable t treatment provided by physical therapists. The secondary problems of d creased joint mobility, skin ulceration, lack of independent mobility, lack « self-care skills, and delayed development of fine and perceptual motor skil can be prevented or ameliorated by physical therapy. Clearly, the depth i which these functions are evaluated is dictated by the setting or circumstance in which the evaluation occurs. In multidisciplinary clinics, the physical the apist is more likely to be screening in order to identify aspects which requir more detailed, diagnostic attention and/or treatment at a later time. In ou patient or inpatient treatment settings, the therapist is more likely to be screen ing all functions while fully assessing some specific areas.

Joint Contractures and Deformities

In screening patients with myelodysplasia for joint contractures and d formities, the presence of malaligned body segments and decreased passiv joint range of motion must be documented. Problem areas can be identified b observing spontaneously assumed postures in supine lying and sitting as we as standing in braces. These observations in combination with a gross asses: ment of passive range of motion can be used to identify the presence of clinicall significant torticollis, scoliosis, kyphosis, lordosis, pelvic obliquity, and ap parent leg length discrepancy. Problems such as genu valgus, talipes calc: neovalgus, as well as other hip, knee, and ankle contractures can also be ide tified in brief screening.

Once malalignment and/or contractures are identified, they should be do umented by goniometry. Next, the extent to which their presence or progre sion can be altered by positioning and therapeutic exercise needs to be dete mined. Of the numerous joint deformities that occur secondary to my lodysplasia defects, only certain types are amenable to nonsurgical treatmen

The deformities that characterize myelodysplasia can be divided into static and dynamic types.[60] Static joint deformities develop as a result of prolonged positioning, while dynamic joint deformities are caused by imbalanced muscular forces. Both types of deformity are initially supple; however, both become fixed or rigid as skeletal and connective tissue structures change in response to prolonged abnormal positioning.

Dynamic joint deformities can be caused by unopposed force from either voluntarily controlled muscle groups or nonfunctional groups with spinal reflex activity intact. One of the most common dynamic deformities associated with unopposed voluntary muscle function is hip dislocation. Equinus deformity of the ankle is frequently caused by reflex activity in nonfunctional gastrocnemius-soleus muscles unopposed by anterior tibialis function.

Static joint deformities can be caused by prolonged intrauterine positioning of the relatively inactive fetus with myelodysplasia. Although they may be supple, soft tissue contractures at some point during intrauterine development, these deformities often involve skeletal change by the time the infant is born. Static joint deformities can also be caused by habitually assumed postures of initially normal joints without muscular imbalance. One of the most commonly occurring static deformity patterns associated with thoracolumbar level myelodysplasia is flexion contracture of the nonfunctional hips and knees. The supine lying and sitting postures assumed by the essentially flaccid lower extremities for prolonged periods of time are responsible for the eventual loss of extension in these joints.

Prolonged joint malalignment during weight bearing can also produce static deformities. Another commonly occurring deformity pattern which can be considered static in nature is the external tibial torsion and genu valgum associated with lower lumbar level myelodysplasia. When an ankle valgus deformity is present, the lack of appropriate orthotic alignment and support of the knee can gradually produce these skeletal changes.[61,62] It is these static joint deformities, developed after birth, which can be prevented by frequent passive range of motion and positioning incorporated into daily activity patterns.[2,63]

The ideal means of treating dynamic joint deformities is surgical redistribution of the available muscle force before skeletal and capsular structures become significantly altered.[63] Although positioning, splinting, and passive exercise can delay the progressive effect of muscle imbalance, they are ultimately unsuccessful. Once mobility of the joint is lost, these nonsurgical methods can prevent or delay further progression of deformity, but they are not effective corrective measures of static or dynamic deformities. The use of braces or splints to decrease joint deformity is contraindicated by the presence of anesthetic skin. Necrosis of that skin is likely to occur before joint mobility is affected.

If full passive range of motion and normal body alignment in recumbent and antigravity positions are found to be present, further evaluation can determine the likelihood of this desirable situation persisting. Through discussion with the patient and caregivers, the variety and distribution of postures or positions used during each day can be determined. A variety of sitting, supine lying, prone lying, and standing positions clearly has more potential than less variability for maintaining the ideal state.

If compromised joint range of motion and/or postural nonalignment are found to be present, more detailed evaluation needs to focus upon determination of the cause. After identifying the specific joints with decreased mobility or inappropriate alignment in certain postures, the therapist needs to identify imbalanced voluntary or involuntary muscular forces associated with those joints. This can be accomplished by manual muscle testing or by facilitating similar movements through play. Movements observed to occur spontaneously or in response to tactile stimulation of the face, neck, arms, or clearly innervated chest area are thought to demonstrate, with fair consistency, use of voluntarily controlled muscle groups. Tactile or painful stimulation to the feet and lower legs are thought to facilitate reflexive, withdrawal movement patterns that can be qualitatively differentiated from controlled, voluntary movement.[1,2] Comparison of spontaneously assumed postures of specific joints in gravity-eliminated positions to those in antigravity positions can help determine the role of extremity weight or weight bearing in the deformity.

Pressure Sores

When screening patients with myelodysplasia for pressure sores, the presence of various stages of anesthetic skin breakdown needs to be identified and documented. The earliest signs of prolonged pressure are redness with, as well as without, swelling. Signs of blistering may precede actual evidence of open sores with partial or full thickness epithelial loss.[63] In screening these patients, all these signs need to be looked for within areas of anesthetic skin. Generally, the areas at high risk for breakdown are those that either bear body weight for prolonged periods or that bear unequally distributed pressure. Activity level, joint mobility, and joint deformity are major factors determining the location of this prolonged or asymmetric pressure distribution. Infants are likely to develop skin breakdown in the area of their original spinal defect. Particularly in cases of lumbar kyphoses, the prolonged recumbent and supported sitting periods they experience make this a susceptible area.

Children attending school are particularly vulnerable to ischial and sacral skin breakdown if they are functionally limited to wheelchair mobility.[63] The prolonged sitting periods dictated by many school settings, as well as the extended periods required for transportation to and from school, increase the vulnerability of these areas. Prolonged periods of wetness with resultant skin maceration, due to ineffective management of incontinence facilitate the development and subsequent infection of these pressure sores. The presence of a pelvic obliquity in association with scoliosis or a unilaterally dislocated hip further increases the vulnerability of sacral and ischial areas by shifting the majority of the upper body's weight to one side.

Braces, splints, and casts can create focused pressure on bony prominences, which is amplified or diminished by body positioning. When lower extremity casts are removed, evidence of pressure on the heel is commonly found as a result of supine lying or straight leg sitting posture that focused pressure to that area. Among children wearing braces, shoes are a common source of pressure that leads to skin breakdown. The inappropriate fit of shoes or malalignment of braces is a recurring source of problems. The small, muscularly imbalanced feet of many ambulatory individuals, however, create an unequal, focused weight distribution that is difficult to accommodate by orthotic adjustments.

If no areas of erythema or skin necrosis are found in screening, further evaluative effort can be directed toward the identification of areas still at risk for this problem. Based on the patient's activity level, means of functional mobility, and the significance of joint contractures or deformity, these areas can be determined. If danger areas are identified, it is necessary to find out the extent to which the patient and caregivers are engaged in preventive measures.

Lack of Independent Mobility and Self-Care Skills

The spinal cord dysfunction characteristic of myelodysplasia dictates the extent to which normal patterns of mobility and self-care skills can develop. Patterns adapted to the upper and lower extremity function available have to be learned in order that independence in mobility, bathing, dressing, and toileting be achieved. On screening for the presence or emergence of these adaptive patterns, the evaluator observes the patient's mobility within the clinic and solicits additional information through questioning.

Functional, age-appropriate mobility can be accomplished by a variety of methods. While upright ambulation with braces and crutches is the goal sought for many, mobility in a wheelchair or prone scooter, as well as by means of an adaptive creeping pattern, may also be considered functional relative to the patient's age and environment.

If space and equipment are available, a child is likely to use his or her most functional, preferred means of mobility in the clinic or department waiting area. If spontaneous mobility is not observed, the patient can be encouraged to get to and from the examination area with as little assistance as possible. While observing mobility, energy cost and quality should be grossly evaluated. Observation of changes in respiratory rate, face coloration, and perspiration can be used to analyze energy expenditure subjectively. The speed and consistency of performance are other factors reflecting endurance relative to energy demands. An individual's control over speed and direction, the smoothness of their movements and their equilibrium control can all be observed as measures of quality. Through questioning and observation, the extent to which the patient can get into and out of this position or means of mobility needs to be determined. If a wheelchair is used, the ability to transfer between it and a bed, toilet, and the floor should be noted. If a 2-year-old uses an adaptive creeping pattern as his or her functional means of exploratory play, the ability to safely get in and out of that creeping position as well as down to the floor needs to be noted.

By discussion with the patient and, if appropriate, the caregiver, the extent to which the following skills have developed needs to be determined: (1) taking off and putting on upper body garments, (2) taking off and putting on lower body garments, (3) taking off and putting on braces and shoes, (4) transferring into and out of the bathtub, (5) bathing and drying, and (6) skin inspection. Depending upon the method of bowel and bladder control used, the extent to which the patient accepts responsibility for assisting with or performing stages of the process needs to be determined. The age means and ranges for achievement of these self-care skills among physically normal children cannot be reasonably applied to the myelodysplasia population. The adaptive patterns learned by children with myelodysplasia generally require more mature levels of cognitive and upper extremity function than their counterparts in normal development. While some developmental information has been reported by Sousa and associates,[59] the age means and ranges for achievement of adaptive mobility and self-care skills are essentially unknown. Based upon knowledge of normal development, individual abilities, and environmental requirements, the therapist needs to make a judgment regarding the age-appropriateness of each patient's adaptive abilities.

If the mobility and self-care skills, which are demonstrated and reported, are determined to be appropriate for age and environmental requirements, the purpose of further evaluation is determination of the extent to which abilities prerequisite for higher levels of skill are being developed. A young child who is independently mobile within the home by use of a prone scooter is not necessarily developing the upright equilibrium responses or upper extremity function that will be needed for upright ambulation or wheelchair transfers. The upper extremity gross motor skills required for most of these adaptive patterns can be evaluated through analysis of the child's ability to perform pull-up and push-up movements in a sitting position. From a stable sitting position, the ability to grasp an overhead support and lift hips off the sitting surface can be observed. The child's ability to lift the body upward using shoulder depression can also be evaluated. From the suspended position, as well as the push-up position, observation of the ability to swing forward and backward can be a source of evaluative information.

During observation of a child's attempts to perform these activities, the evaluator's attention needs to be directed toward the rate and smoothness of movement; the length of time the hip elevation can be maintained; the amount of extraneous movement present; and the symmetry of the upper extremity efforts. If not evident during these activities, identification of the level to which postural reactions have developed is worthwhile. Postural adjustment and protective upper extremity responses in sitting should be specifically evaluated. If appropriate to the child's level of function, they should be evaluated in standing with braces and crutches.

If the mobility and self-care skills identified are determined to be inadequate for age or environmental requirements, the purpose of further evaluation is determination of the limiting factors. The gross upper extremity function prerequisite for most of these activities can be determined as described in the above paragraph. The child's attempt to perform the mobility or self-care tasks of concern should be observed to isolate specific problem areas. Causes of inadequate function are commonly found in the method or movement pattern used by the child. For example, hand placement used for sliding board transfers may be such that weight shifting is made more difficult than necessary. Erroneous learning of hand placement can simply be corrected and remediated by practice in an appropriate position. Problems with motor planning, however, can be present and should be anticipated. The inability to shift or advance body weight can reflect lack of upper extremity strength or inability to coordinate use of neck and shoulder musculature to move the trunk. Poorly developed equilibrium responses often account for inadequate mobility skills. Lack of sensory input from the lower extremities as well as lack of lower extremity participation in the movement response significantly alter the development of upright postural control.

Joint contractures or deformities may also be a limiting factor. The limitations created by assistive devices need to be considered. Wheelchairs that are ill-fitting or without removable arm rests can hinder transfer function as can braces that are malaligned or with debris-clogged ankle joints. Other factors relative to adaptive mobility and self-care skills that need to be considered are motivation and opportunity for practice.

Deficient Development of Fine Motor and Perceptual-Motor Skills

This area of concern in evaluation encompasses the wide range of skills for which children with myelodysplasia generally use normal upper extremity movement patterns. These skills include such basic movements as directed reaching and pincer grasping, as well as complex patterns such as cutting with scissors and writing. They include functional skills such as self-feeding, buttoning, and snapping upper body garments. This group of skills is in contrast with the self-care skills, such as applying braces, which involve complex, sensorimotor abilities that are not required of physically normal children.

The primary focus of screening for deficient development of fine and perceptual motor skills is documentation of the presence or absence of age appropriate milestones in these areas. Unfortunately, a standardized, norm-referenced measure designed to validly screen this range of skills in the myelodysplasia population does not exist. In order to avoid the time required for use of detailed diagnostic tests and to obtain the reliability afforded by use of standardized tests, the Denver Developmental Screening Test (DDST) can be used.[64] Although intended for use with "apparently well" children, the DDST can be used to monitor the apparently normal development of skills that do not involve the lower extremities. The standardized administration and scoring criteria can be implemented without modification in the personal-social, fine motor-adaptive, and language sections of the test. As stated in the manual, an evaluation that reveals a DDST section with two or more delayed test items, in addition to the gross motor section, should be classified as "abnormal." An evaluation that reveals a section with one delayed item and no age-appropriate items passed, in addition to the gross motor section, should be classified as "questionable." An evaluation which reveals no delays in any of the sections, other than the gross motor, should be classified as "normal." Clearly, the DDST needs to be administered to this population with consideration given to the quality of their responses. The labels of "abnormal, questionable, and normal" should be used only to help determine the need for further evaluation and not for literal interpretation to anyone.

One element of quality that can easily be observed while administering the DDST is hand preference. The age at which hand preference or dominance is established within the neurologically normal population is relative to specific skills and a topic of continued debate.[65] It can, nevertheless, be a revealing area to use in screening 4- to 6-year-olds for upper extremity dysfunction. In two studies of myelodysplastic, hydrocephalic children from 6 to 10 years of age, 30 percent were found to demonstrate mixed handedness in contrast with 2 to 5 percent in control groups.[66] While no significant link has been established between lack of hand preference and low IQ or neurologic dysfunction, its relationship to delayed manual skill development seems apparent.[66] Absolute dependence upon one upper extremity for skilled activity, however, is significantly predictive of neurologic dysfunction.

After the age of 6 years, use of the DDST for screening becomes inappropriate.[65] There is no single valid standardized screening test that samples the full range of complex fine and perceptual motor skills in the school-age population. Portions of standardized, norm-referenced tests can, however, be useful as objective screening measures if interpreted judiciously.

Although in need of further validation, Cornish[67] has described an 11-item screening test for age-appropriate motor planning ability from 6 to 12 years of age. Of the 11 items, only 5 can be uniformly administered to children with myelodysplasia because of lower extremity function requirements. Those five items that can be used are (1) a vertical throw, hand clap, and catch sequence repeated as rapidly as possible with a tennis ball for 30 seconds, (2) and (3) a peg placement test using dominant and nondominant hands, and (4) and (5) a grip strength measurement using dominant and nondominant hands. Mean scores and standard deviations for these five items, which are based on their administration to 210 normal children, are reported. Failure of a child with myelodysplasia to score within the ranges reported for his or her age on these test items can be cautiously interpreted as an indication for further diagnostic evaluation.

Another screening measurement can be adopted from a study comparing the performance of 8-year-olds with and without diagnosed learning disabilities on measures of fine motor activity speed. After analyzing the responses of 50 children, 25 control subjects, and 25 with learning disabilities, Kendrick and Hanten[68] reported that rapid sequence opposition between the thumb and index finger differentiated between the two groups. During a second testing period, the normal children touched 38.4 ± 3.8 times in comparison to the learning disabled children's 30.6 ± 4.5 ($p < 0.01$). Keeping in mind that predictive validity of this item remains to be proven, it could be administered to 8-year-old patients with myelodysplasia and interpreted in terms of speed within the normal range, smoothness, rhythm consistency, and elimination of extraneous movement. Lack of speed within the normal limits or subjectively poor response quality could be used as indications for further evaluation.

If no deficiency is suggested by screening test items, no deficiency perceived by the quality of responses, and no significant frustrations expressed by the child or caregivers, further evaluation of perceptual and fine motor skills may be deemed unnecessary or of low priority. From a preventive perspective, however, further evaluation can be directed toward determination of the experiential opportunities available to the child for further expansion of these abilities. Of specific concern with the infant and young toddler are opportunities for independent exploration of space and for two-handed play in a stable upright posture.[69]

If deficiency is suggested by screening test items, by diminished quality of performance perceived by the examiner, or by concerns expressed in caregiver-child interviews, further diagnostic evaluation can branch out in several directions. When concerns are based primarily on screening test results, those tests need to be readministered at a later date to determine whether or not the pattern of delay persists. Delayed development specific to the language section of the DDST is appropriately investigated further by a speech pathologist. Consistently delayed development throughout all sections of the DDST may be indicative of mental retardation. This is appropriately evaluated further by individuals skilled in the administration of standardized, norm-referenced tests of learning potential or intelligence. Although not highly predictive of later scores on the Stanford-Binet Intelligence Test, the Bayley Scales of Infant Development (BSID) Mental Scale is a well-standardized test that can reliably describe a child's learning or developmental level relative to the general population.[70] Due to the gross motor nature of the items throughout the Psychomotor Scale of the BSID, this portion of the test is inappropriate for use with the myelodysplasia population. The Mental Scale of the BSID, however, can describe learning level as well as basic fine and perceptual motor skill development among this group.

Delays in development of fine motor and/or personal-social abilities identified on the DDST or by other screening methods require further evaluation of upper extremity functional abilities as well as refined coordination capacity. In order to explore upper extremity functional activities in detail, relevant sections from the numerous standardized developmental profiles can be used for preschool levels. The Callier-Azusa Scale is one such profile that has subscales for fine motor, visual motor, feeding skills, and perceptual abilities.[71] The perceptual abilities subscale is further divided into responses to visual, auditory, and tactile input.

Four of the eight subtests that make up the Bruininks-Oseretsky Test of Motor Proficiency (BOTMP) are appropriate for administration to 4.5- through 14.5-year-olds affected by myelodysplasia.[72] For evaluation of refined visual motor coordination skills of the upper extremities, three subtests from the

BOTMP can be helpful as well as subtests from Touwen's protocol for evaluation of children with minor neurologic dysfunction.[65,72] Seven of the nine test items Touwen includes in his assessment of coordination and associated movements can be administered to this group with the only modification being use of a sitting rather than a standing posture. Administration, recording, and interpretation criteria are explained for each of these items, which are thought by Touwen to reflect central nervous system maturation and "proprioceptive system" function.[65] Visual pursuit, scanning, and fixation limitations may appear to be a source of visual motor problems. If this is the case, the relatively quick assessment of these factors outlined by Touwen can be helpful.

Neonatal Assessment

Physical therapy evaluation of a neonate with myelodysplasia should serve the same primary purpose as assessment of a child or adolescent. The limited response capacity of neonates, however, places assessment of their problems in a distinct category. Differentiating between voluntary and involuntary lower extremity movement responses for purposes of anticipatory management can be quite a challenge. Voluntary movement is more likely to be observed in the lower extremities when the infant is alert and actively moving the arms.[2] Lower extremity movement responses to stimulation around the face and chest and shoulders are likely to be voluntary in nature.[2,4] The reflexive character and stimulus dependency of involuntary muscle responses help to distinguish them from voluntary movement. Tactile stimulation of skin over the hip flexor, knee flexor, and all ankle and toe musculature can produce contractile responses in physically normal neonates.[73] These same responses can be elicited when only segmental spinal cord function is present. Consequently, they alone should not be interpreted as evidence of corticospinal tract integrity.[4] While one to two beats of ankle clonus is within normal limits for the immature central nervous system of any neonate, sustained or easily elicited ankle clonus is suggestive of involuntary function of the gastrocnemius-soleus muscles. Similar clonic responses as well as resistance to quick lengthening may also be detected in the lateral hamstrings and toe flexors. If quick stretching of a muscle group on one leg elicits not only a contraction response of that muscle, but of the same muscle(s) on the other leg as well, a crossed stretch reflex has been elicited. This is characteristic of isolated spinal cord segment function and should not be confused with spontaneous, voluntary movement.[4] Stimulus-dependent flexor withdrawal is a primary pattern associated with involuntary movement. The time span between stimulus and onset of movement as well as between onset and completion of withdrawal movement, is reported to vary within a wide range.[3,4] Consequently, a smooth, slow, but stimulus-dependent flexor withdrawal movement is no more indicative of spinal cord integrity than a jerky, brisk withdrawal to stimulation. Stark and Baker[4] report that crossed extensor reflexes are seldom present when corticospinal tract function is not present; however, Brocklehurst[3] includes this response among those that can be elicited when no voluntary control of the extensor muscle groups is present. Electrical stimulation of muscle groups has been used by Sharrard[2] as a means of confirming lower motoneuron innervation; however, the usefulness of the process has been described as minimal by several other authors.[3,63,74]

Determination of the level of intact sensation is probably more difficult and subjective than determination of motor function, but is important for preventive management. When an infant is in a drowsy or quiet state, noxious stimulation can be administered to the areas of skin innervated by the sacral and distal lumbar cord segments. By progressing from most distal to proximal segments, the examiner can usually determine which areas produce cry, grimace, or startle responses distinguishable from spinal cord level withdrawal responses.[2,3]

The primary functional skill to be evaluated in neonates with myelodysplasia is nipple feeding ability. Since these neonates are at risk for cranial nerve damage from an Arnold-Chiari malformation, a feeding evaluation should focus on components of suck, swallow, and respiration, as well as the function of each cranial nerve. The neonatal assessment of sensorimotor function should provide a basis for planning treatment measures that prevent or improve joint contractures, pressure sores, and oral motor dysfunction.

Observation of Complications

Therapists caring for myelodysplastic-hydrocephalic patients should be well aware of the signs of shunt malfunction and neuropathic fractures. These are not only signs that should be considered during designated evaluation periods, but that should also be monitored in any treatment setting. The initial signs of acute shunt obstruction and/or infection mimic those of a viral illness. They are headache, irritability, lethargy, and vomiting.[3] The initial sign of a fracture is often a fever.[75] As is often the case, no traumatic event can be recalled, and the fever is logically attributed to a urinary tract infection.

PHYSICAL THERAPY

The facilitation of both the development and maintenance of as optimal a level of independent function as possible is the general goal shared by the medical team members involved in care of each individual with myelodysplasia. More specifically, the overall goals of physical therapy for an individual with myelodysplasia are to facilitate as normal a sequence of sensorimotor development as possible and to prevent the development of secondary joint deformities and skin ulceration. These goals are ideally pursued through a combination of direct, therapist-provided patient care coordinated with an ongoing home care program. The specific methods for adaptive function and developmental facilitation appropriate for each patient's age and ability need to be taught by the therapist to that patient and caregivers. Once these methods are correctly learned, they should be incorporated into the daily care routines or play within the home environment. The actual refinement of adaptive self-care and mobility skills should be the result of practice that meets the caretaking and play activity needs of the child and family. The parents or primary caregivers of a physically normal child generally feel competent to provide for the needs of that child. For the caregiver of a child with myelodysplasia, however, this sense of competence needs to be fostered rather than diminished by the treatment-related activities carried out at home.

Joint Contractures and Deformities

Physical therapy is directed toward the goals of preventing static joint deformities; resolving minor static joint deformities; preventing the rapid deterioration of dynamic deformities; and minimizing the risk of neuropathic fractures. The primary methods for accomplishing these goals are passive range-of-motion exercises, positioning, and splinting.

Full passive joint mobility throughout the body is ideally the goal of treatment. Mobility that allows stable joint alignment for standing, sitting, and transfers, however, is often accepted as a more realistic guide for both physical therapy and orthopedic management. In an upright position, the cervical and upper thoracic spine need to be centered over the pelvis. The pelvis must be level for equal weight distribution in sitting. Hips and knees should flex to at least 90 degrees for sitting and transferring without increasing the risk of neuropathic fractures. For standing, the hips should extend to neutral without significant rotation or adduction. If this hip range is not present, development of knee flexion contractures and lumbar lordosis can be facilitated. When standing with hip flexion contractures, tightened iliopsoas muscles can exert an amplified dislocating force on the hip joint.[74] Standing and, especially, ambulation are limited in their functional value if hip extension to neutral or beyond is not present. With locked long leg braces in place, hip flexion tightness precludes sufficient shifting of the center of gravity over the feet to produce a balanced stance and allow upper extremity freedom from weight bearing. Knees should reach essentially full extension for functional dressing skills, if not for standing and ambulation. In standing, the presence of knee flexion contractures dictates positions of hip flexion and ankle dorsiflexion if balance is to be achieved. Lack of essentially complete hip and knee extension limit bed mobility and the variety of lying positions which are comfortable. In standing, the joints of the ankle and foot should provide a plantigrade surface across which body weight can be equally distributed. While a neutral ankle is adequate for standing, approximately 10 degrees of ankle dorsiflexion is needed for forward progression. In the absence of gastrocnemius-soleus muscle function, dorsiflexion of approximately 10 degrees may be all that is desirable. Dias has noted that 20–30 degrees dorsiflexion, in the absence of plantarflexion control, facilitates development of ankle valgus, external tibial torsion and genu valgum.[62] If not for standing purposes, the ankle and foot should have unrestricted passive mobility into a neutral position so that shoes and wheelchair pedals do not create pressure sores.

Passive range of motion can be performed for patients with myelodysplasia using any of the methods appropriate for soft tissue tightness. Since the risk of neuropathic fractures is present, considerable attention should be directed toward secure stabilization both proximal and distal to the joint being treated. The range of single joints should be attended to before two-joint muscle groups receive passive stretching. While maintenance of joint mobility in the lower extremities is a ubiquitous component of physical therapy for patients with myelodysplasia, neck mobility is often overlooked in hydrocephalic patients until torticollis is evident. Neither the incidence nor the etiology of this problem have been investigated. Habitual prone positioning, shunt tubing adhesions, irritation of cervical soft tissue by tubing, and/or compensation for spinal deformity, however, are possibilities. As with torticollis in otherwise normal children, neck mobility and facial symmetry can be maintained and restored by exercise and positioning if initiated soon enough.[76]

The amount of time that should be invested in range of motion exercises for torticollis or other contractures, or for preventive purposes, has not been established by clinical research. Kopits[74] recommends that all joints without complete sensorimotor function receive full range two to four times each day. Menelaus,[63] on the other hand, considers it "improper to impose on the parents" the responsibility of passive range of motion exercises. Perhaps the number of variables that complicate each individual situation will cause this to remain an intuitive decision mutually agreeable to the child, parent, and therapist.

Although maximum available range can be achieved for brief periods during passive exercise, positioning can be used to maintain functional ranges for longer periods of time. Prone lying and standing are the two positions most frequently used to counteract the hip and knee flexion postures characteristic of supine lying and sitting. One position, recommended by Drennan,[77] consists of prone lying with placement of the feet off the end of a mattress or cushion and swaddling of the legs together. The foot position eliminates pressure from their dorsal aspect and allows them to assume a relatively plantigrade position. By use of a towel, diaper, or, as Menelaus[63] recommends, a section of "Tubigrip," the legs are held together, preventing hip abduction and lateral rotation. While this position is designed to prevent tightening of the iliotibial bands, it may be contraindicated for children having unstable hips with muscular imbalance. Lack of mobility in the hips or knees may also preclude the use of a flat, prone position.

When hip, knee, and ankle mobility are sufficient, periods of standing can be used to maintain lower extremity joint ranges. Obviously, orthoses of appropriate fit and sufficient support are required for this. For the individual without ambulation skill, standing in braces can be a frightening, as well as boring, situation. A standing table that provides additional external stability and a play surface can resolve this problem. Various forms of supervised standing play can be used to encourage functional upper extremity skills.

Regardless of the specific position used to maintain mobility, anesthetic joints should not be forced to their maximum range in that position. In order to prevent joint damage, fractures, and skin breakdown, these joints should be maintained in positions within the limits of free mobility.

The splints used for treatment of myelodysplasia generally serve the purposes of slowing the progression of dynamic deformities, halting the progression of static deformities, or preventing the recurrence of deformities after surgical correction. The role of lower extremity splints in the early management of hips at risk for dislocation due to muscle imbalance is still a topic of debate among orthopedists. McKibbon,[78] who originally proposed their use, considers a splint that holds both hips in extension, abduction, and slight medial rotation to be useful in maintaining hip reduction and preventing hip flexion contracture development. Various heat and vacuum-formed plastic splints have been designed to serve this purpose. While avoiding the cost and pressure-point problems associated with these rigid splints, Jaeger[79] has reported successful use of a foam wedge splint placed between the legs and held in place by foam straps that control hip rotation.

The recurrent nature of knee flexion contractures and equinovarus deformities have made them a focus of splinting efforts. The dynamic nature of most of these knee or ankle contractures limits the initial preventive role of splints. After soft tissue release, however, posterior splints for use during sleep are considered appropriate preventive measures by Menelaus.[63] The creation of splints that cover areas of anesthetic skin is clearly a refined skill that has to be developed through experience. Basically, however, the splint must conform closely to the body in order to distribute pressure evenly rather than focus it on high-risk areas. To avoid shearing forces on the skin, the splints should fit tightly enough to prevent slipping movement. Thin cotton stockinette is frequently used to separate the splint from direct contact with the skin. Splint use should be completely discontinued when redness is noted from pressure. Once the erythema has completely resolved and the splint has been altered, splint use can be gradually resumed if the signs of pressure do not return. Pressure sore development is such a common complication of splint use over anesthetic skin that their use is considered altogether inappropriate by some physicians.[2] As with range of motion exercises and positioning, no valid formula exists for determination of how long splints should be worn each day or how long daily use should be continued. Even if there were such a formula, it would have to accommodate the same factors of tolerance level and individual motivation currently guiding these decisions.

Approximately 20 percent of individuals with myelodysplasia experience neuropathic fractures.[63] A high percentage of these fractures follow postoperative cast immobilization. Avoiding prolonged immobilization periods is one preventive method that is being implemented more frequently by surgeons. After a fracture itself or corrective orthopedic surgery, initiation of weight bearing as soon as stability is confirmed is another measure thought to prevent fractures.[63,74] Lack of proper stabilization during transfers or too vigorous an effort during therapeutic exercise are possible causes of neuropathic fractures. While whirlpools are very useful in skin care after cast removal, the poorly controlled movement of buoyant legs need to be minimized. Bivalved casts or supportive splints can be used to cradle the vulnerable leg(s) during transfers until functional joint mobility has been gently reestablished.[63]

Pressure Sores

Whether treating pressure sores that have already developed or designing a program to prevent their occurrence, physical therapy is directed at controlling the factors that facilitate skin breakdown. These factors are sustained local pressure, friction, shearing force, skin maceration, and infection.[80] Once skin necrosis has developed, the effects of these factors need to be eliminated for complete healing to occur. Since total elimination of these factors is not conducive to a functional lifestyle, preventive programs are directed toward minimizing and counteracting their effects.

Sustained local pressure over ischial or sacral areas of skin breakdown can only be eliminated for healing purposes by discontinuing wheelchair use and sitting. This requires a closely followed program of prone lying, sidelying, and, if appropriate, standing to allow for healing while preventing the development of skin breakdown in other areas. If standing with braces is not feasible, prone standing devices can be used.

In theory, the location of focused pressure can be changed by increasing the area over which force is distributed or increasing the distance between points of force.[80] One treatment method that applies this theory to the treatment of pressure sores on the feet is total contact plastering. Positioning the foot and ankle in as functional a position as possible, plaster is applied to conform closely to lower extremity contours. This method of casting can prevent further shearing and friction injury, distribute pressure, and facilitate deep tissue healing. Sharrard[2] reports complete healing of significant sores on the feet of myelodysplasia patients within 6 weeks by use of this below-knee casting technique.

Although costly and supported primarily by uncontrolled clinical trials, hyperbaric oxygen therapy is another means of treating pressure sores that may prove to be a valuable addition for the care of patients with myelodysplasia. Fischer[81] reports complete healing of 26 cases of previously "resistant" pressure sores following this type of treatment.

Once healing has occurred or prior to the ulceration of skin in anesthetic areas, programs for alternating body positions during the day need to be developed in collaboration with the patient and caregivers. These positioning periods correspond with those already discussed as needed for the prevention of flexion contractures. Particular attention needs to be directed toward the school-age patient who spends long periods of time in a wheelchair. The ongoing facilitation of prone or standing periods for primarily wheelchair-limited children during school hours can be a very worthwhile, preventive role for school-system therapists to fulfill. Teaching and encouraging these individuals to do push-ups and shift their weight from side to side in the wheelchair are commonly implemented preventive measures. These practices, however, do not seem to preclude the need for periods when pressure is totally removed from the ischial-sacral area. Clinical research validating the usefulness of wheelchair push-ups and lateral weight shifting in terms of temperature or circulatory changes in the posterior skin is lacking.

Particular attention needs to be directed toward the individual with ambulatory skill sufficient for community mobility. Periods that provide for complete elimination of weight bearing and prevention of venous stasis should be planned within daily routines. Correctly fitting shoes and braces are crucial to these individuals. With varying degrees of success, numerous modifications of shoes, such as cut-outs and shoes that unlace their entire length have been tried in order to distribute pressure as well as ensure that the foot is positioned correctly.

Wheelchair cushions are one of the primary means of distributing body weight away from the sacral and ischial areas during sitting. Because of its availability and relatively low cost, polyurethane foam is one of the most commonly used materials for wheelchair cushions. Loss of load-bearing capacity is one of the factors that limits the useful life-span of these cushions. Through static and dynamic fatigue testing, McFadyen and Stoner[82] have confirmed that a patient's weight and the duration of sitting periods are prime factors determining the length of time a polyurethane foam pad can serve a protective function. They also determined that during 24-hour periods without compression, these pads recovered an average of 80 percent of their indentation load deflection capacity. Consequently, they recommend the purchase of two cushions that can be used on alternate days.

Investigating the heat and humidity-dissipation capacity of various types of padding, Stewart and associates[83] noted a moisture-absorbing ability relatively unique to polyurethane. The heat-absorbing capacity of this type of pad, however, was found to be poor and a cause of increased local skin temperature among subjects. On the other hand, they found that humidity remained at a relatively low level during use as long as the pad was covered with a porous material. This humidity-controlling effect was lost when vinyl covered the foam.

Because of their increased load-bearing capacity, wheelchair cushions made of gel materials are generally thought to be superior to foam cushions. Results from the investigation of Stewart and associates[83] point out the limitations of gel cushions in controlling heat and humidity. They found that gel material had very little if any capacity for dissipating moisture. They found that this material was effective for approximately 2 hours in controlling skin temperature because of its capacity to absorb heat. Due to an apparent loss of heat-absorbing ability and the presence of high humidity, the authors recommended that gel cushions be used for no more than 3 hours without permitting them to cool. Similarly, water flotation cushions were found to reduce skin temperature, at least initially. Due to their nonporous structure, flotation pads were found to control humidity poorly.[83]

Clearly, the ideal wheelchair cushion capable of compensating for lack of sensation and mobility under all circumstances has not been developed. When programs for the prevention of pressure sores are being outlined, these load-bearing, heat and humidity-dissipating characteristics of cushions need to be considered. The cost, availability, and durability need to be considered in light of the limited capacity of any wheelchair cushion to provide protection when used all day every day.

Friction and shearing forces need to be controlled in addition to static pressure in order for pressure sores to heal or be prevented. Friction is primarily a force abrading superficial epithelial tissue. Shearing, however, refers to the tangential force caused by gliding of superficial over deeper tissues, which results in obstructed circulation and relatively deep trauma.[84] Skin damage due to friction is controlled in the lower extremities by eliminating significant movement within shoes and braces during ambulation and standing transfers. When pressure sores are on the feet, even the abrasion produced by bed sheets may have to be eliminated.[63] Sitting transfers are a main source of friction and shearing to the ischial-sacral area. Moist skin, clothing, or wheelchair cushions are sources of friction that complicate sliding transfers. Shoulder depression ability that is insufficient to shift weight off the ischial-sacral area during transfers is another factor contributing to skin breakdown. To prevent skin breakdown, measures should be taken to improve the quality of these sitting transfers. A tightly fitting pelvic band that pulls sacral area skin upward during stationary sitting or sitting transfers can be a source of shearing damage to the sacral area. A tightly fitting calf band that pulls skin upward as ankle dorsiflexion occurs during standing or ambulation can be a source of shearing damage to the heel area. Such situations can be altered by proper fitting of braces and the use of long socks or other thin, conforming articles of clothing between braces and skin.

The effects of maceration and infection also need to be eliminated for ulceration healing and controlled for prevention.[84] Maceration describes the damage to superficial skin that occurs when an area is kept moist for a prolonged period by excessive perspiration or incontinence. In the absence of open sores, hair follicles and pores can become infected due to poor circulation and incontinence. Maceration and infection facilitate the presence of each other, as well as make skin more vulnerable to the effects of prolonged pressure, shearing and friction. In order to free open sores of infectious organisms and necrotic tissue, whirlpools are frequently used in conjunction with topical or systemic antibiotics. Of particular importance to both preventive and corrective treatment is an effective bowel and bladder management pattern that is appropriate for home as well as school.

In summary, the prevention or healing of pressure sores requires development of positioning programs and effective management of incontinence. It can require the modification of braces, wheelchairs and their accessories, as well as techniques used for ambulation and transfers. Programs for preventive care are incomplete without establishment of a routine skin inspection method.

Lack of Independent Mobility and Self-Care Skills

Numerous studies of the mobility skills achieved by patients with myelodysplasia lesions at varying levels have provided information upon which predictions of functional mobility in child and adulthood can be based.[85-87]

From these results, the goal of therapeutic ambulation for any myelodysplasia patient without major brain damage is justified as realistic during childhood. While therapeutic ambulation serves many purposes, it often does not meet the child's need for mobility during the preschool or school years. The therapist must keep a realistic perspective on the potential for ambulation to actually fulfill each child's need for functional mobility. When time, teaching, and financial resources are applied only to the development of walking skill in early childhood, the unfortunate result can be a 5-year-old child with ability to independently walk 100 feet in 10 minutes, but lack of the transfer and wheelchair mobility skills needed for a school setting.

Longitudinal studies of mobility skills among people with myelodysplasia defects use the terms community, household, therapeutic, and wheelchair to describe levels of skill. *Community* ambulation describes the ability to walk with or without braces and other assistive devices indoors and outdoors as well as to negotiate most natural and architectural barriers.[87] Ability to functionally ambulate within a community implies that the person has endurance sufficient to the energy demands presented by their gait pattern and environment. *Household* ambulation describes the ability to walk with or without assistive devices and braces on level surfaces of varying textures as well as negotiate doorway and other minor architectural barriers found indoors.[87] While household ambulation imposes lower endurance demands than community ambulation, both require ability to transfer independently between sitting and standing positions. *Therapeutic* and exercise ambulation are terms used interchangeably with nonfunctional ambulation. While a therapeutic ambulator may be able to ambulate independently with braces and assistive devices, assistance is required to transfer between sitting and standing.[87] The energy demands of the gait pattern often limit the range of their ambulation to relatively short distances. *Wheelchair* mobility describes the ability to independently propel from one point to a destination. The label of functional wheelchair mobility implies the ability to transfer in and out of the chair and to negotiate doorways and other minor barriers.

These studies of mobility skill achievement consistently demonstrate an eventual transition from ambulation to wheelchair mobility among all but the population with L5 and S1 lesion levels.[85–87] Individuals with loss of function below the T2 through T12 level are able, as a general rule, to develop therapeutic ambulation skill in childhood. The majority of them, however, use a wheelchair as their primary means of mobility throughout childhood and adulthood. Children born with a loss of sensorimotor function below L1 and L2 generally develop therapeutic or household ambulation skills. Their primary means of mobility, however, remains the wheelchair throughout childhood and adulthood. Loss of sensorimotor function below L3 or L4 generally predicts the ability to develop household ambulation skills, if not communitywide skill, in childhood. During adolescence, these individuals generally convert to use of a wheelchair for community and household mobility. This is due, in part, to the energy demands of ambulation, which rise in proportion to increases in their height and weight. The majority of people with L5 and S1 levels of sensorimotor function develop community ambulation skill in childhood and maintain that ability throughout adulthood.

Horizontal mobility is normally achieved between 8 and 10 months of age by a child's development of the ability to crawl on the abdomen and creep on hands and knees.[70] With this horizontal mobility, the child explores the surrounding environment and begins to delight in a sense of emerging independence. This activity also provides opportunities for development of upper body strength, coordination, endurance, and equilibrium responses. Horizontal mobility must be facilitated among infants with myelodysplasia in order to provide similar experience in preparation for other mobility skills. Although many children with partially functioning lower extremities are able to learn adaptive creeping patterns (side-hitching and rabbit hopping), these patterns may reinforce imbalanced muscle control or joint deformities already present. Before facilitating the development of adaptive creeping skill, therapists and caregivers should determine the extent to which that skill will contribute to hip and knee flexion contractures, equinus foot deformities, scoliosis, and increased lumbar lordosis or kyphosis. If introduced before a child learns an adaptive creeping pattern, prone scooter boards and hand-propelled sitting carts (chariots) can provide less deforming alternatives.

Hand-propelled carts that support the child in a long sitting position are generally more popular with young children than prone scooters. Although they provide household mobility and are simple to operate, they have disadvantages which should be considered. The more complex upper extremity movement patterns required for ambulation and transfers are not well facilitated during use of these carts. Prolonged periods of hip flexion and ischial-sacral pressure occur as the child becomes adept with its use. While prone scooters have none of these disadvantages, the determined resistance of some myelodysplasia children to them is a commonly encountered problem. Whether this is due to lack of experience, to a feeling of helplessness in prone, or to some type of vestibular system dysfunction, the benefits of prone scooter mobility make consistent, patient teaching efforts worthwhile. The prone scooter should be introduced to a child when he or she has the ability to roll and pivot in prone lying as well as support weight and balance on one extended arm in prone while reaching with the other. In order to make initial encounters with the scooter positive, the child can be encouraged to play with it while not on it. The child can put toys on it and move the scooter about in order to feel its motion. Seeing other children scooting in prone on it is helpful. When the child is on the scooter, he or she can be reinforced for staying on it for periods of stationary prone play or for periods of back and forth rocking. Once the child enjoys this, slow rides on the scooter can be provided to familiarize the child with the motion.

As with ambulation, progression on smooth, polished surfaces should be achieved prior to textured surfaces. As in the normal prone progression sequence, backward movement on the scooter is more quickly learned than forward. As an initial step, the child on the scooter, supporting weight on extended arms, can be slowly rocked back and forth by another person. The child can be assisted in pushing backward in order to obtain a toy placed under the scooter. A play partner sitting in front of the child on the scooter can hold hands with that child and encourage pushing and pulling movements. With this activity, as well as backward, pivoting, and forward movement, the amount of assistance provided can be decreased as the child gains control.

Prone scooters are available through many medical equipment companies; however, parents and staff in institutions often choose to build their own. Detailed plans for a prone scooter suitable for use by any child with myelodysplasia, but designed for a 5-year-old child in a double spica cast, are presented in an article by Streissguth and Streissguth.[88]

The ability of most patients with myelodysplasia to achieve at least a therapeutic level of ambulation skill is supported by studies of relatively large populations; however, the value of this ability has been and continues to be questioned.[85–87] Hoffer and colleagues[87] reported that a child with an open myelomeningocele defect will achieve his or her maximal level of ambulation ability by the age of 9 years. Correspondingly, other authors report 10 to 13 years as the ages when children with lumbar level defects begin to discard crutches and braces for wheelchair mobility within their community if not their home.[74] These trends raise valid questions about the benefits realized in relationships to the time, effort, and expense required for these children with thoracic and lumbar lesions to ambulate for a relatively brief period. In response to this questioning, the following list of beneficial effects directly related to childhood ambulation and standing has been proposed in current literature:[3,63,74,88–90]

1. Improved bowel and bladder drainage
2. Prevention of osteoporosis and facilitation of osteoblastic activity
3. Improved cardiopulmonary endurance
4. Prevention of ischial-sacral pressure sores
5. Maintenance of hip and knee joint extension and ankle dorsiflexion
6. Improved interaction with the environment
7. Improved upper extremity strength, coordination, and endurance

Clinical studies supporting these proposed benefits are still lacking. If these effects do occur, they clearly facilitate the development of functional wheelchair skills as well as ambulatory capacity.

Although some people with low lumbar level lesions are able to ambulate without braces in adolescence and adulthood, bracing is required in at least the initial stages of gait training for the majority of children with myelodysplasia. Double upright, metal braces with hinged joints are still the most common type of orthosis used for individuals with myelodysplasia. The ankle joints of long and short leg orthoses should have their free motion limited to approximately 10 degrees.[62,89] Dorsiflexion or anterior ankle stops, in combination with rigid sole plates extending to the metatarsophalangeal joints, should counteract the knee flexion tendency imposed by lack of or weakened gastrocnemius-soleus function.[91,92] If functional dorsiflexion is not present, a posterior or plantar flexion stop should simulate toe pick-up and prevent a foot drop pattern from interfering with forward progression.[91] Posterior calf bands of short or long braces should be located as high on the calf as possible without interfering with knee movement or creating pressure on the neural or vascular structures.[93] High placement decreases the amount of pressure exerted on the calf by this band, as it helps control ankle plantar flexion during swing phase. This band should also prevent the lower leg and knee from moving posteriorly in the brace and should play a significant role in maintaining the brace aligned with the leg when a long leg brace is unlocked and flexed during sitting.[91] For long leg braces, the knee straightening force supplied by knee pads or straps should be applied as close to the knee as possible, with greater force applied below the knee than above. Ideally, the force should be carried by two straps applied over the suprapatellar and patellar tendon areas, rather than a single wide knee pad that allows focused pressure on the patella itself.[91] The posterior upper thigh band is appropriately located 1 to 1.5 inches from the ischium during standing and walking.

All orthotic joints should be matched with their anatomic or functional counterparts on the legs. Correct alignment of the orthotic knee and the functional knee joint axis of the person is important for prevention of pressure, friction, and shearing points during ambulation. As children grow and minor lengthening adjustments are made on their braces, the knee joint is easily displaced. Since the functional axis of the human knee changes during movement from full extension to full flexion, the functional axis of the knee in extension is usually the starting point for orthotic knee joint alignment. When the orthotic knee axis is posterior to or behind the human knee axis in extension, flexion of the knee will increase pressure from the posterior thigh and calf bands as well as shift the entire brace distally.[94] Each time the child sits down, the heels will tend to come out of the shoes and pressure will be increased over the dorsum of the foot. Location of the axis anterior to or in front of the extended knee's functional axis produces the opposite effect.[94] This problem can produce the groin pressure that occurs when some children sit from standing. Location of the axis distally or below the knee's functional joint in extension creates a similar shifting of the brace into the groin. The pressure of the calf band against the posterior lower leg is increased and a shearing force affecting the calf and heel areas can result. The opposite effect occurs when the orthotic knee axis is proximal to or above the extended knee axis in standing.[94] Orthotic uprights and knee joints may be deliberately aligned in lateral or medial rotation relative to the anatomic knee in order to counteract slight genu valgus or varus. If excessive rotation is present, however, pressure from the uprights against the thigh can occur in standing or sitting. These uprights not only create static pressure points but also rotational shearing forces. Consequently, this is not a situation that should be allowed to persist.

The use of pelvic bands and lockable orthotic hip joints with paraplegics is a subject of controversy. Electrogoniometric studies have shown that posterior pelvic tilt is not maintained and lumbar movement is actually increased in the presence of locked orthotic hips and a pelvic band.[89,91] Unless extension force is applied at the sternum by more elaborate thoracic bracing methods, hip flexion and lumbar lordosis will probably persist with orthotic hip joints locked. If present, however, a pelvic band with hip joint locks should significantly limit the amount of hip rotation or lateral movement that can occur. The additional bracing should also increase the child's sense of security and balance.

While these standard, double upright, metal braces are the most commonly used orthoses with the myelodysplasia population, numerous other types have been developed as a result of improvement efforts. The parapodium, introduced by Motlock, is one of the more frequently used orthoses developed for the specific problems associated with myelodysplasia.[63] This brace succeeds in providing such a stable base of support that children with thoracic and lumbar lesions can stand without assistive devices. Although not the ideal situation, the parapodium has been modified to accommodate joint contractures and deformities more safely than conventional long leg braces.

Taylor and Sand[95] report favorable gait training results using a modification of the parapodium called the Verlo brace or vertical loading orthosis. With this orthosis, the angle the base or standing plate makes with the uprights supporting the legs can be adjusted to vary the child's ankle position and projection of the center of gravity. With placement of the ankles in slight dorsiflexion with the center of gravity forward, locomotion is made less laborious than with a fixed baseplace that maintains neutral ankle position. These authors report that 16 patients from 3 to 10 years of age, with lesions from T8 to L3, were fitted with a Verlo brace.[95] Of those 16, only one 3-year-old child failed to learn either a pivot or swing-to gait pattern. Lack of gait training opportunities, illness, and central nervous system dysfunction accounted for the four children that were unable to progress from a pivot to a swing-to gait pattern.

Rose and associates[96] report favorable gait training results using a "hip guidance orthosis" with 27 myelodysplasia patients between the ages of 5 years 8 months and 15 years 7 months.[125] The rigid bilateral long leg braces are attached to an essentially rigid thoracic support with a specific type of orthotic hip joint which permits no more than 5° of adduction. As the child shifts weight off one lower extremity by a lateral movement, that free extremity moves forward under the influence of gravity. Of the 27 myelodysplasia patients fitted with this hip guidance orthosis, 13 improved from therapeutic to household, or household to community, ambulation status. In comparison with their previous bracing, the 27 subjects had a mean increase in ambulation speed of 87.3 percent.

The parapodium, Verlo, and hip guidance orthoses are primarily designed to assist patients with thoracic and high lumbar lesions. Methods of bracing reported by Lindseth and Glancy[97] and by Nuzzo[98] are of particular use among patients with L3 to L5 function. A polypropylene ankle-foot orthosis based upon the principles of the SACH foot prosthesis is described by Lindseth and Glancy.[97] Using the solid ankle of this molded orthosis to facilitate knee extension control, the authors report significantly improved gait quality for 43 of 74 subjects. Nuzzo[98] describes the use of ankle-foot orthoses connected to a pelvic belt by elastic strapping that is wrapped around the thigh in various helical patterns. By variation in the location of the strap's attachments and their circumferential wrapping patterns, hip extension, and abduction can be assisted in combination with knee flexion, knee extension, and hip medial or lateral rotation.

Regardless of the type of orthosis used, tolerance to wearing it for both non-weight-bearing and weight-bearing periods must be gradually developed. The need for families beginning brace-wearing programs to be taught a correct and safe method of putting them on and taking them off should be clear. Methods for safe use of standing tables or simply providing support in standing should also be carefully taught. The child's initial experiences wearing braces and standing should be well planned to emphasize their positive aspects. If the child has developed the ability to roll, sit and come to a sitting position, the accommodation of these skills to the weight of braces should be facilitated. Through play on the floor, the caregiver can assist and encourage these movements. By development of mobility in braces, the child not only improves upper body strength and control, but also decreases the helpless or trapped perception many of them experience. While standing in the braces, the child can be introduced to activities that necessitate standing. Playing in upper level drawers, looking out windows, and playing with water in a sink are examples of such activities.

In preparation for gait training or the learning of transfer techniques, children with myelodysplasia lesions need to develop trunk control and strength in their arms. Development of these general prerequisites clearly make the initial learning period less frustrating and more enjoyable for everyone involved. A child's directed reaching efforts can be used in play to challenge their postural adjustment abilities as the center of gravity is altered. These balance activities can be initiated when the child is in a stable sitting position using the surfaces of low tables or the floor for play. Once mastered in sitting, activities can be pursued on the surface of a standing table or at a table that is approximately at the child's waist level. Trunk equilibrium responses in sitting can be further challenged on tilting boards or large therapeutic balls. "Bucking broncho" rides while sitting on an adult's lap can provide a similar challenge to the child's postural control responses.

In order to have sufficient upper extremity strength and endurance for successful ambulation and transfers, development of the upper extremities must begin at a young age. Learning to maneuver a prone scooter or sitting cart as well as use an adaptive creeping pattern contributes to this developmental process. Pull-up and push-up arm activities can be incorporated into home routines in numerous ways to develop these movement patterns. Using the hands of an adult, a child can be encouraged to pull up from supine lying into sitting. From a sitting position, the child can lift the hips off the floor or bed in a similar manner. The difficulty of sitting pull-ups can be increased by replacing the adult's hands with a vertically held broom handle or knotted rope, encouraging use of one arm only, or by positioning the handle or rope off to one side. Children who are able to do sitting pull-ups usually enjoy swinging from that position while holding onto an adult's hands. The amount of swinging provided by the adult can be gradually decreased as the child learns to control it by upper body movements. Once mastered in a sitting position, these same pull-up and swinging patterns can be encouraged in standing during brace-wearing periods.

As is the case in the developmental sequence of physically normal children, push-up movement patterns in the upper extremities need to develop in prone lying before sitting. An adult can assist prone push-up patterns by supporting a child at the hips and lower trunk while reducing the amount of body weight the child supports with the arms. While the child pushes the body upward, trucks or balls can be rolled through the space under the elevated chest to add an element of play. From a prone position, wheelbarrow or hand walking can be facilitated by an adult supporting the lower extremities and, if necessary, the trunk. Forward, backward, and lateral hand walking can be encouraged, as well as "races" with playmates.

While a child is learning to do sitting push-ups, the body lifting component needs to be assisted. Once the child is able to control a degree of upward movement, the adult can help move the pelvis backward in order to produce a backward scooting movement pattern. This backward scooting movement is generally mastered by children with myelodysplasia before forward and lateral scooting. The learning of all these scooting patterns is facilitated in a bathtub or inflatable wading pool. The slick surface and buoyancy provided by waist-deep water can decrease the energy requirements and increase the element of play involved in developing these skills. Scooting on a smooth floor is more easily learned with braces off and clothing covering the legs. As soon as the movement pattern is learned, however, it should be practiced with braces on. While this requires more strength, and may initially shorten play periods in this position, braces protect the legs from abrasions and fracture-producing forces. The alignment maintained by braces can improve the efficiency of forward scooting once sufficient upper extremity strength is developed.

Concensus is lacking among physical therapists concerning an optimal sequence or protocol for gait training of patients with myelodysplasia. General agreement does seem to exist, however, on some main principles. First, gait training is ideally begun as soon as the child is maturationally ready in terms of prerequisite skills. Second, the sequence of gait training should represent a progressive increase in requisite energy expenditures, as well as in upper extremity and trunk coordination and equilibrium responses. And third, once a child becomes skilled at any method of ambulation, a preference for that method and resistance to other methods naturally develops.

Determining that a child is maturationally ready to begin gait training remains a fairly intuitive matter. Menelaus[63] recommends that a child's attempts to pull up into a standing position be used as a criterion for beginning a standing and gait training program. Others use the age of 1 year as a time to begin standing programs and 18 months for gait training.[74] Many therapists use the presence of head and trunk control while standing in braces, as well as protective equilibrium responses in sitting, as prerequisite skills or criteria for initiation of gait training. Very helpful information is provided by Taylor and

Sand's[99] study designed to determine the chronologic age at which normal children could learn to ambulate independently in a Verlo brace with a minimum number of training sessions. The authors found 24 months to be the age or developmental level at which independent ambulation with a "walkerette" could be achieved within a reasonable period of training. After 22 months, however, they found that more children were strongly resistant to putting on the brace. The youngest children, between 11 and 15 months, were the group that most readily accepted the brace's confinement. For these reasons, they recommend that braces be provided to children for standing purposes when they are 11 to 15 months old, or of that developmental equivalent, in order to avoid the risk of brace rejection.

In general, a progression of difficulty is reflected in the range of gait patterns which begins with a swivel movement and progresses to a four-point or swing-to pattern. The swing-to pattern is followed by the actual swing-through pattern. In the progression of difficulty, a four-point pattern with locked orthotic knees is followed by the unlocking of one side, then the unlocking of both. This ideally precedes the introduction of short leg braces unless full knee function is present. The swivel gait, used with parapodiums or hip-knee-ankle-foot orthoses, requires primarily weight shifting and trunk rotation ability when used with various assistive devices. While a four-point gait pattern requires that both hip joints move freely, a modified gait which requires only one unlocked hip can be taught as an intermediate step. The modified four-point pattern requires unilateral hip flexion with pelvic-hip stability assisted by the locked orthotic hip joint. Alternating hip flexion, with no anterior-posterior hip stability assistance provided by the braces, is required for the conventional four-point pattern. The swing-to pattern and, to a greater extent, the swing-through pattern, require strength in the upper extremities sufficient to support body plus brace weight, as well as equilibrium and coordination sufficient to produce a swinging movement. While the upper extremity demands of four-point patterns are less, the extent to which they perpetuate hip dislocation by strengthening the deforming hip flexors should be considered before these patterns are taught.

A progression of increasing difficulty, or decreasing support, is also reflected in the range of assistive devices used for gait training. The sequence begins with parallel bars, progresses to a walker with front wheels or other means of assisting forward progression, then to a standard walker, to "quad" canes and finally to forearm crutches.

Obviously, the gait patterns taught and the assistive devices used with myelodysplasia patients should be chosen and changed on the basis of the individual's current ability and projected level of achievement. The transition from one assistive device to a less supportive device should not be concurrent with a transition from one gait pattern to a more demanding one.

A significant determinant of gait training success appears to be the type of reinforcement received by a child for his or her efforts. Frequently, a logical explanation of treatment goals to a child is the initial method of persuasion used by therapists. Once resistance or actual negative behavior patterns develop in response to the prospect of practicing ambulation, these negative responses may become the focus of considerable reinforcing attention. Hester[100] has demonstrated with a profoundly retarded child, and Manella and Varni[101] with a myelodysplasic child, the benefits of the incorporation of behavior modification techniques into gait training. Within a period of 3 weeks, the transition from nonambulatory status and temper tantrums at the prospect of gait training, to independent assumption of standing and walking for 300 feet is reported by Manella and Varni.[101] Before "tantrum" patterns of behavior develop, it is obviously important to provide children with reinforcement that they comprehend as a reward rather than logical adult explanations. Once these disruptive patterns occur, however, behavior modification techniques appear to be a means of reversing them.

A variety of guidelines are used among physical therapists and orthopedists concerning the optimal time to provide a child with a wheelchair. Once a child masters the ability to propel a wheelchair, interest in gait training declines in direct proportion to the laboriousness of that child's ambulation. One guideline that can aid this decision-making process stems from the goal to facilitate as normal a sequence of development as possible. When a child's continued cognitive and psychosocial development is limited by that child's lack of efficient independent community mobility, the learning of functional wheelchair skills becomes more important than maintenance of marginally functional ambulation skills. In addition to providing a means of independent mobility, the advantages of wheelchair use are believed to be (1) provision of a less energy-consuming means of mobility than their ambulation pattern, (2) increased freedom for hand use, (3) ability to move at a speed more closely resembling that of ambulatory people, (4) increased ability to carry or transport objects, and (5) increased potential for recreational activities.[102] The disadvantages are (1) increased risk for development of ischial-sacral pressure sores, (2) increased risk for development of hip and knee flexion contractures, and (3) risk of spinal deformity deterioration.[102]

In order to accentuate the advantages and diminish the disadvantages of wheelchair use, several specific items should be considered when ordering a wheelchair. Appropriate dimensions of a wheelchair seat are crucial to decreasing the risk of pressure sores and spinal deformity deterioration. The height of the seat should be set in relation to the footrests in order to provide 80–90 degrees of flexion at the hips and knees.[103] If the footrests are low, the person tends to slide forward in the seat and create an ischial-sacral friction or shearing force. Increased pressure on the posterior thighs from the front edge of the seat can interfere with lower extremity circulation. If the footrests are high, increased weight is shifted onto the ischial-sacral area and a gravity-assisted abduction-lateral rotation posture of the hips is facilitated. A child who has developed therapeutic ambulation skill, but demonstrates little potential for household ambulation, should have a wheelchair seat essentially level in height with the beds and chairs to which he or she will learn to transfer. This may require placement of footrests fairly high off the floor to maintain their correct relationship with the seat. On the other hand, to maintain household ambulation ability, the seat of the wheelchair should be low enough to facilitate standing transfers. For this purpose, the foot-pedals should be no less than and as close to 2 inches off the floor while the correct relationship with seat height is maintained. The width of a wheelchair seat should allow only 1 to 2 inches between the person's lateral thighs and the edge of the seat.[103] Since long leg braces occupy considerable chair space, the seat width should be planned to accommodate them if warranted by sufficient wearing time. Both propulsion strength and endurance are compromised, as well as the work of wheelchair mobility increased, by an excessively wide seat. The depth of the wheelchair seat needs to be sufficient to prevent a gap forming at the back that traps sacral tissue causing friction and shearing forces. On the other hand, a seat which is too deep can create pressure in the popliteal area that compromises lower extremity circulation. In order to facilitate transfers in and out of the wheelchair, specific types of armrests and footrests, as well as variations in wheel diameter, can be provided.

Two aspects need consideration when determining the diameter of wheels for a chair. The smallest diameter wheel, 20 inches, does not rise above the chair seat and obstruct sitting transfers to the extent that larger wheels do. The smaller the wheel diameter, however, the more force the person has to generate to initiate and maintain forward movement.[103] The overall efficiency of propelling is greater with larger rimmed wheels.[103] For this reason larger wheels are usually thought of as helpful to people with short or weak arms. Handrims with a rubber or plastic coating to increase the ease of grasping and propelling the chair are helpful.

"Growing" chairs, which can increase in size as reupholstering is done, are generally considered cost effective for chronically involved children. These chairs generally expand from a size appropriate for an average 6- to 8-year-old to that of an average 12-year-old.[103] Consideration should be given during the ordering process to the level of maintenance required and use the wheelchair will receive. Without an ongoing maintenance program, this wheelchair is unlikely to survive the 4 to 6 years of active use that makes it seem a wise investment. The level of maintenance care any wheelchair receives is a primary factor determining its useful life-span and the extent to which appropriate fit can be retained.

Currently, insufficient information exists about the development of physically normal children, or those with myelodysplasia, to determine an age younger than which wheelchair mobility and transfer skill are unrealistic. The teaching of these skills, however, is frequently not initiated until the person with myelodysplasia becomes too heavy for their caregivers to lift. Clearly, there is a stage prior to this regretable situation when mobility and transfer training can and should be initiated. Once a child has developed the ability to assist with push-up and pull-up movement patterns, he or she should begin assisting with transfers on and off a prone scooter or sitting cart. Once wheelchair propulsion has been learned, the child's assistive role getting into and out of the chair needs to begin and the passive role needs to end.

Corresponding with the tendency to equate myelodysplasia with paraplegia, the shoulder depression, push-up transfers used by paraplegics are generally the focus of the myelodysplasia patient's transfer training; however, the normal proportional relationship between lower extremity and trunk length characteristic of paraplegics is often not the case with this group. The normal neurologic function and capacity for strength and endurance gains in the upper body of paraplegics may not be present in the child with myelodysplasia either. The possibility that a young child may not have the central nervous system maturation required to execute these transfers also needs to be considered. For these reasons, the pull-up transfers taught more frequently to quadriplegics, using overhead loops or a trapeze, can be a more realistic starting point for transfer training of children with myelodysplasia. The child can initially practice the necessary wheelchair and body movement patterns, as well as participate in transfers by using an adult's hands as a support from which to pull upward. Ideally, an overhead trapeze can be attached to the child's bed at home so that at least one transfer is fully independent at a young age.

Because of the shortness of children's legs, particularly those with myelodysplasia, front-approach transfers can be much safer than side approach. If knee flexion contractures are not a significant problem, the child can assume a long-sitting position while facing the side of the bed from the wheelchair with the lower portion of both legs on the bed. From this position, the child can use pull-up assistance to move the hips laterally onto the bed or other surface. This transfer pattern, as well as more complex methods used by quadriplegics but modifiable for myelodysplasia patients, are throughly described and illustrated in other texts.[104,105]

The endurance required for functional, communitywide wheelchair mobility is often given inadequate attention in treatment. While wheelchair mobility is less energy consuming than ambulation with assistive devices, Glaser and associates[106] have found that, in general, wheelchair locomotion requires a higher maintained heart rate than ambulation by a physically normal individual. Similar studies of the cardiovascular responses of children during wheelchair locomotion have not been published. Given the size and strength of a child's upper body relative to the size and weight of a wheelchair, it seems logical that a similar, if not greater, increase in heart rate occurs. Glaser and associates[106] have identified four primary factors that influence cardiovascular responses during wheelchair propulsion. The characteristics of the wheelchair itself and the velocity at which it is propelled are two of those factors. Stability of the wheels and axle mechanism, as well as the wheel diameter, are examples of characteristics that influence the speed and efficiency with which locomotion can occur. Architectural conditions are a third factor that can increase the resistance to rolling and thereby increase energy expenditure. Increased ventilatory requirements and heart rate responses are reported to occur with propulsion across even low pile carpet.[106] The fourth factor is the fitness level of the individual for upper extremity work. Hildebrandt and associates[107] have pointed out that average daily wheelchair use may not be of sufficient intensity or duration to have a training effect for the individual. Since average wheelchair use may not prepare a person for functional community mobility, the benefits of conditioning programs have been proposed and supported in work by Glaser and his associates.[108] Using apparatus that simulates wheelchair propulsion, they have demonstrated that a 5-week training program can improve cardiovascular responses of normal subject to a heavy work load.[108] The extent to which these results can be duplicated in groups of younger and/or physically disabled subjects remains to be determined.

Similar to the problems that children with myelodysplasia encounter in learning wheelchair locomotion and transfers, their delayed development of self-care skills can be due to several interrelated factors. Obviously, the extent of spinal cord and/or brain damage is a primary factor limiting the rate of, if not overall capacity for, skill development. Parental attitudes are another major factor. Acceptance of their child's physical limitations as permanent is prerequisite to parental readiness for learning and reinforcing any of the self-care techniques. The child's attitude toward independence in dressing, bathing, and toileting is another major factor. The prospect of independence in an activity must provide more prospective if not immediate rewards than continued dependence.

Successful development of ability to maneuver clothing or braces on and off the body requires certain characteristics of the braces, as well as of the person's motor skills. The lightness in weight and freedom of orthotic joint movement that facilitate ambulation and standing transfers also make the taking off and putting on of braces easier. The fewer straps and less bracing the child has to deal with, the easier the application process is. The motor skills required for development of dressing skills are ability to position legs, roll from side to side, sit up from a lying position, sit stably with at least one arm free, and shift weight using push-up or pull-up maneuvers.

In preparation for dressing practice, several play activities can be used to facilitate the learning process. The child can be encouraged to place rings made of various articles on the arms and legs. These rings can be made from buckled belts, knotted scarves, or colorful embroidery hoops. The more rigid the loops are, the more easily they can be maneuvered on and off an extremity. The more lax they are, however, the more closely the loops resemble clothing. Large loops of stretchable material can be manipulated from overhead to off the feet or the reverse. Initial dressing practice can be done with large stretchable garments that require the same motor patterns without the constraint of appropriately fitting clothes. This can be turned into a creative game of "dress-ups" in mother's or father's clothes. Although the ages at which physically normal children accomplish independent dressing skills cannot serve as guidelines for the myelodysplasia population, the general trends of this normal sequence can. Positioning the body in order to help with dressing or undressing is the first independent step that occurs. After that, the ability to take off articles of clothing precedes the ability to put on the same article. Ability to open or release fasteners generally precedes the ability to secure or close them.[109]

Development of independent bathing and toileting skills are closely related to transfer skill development. Transfers between a wheelchair and bathtub or toilet represent two of the more challenging transfer situations which a child with myelodysplasia has to manage. The relatively short arms of a child, in relationship to the width of a standard bathtub, are a factor that complicates tub transfers. For this reason, as well as others previously stated, both the methods and the apparatus used by quadriplegics for tub transfers can be utilized by children with myelodysplasia. Bath transfers are made safer and more easily negotiated if a secure stool is placed at the back of the tub. This stool should be essentially level with the tub edge so that the individual can transfer onto it, then lower themselves down into the tub. A second step, providing an intermediate level, can be especially helpful in the process of getting out of the tub. Prerequisite to learning bathtub transfers, the child should be able to move up and down steps from a sitting position. Depending upon the ability of the child, this up and down movement can be initially facilitated by assisting the child's push-up or pull-up efforts. For practice of a less demanding level of this skill, scooting up and down an incline can be incorporated into play.

Transfers on and off of a toilet do not require a specific technique of movement that is difficult to master. These transfers, however, do require apparatus that alters the level of the toilet seat, reduces the size of the toilet opening and provides places from which the child can securely control body movement. With some exceptions, the apparatus used for these purposes is essentially the same as that used by adult spinal cord injured patients. If a child is doing a standing transfer to a toilet, an elevated platform may be required to reduce the proportionate height of the toilet. For wheelchair transfers, the seat has to be elevated to the level of the wheelchair. While some commercially available seat attachments can be adjusted to the height of a child's wheelchair many are too high. The small size of a child, plus the lack of posterior hip and thigh sensation, dictates the need for a smaller seat opening than is present in many of these seat attachments. Since the wall or back of a toilet is generally too far behind a child to provide sitting support, additional back support may be needed. Because of these specific needs, several designs for "homemade" adaptations have been published.[104]

Successful development of independence in bowel and bladder management is probably more dependent upon parental acceptance levels than are the development of dressing and bathing skills. By providing a well planned teaching program and consistent supportive guidance to parents, Hannigan[34] has demonstrated that clean intermittent catheterization can be taught to young children. Using practice dolls and magnifying mirrors, four children with myelodysplasia and mental ages of 5 years were able to achieve independence or to require minimal assistance with clean intermittent catheterization in the home as well as the school setting. Although this is a very small group of children, the results are encouraging. No studies are available which help to determine the mental age at which a child could be expected to assist with or accept full responsibility for skin inspection, a bowel evacuation program, or care of various urine collection devices. With the continued efforts of pediatric nurses to provide well-planned, consistent teaching programs, it seems reaonable to anticipate that most children with myelodysplasia can achieve independence with these toileting skills also.

Deficient Development of Fine Motor and Perceptual Motor Skills

Current research documents the presence of delayed or deficient development of fine and perceptual motor skills among children with myelodysplasia and hydrocephalus.[42,46] The extent to which these delays or deficiences can be attributed to brain damage as opposed to lack of experience remains to be determined. Although the child's need for assistance from others in gaining fine and perceptual motor experiences at a relatively normal age seems apparent, the actual benefits of the intervention have not been proven. Prevention of or compensation for delays in development of these skills seem logical to expect, but the short- and long-term results of intervention programs for children with myelodysplasia and hydrocephalus are not known.

Early intervention programs for children with myelodysplasia are directed toward facilitation of fine and perceptual motor skills with as normal a rate and sequence as possible. They are also directed toward compensation for the lack of early sitting and mobility skills. While most of the goal-directed, early intervention programs which have been published can be modified for use by children with myelodysplasia, some have been designed specifically for them. Rosenbaum and coauthors[69] have outlined a progression of play activities designed to facilitate visually directed hand function during the first year of development. Though less specific, Anderson and Spain[66] have described a progression of play which spans the preschool period. In addition to activities for facilitation of visually directed hand function, they provide play suggestions that facilitate body and tactile awareness, form and space perception, manual dexterity, number concepts, and attending or concentration ability. Nakos and Taylor[110] describe the rationale and protocol for an 8-week myelodysplasia infant treatment group. While including activities that teach parents about the facilitation of sensorimotor development, they have developed a program which also facilitates supportive interaction among the parents.

Numerous devices have been developed to assist young children to maintain a sitting position or attain mobility. Bean bag chairs can be used to support small infants in upright or to provide a sense of security to children learning to sit alone. When a child reaches the age of 6 to 8 months without the ability to maintain a sitting posture with their hands free, Menelaus[63] recommends the use of a sitting orthosis. By molding polypropylene to fit the trunk and buttocks area, a means of support is provided that frees the hands for play and can be used on the floor, in a high chair, or any place the child desires to be. The use of prone scooters and long sitting push carts to facilitate early mobility have already been described. Regardless of the type of apparatus used to aid sitting or mobility, the child has to gradually accept it and feel securely supported by it. If this is not the case, the child will not engage in the developmental play that the equipment was originally designed to facilitate.

Based on a review of the results reported from preschool programs available for children with myelodysplasia in Great Britain, Anderson and Spain[66] summarized the advantages and disadvantages of these programs. They concluded that social and emotional development was improved in terms of interaction skills and desire for independence. Motor skills improved, at least in terms of increased motivation to engage with other children in play activities requiring mobility. These factors enabled the children attending preschool programs to make a smoother transition into school settings. The authors also concluded that these programs gave the children's mothers a source of support, as well as relief from responsibility for predictable time periods. The mothers also gained a more realistic perception and acceptance of their child's strengths and weaknesses. The disadvantages that Anderson and Spain found were the cost and difficulty of transporting the child to and from the program site. The handling of feeding and clothing articles, as well as braces or other equipment, in addition to the child, was a problem particularly for the mothers of 4- and 5-year-olds.

Although the perceptual motor problems of children with myelodysplasia and hydrocephalus have been documented by numerous studies, little information has been published about treatment and remediation methods, or their results, with this group. Gluckman and Barling[111] have reported results from use of the Frostig Program for the Development of Visual Perception during a 6-week period for 12 children with hydrocephalus and myelodysplasia. Using the Frostig Developmental Test of Visual Perception as a pre- and posttest they found that the treatment group made gains in contrast to 12 children in an attention placebo group and 12 in a control group; however, the authors report insufficient data for the reader to determine the significance of the nine point average increase in scores among the treatment group. The treatment program used in this study, as well as other less formally evaluated programs demonstrates a problem that is yet to be resolved. The test items used to measure perceptual motor skills are very similar to the treatment or remediation activities used in many programs. When this is the case, there is considerable risk of teaching the child how to take the test more adeptly, rather than developing new skills that are transferable to functional skills such as reading and writing.

Several authors[45,46,52] have used portions of Ayres' Southern California Sensory Integration Test to measure perceptual motor problems among children with hydrocephalus and myelodysplasia. Minimal information, however, has been published regarding the results or methods of implementing the techniques specific to Ayres' approach to sensory integrative treatment with these children. The role that vestibular stimulation techniques might play in the treatment of hydrocephalic children with either a low tolerance for movement in space or a low threshold to the stimulus of that movement is unknown.

TREATMENT WITHIN THE PUBLIC SCHOOL SYSTEM

Because of the complexity of the problems associated with myelodysplasia and hydrocephalus, numerous specific needs should be considered when planning for school placement. This group has a broad range of educational needs

While most benefit from the stimulation of being with cognitively normal children, some of the children with myelodysplasia clearly require the services of specialists in learning disorders to acquire basic academic skills. The expertise of both special educators and occupational therapists is frequently needed in order to provide a program sufficient to facilitate academic as well as specific fine motor and perceptual motor development. Although a less prevalent problem, delayed development of communication skills may require the services of a speech pathologist. Because of pressure sores, urinary tract infections, fractures, and other assorted medical complications, the school absentee rate of children with myelodysplasia is high. In order to prevent significant disruption of the child's learning program, homebound or hospitalbound teachers need to be available within the school system.

In order to prevent additional absenteeism, appropriate transportation to and from school needs to be arranged. Vehicles designed to accommodate wheelchairs, as well as the limitations of people ambulating with assistive devices, are needed. Whether the child uses a wheelchair or assistive devices for mobility, architectural barriers should not hinder their movement in and out of the school, between classrooms and in and out of a bathroom. Children with myelodysplasia require bathrooms with sufficient space in which to maneuver a wheelchair, as well as stable support bars to assist with transfers. They need to have a consistently present, knowledgeable person to assist, as needed, with bowel and bladder management. In addition to assistance, they need privacy and sufficient time to attend to these self-care needs.

The extent to which a therapist can provide specific treatment for individual children varies in accordance with each school system's perception of the role of physical therapy in education. The ease with which many children fit into the school setting can be increased by individualized physical therapy directed toward increasing their transfer or locomotion skills. Improving the speed or dexterity with which toilet transfers are accomplished can simplify the child's assistive needs. The speed or quality of toileting, dressing and self-feeding skills can be increased by individualized occupational therapy. Teaching children and their teachers how to perform transfers on and off the floor can increase a young child's ability to participate in some classroom activities. Increasing the endurance of a child in ambulation or wheelchair locomotion can alter the ability to participate in activities with physically normal children. Whether working with individual children or supervising groups of them, prevention of the side effects of prolonged wheelchair sitting can be a major concern for physical therapists to address. Pressure sores and flexion contractures need not be the price that has to be paid for mainstream educational opportunities. If daily activity periods could be planned when these children would study or play in prone lying or standing positions, many of these secondary problems could be prevented.

School placement decisions for children with myelodysplasia are usually a compromise between efforts to normalize their environments and efforts to provide special services. Ideally, these special services would be available to each child regardless of the location of their school. In reality, the funding available for the services of special education teachers, hygiene assistants, transportation assistants, physical and occupational therapists, and other related personnel has been limited. It seems apparent that the child whose self-care and mobility skills most closely approximate those of physically normal children has the greatest opportunity for educational placement based on cognitive ability and school proximity. As long as this is the case, the focus of habilitation is shifted to the preschool period and the scope of that habilitation is widened from therapeutic ambulation to a broader perspective of functional goals.

REFERENCES

1. Freeman JM (ed): Practical Management of Meningomyelocele. University Park Press, Baltimore, 1974.
2. Sharrard WJW: Congenital and developmental abnormalities of the neuraxis. In Sharrard WJW (ed): Paediatric Orthopaedics and Fractures. Vol 2. 2nd Ed. Blackwell Scientific, Oxford, 1979.
3. Brocklehurst G (ed): Spina Bifida for the Clinician. Clinics in Developmental Medicine, No. 57. Lippincott, Philadelphia, 1976.
4. Stark GD, Baker GCW: The neurological involvement of the lower limbs in myelomeningocele. Dev Med Child Neurol 9:732, 1967.
5. Stark GD: Spina Bifida: Problems and Management. Blackwell, London, 1977.
6. Laws ER: Neurosurgical management of meningomyelocele. In Freeman JM (ed): Practical Management of Meningomyelocele. University Park Press, Baltimore, 1974.
7. Stein SC, Schut L: Hydrocephalus in myelomeningocele. Child Brain 5:413, 1979.
8. Gardner WJ: Etiology and pathogenesis of the development of myelomeningocele. In McLaurin RL (ed): Myelomeningocele. Grune and Stratton, New York, 1977.
9. Padget DH: Neuroschisis and human embryonic maldevelopment: New evidence on anencephaly, spina bifida and diverse mammalian defects. J Neuropathol Exp Neurol 29:192, 1970.
10. Williams B: Further thoughts on the valvular action of the Arnold-Chiari malformation. Dev Med Child Neurol suppl 25:105, 1971.
11. Gardner WJ: Hydrodynamic mechanisms of syringomyelia: Its relationship to myelocele. J Neurol Neurosurg Psychiatry 28:247, 1965.
12. Carter CO, Evans K: Spina bifida and anencephalus in greater London. J Med Genet 10:209, 1973.
13. Renwick JH: Hypothesis: Anencephaly and spina bifida are usually preventable by avoidance of specific but unidentified substance present in certain potato tubers. Br J Prev Soc Med 26:67, 1972.
14. Knox EG: Anencephalus and dietary intakes. Br J Prev Soc Med 26:219, 1972.
15. Fedrick J: Anencephalus and tea drinking. Proc R Soc Med 67:356, 1974.
16. Carter CO, David PA, Laurence KM: A family study of major central nervous system malformations in South Wales. J Med Genet 5:81, 1968.
17. Naggan L: Anencephaly and spina bifida in Israel. Pediatrics 47:577, 1971.
18. Naggan L, McMahon B: Ethnic differences in the prevalence of anencephaly and spina bifida in Boston, Mass. N Engl J Med 277:1119, 1967.
19. Alter M: Anencephalus, hydrocephalus and spina bifida. Epidemiology, with special reference to a survey in Charleston, SC. Arch Neurol 7:411, 1962.

20. Smithells RW, D'Arcy EE, McAllister EF: The outcome of pregnancies before and after the birth of infants with nervous system malformations. Dev Med Child Neurol suppl 15:6, 1968.

21. Laurence KM: The recurrence risk in spina bifida cystica and anencephaly. Dev Med Child Neurol suppl 20:23, 1969.

22. Congenital Malformation Surveillance Report, January–December, 1979. Center for Disease Control, Atlanta, GA, 1980.

23. Windham GC, Edmonds LD: Current trends in the incidence of neural tube defects. Pediatrics 70:333, 1982.

24. Brock DJH, Sutcliffe RG: Alpha-fetoprotein in the antenatal diagnosis of anencephaly and spina bifida. Lancet 2:197, 1972.

25. Brock DJH, Bolton AE, Monaghan JM: Prenatal diagnosis of anencephaly through maternal serum alpha-fetoprotein measurements. Lancet 2:923, 1973.

26. Bennett MJ, Blau K, Johnson RD, et al: Some problems of alpha-fetoprotein screening. Lancet 2:1296, 1978.

27. Marci JN, Haddow JE, Weiss RR: Screening for neural tube defects in the United States. Am J Obstet Gynecol 133:119, 1979.

28. Haddow JE, Marci JN: Prenatal screening for neural tube defects. JAMA 242 (6):515, 1979.

29. McLone DG: Technique for closure of myelomeningocele. Child Brain 6:65, 1980.

30. Hall P, Lindseth R, Campbell R, et al: Scoliosis and hydrocephalus in myelocele patients. J Neurosurg 50:174, 1979.

31. Bergman EW, Freeman JM, Epstein MH: Treatment of infantile hydrocephalus with acetazolamide and furosemide: three to four years follow-up. Ann Neurol 8:227, 1980.

32. Smith HP, Russell JM, Boyce WH, et al: Results of urinary diversion in patients with myelomeningocele. J Neurosurg 50:773, 1979.

33. Enrile BG, Crooks KK: Clean intermittent catheterization for home management in children with myelomeningocele. Clin Pediatr 19:743, 1980.

34. Hannigan KF: Teaching intermittent self-catheterization to young children with myelodysplasis. Dev Med Child Neurol 21:365, 1979.

35. Action Committee on Myelodysplasia, Section on Urology: Current approaches to evaluation and management of children with myelomeningocele. Pediatrics 63:663, 1979.

36. Drummond DS, Moreau M, Cruess RL: The results and complications of surgery for the paralytic hip and spine in myelomeningocele. J Bone Jt Surg 62B:49, 1980.

37. Feiwell E: Surgery of the hip in myelomeningocele as related to adult goals. Clin Orthop 148:87, 1980.

38. Menelaus MB: Progress in the management of the paralytic hip in myelomeningocele. Orthop Clin North Am 11:17, 1980.

39. Allen BL, Ferguson RL: The operative treatment of myelomeningocele spinal deformity—1979. Orthop Clin North Am 10:845, 1979.

40. Hall JE: Dwyer Instrumentation in anterior fusion of the spine. J Bone Jt Surg 63A:1188, 1981.

41. Allen BL: Anterior-posterior plating for congenital myelomeningocele kyphosis. Orthop Trans 2:68, 1978.

42. Wallace SJ: The effect of upper-limb function on mobility of children with myelomeningocele. Dev Med Child Neurol, suppl 15 29:84, 1973.

43. Anderson EM, Plewis I: Impairment of a motor skill in children with spina bifida cystica and hydrocephalus. Br J Psychol 68:61, 1977.

44. Sand PL, Taylor N, Hill M, et al: Hand function in children with myelomeningocele. Am J Occup Ther 28:87, 1974.
45. Grimm RA: Hand function and tactile perception in a sample of children with myelomeningocele. Am J Occup Ther 30:234, 1976.
46. Brunt D: Characteristics of upper limb movements in a sample of meningomyelocele children. Percept Mot Skills 51:431, 1980.
47. Emery JL, Lendon RG: Clinical implications of cord lesions in neurospinal dysraphism. Dev Med Child Neurol, suppl 14 27:45, 1972.
48. Variend S, Emery JL: The pathology of the central lobes of the cerebellum in children with myelomeningocele. Dev Med Child Neurol, suppl 32:99, 1974.
49. Badell-Ribera A, Shulman K, Paddock N: The relationship of non-progressive hydrocephalus to intellectual functioning in children with spina bifida Cystica. Pediatrics 37:787, 1966.
50. Tew B, Laurence KM: The effects of hydrocephalus on intelligence, visual perception and school attainment. Dev Med Child Neurol, suppl 17 35:129, 1975.
51. Miller E, Sethi L: The effect of hydrocephalus on perception. Dev Med Child Neurol, suppl 13 25:77, 1971.
52. Gressang JD: Perceptual processes of children with myelomeningocele and hydrocephalus. Am J Occup Ther 28:266, 1974.
53. Tew B: The 'Cocktail Party Syndrome' in children with hydrocephalus and spina bifida. Br J Disord Commun 14:89, 1979.
54. Tew B, Laurence KM: The ability and attainments of spina bifida patients born in South Wales between 1956 and 1962. Dev Med Child Neurol, suppl 14 27:124, 1972.
55. Spain B: Verbal and performance ability in pre-school children with spina bifida. Dev Med Child Neurol 16:773, 1974.
56. Quinton D, Rutter M: Early hospital admissions and later disturbances of behavior. Dev Med Child Neurol 18:447, 1976.
57. Douglas J: Early hospital admissions and later disturbances of behavior and learning. Dev Med Child Neurol 17:426, 1975.
58. Hayden PW, Davenport SLH, Campbell MM: Adolescents with myelodysplasia Impact of physical disability on emotional maturation. Pediatrics 64:53, 1979.
59. Sousa JC, Gordon LH, Shurtleff DB: Assessing the development of daily living skills in patients with spina bifida. Dev Med Child Neurol, suppl 18 37:134, 1976.
60. Tzimas NA: Myelodysplasia: Combined orthopedic and physiatric management part II. In American Academy for Cerebral Palsy, 28th annual meeting: Syllabus of Instructional Courses. 1974.
61. Lusskin R: The influence of errors in bracing upon deformity of the lower extremity. Arch Phys Med Rehabil 47:520, 1966.
62. Dias LS: Ankle valgus in children with myelomeningocele. Dev Med Child Neuro 20:627, 1978.
63. Menelaus MB: The Orthopaedic Management of Spina Bifida Cystica. 2nd Ed Churchill Livingstone, Edinburgh, 1980.
64. Frankenburg WK, Dobbs JB, Fandal A: The Revised Denver Developmental Screening Test Manual. University of Colorado Press, Denver, 1970.
65. Touwen BCL: Examination of the Child with Minor Neurological dysfunction 2nd edition. Clinics in Developmental Medicine, No 71. Lippincott, Philadelphia 1979.
66. Anderson EM, Spain B: The child with spina bifida. Methuen, London, 1977.
67. Cornish SV: Development of a test of motor-planning ability. Phys Ther 60:1129 1980.

68. Kendrick KA, Hanten WP: Differentiation of learning disabled children from normal children using four coordination tasks. Phys Ther 60:784, 1980.
69. Rosenbaum P, Barnitt R, Brand L: A developmental intervention programme designed to overcome the effects of impaired movement in spina bifida infants. In Holt K (ed): Movement and Child Development. Clinics in Developmental Medicine, No 55. Lippincott, Philadelphia, 1975.
70. Bayley N: Manual for the Bayley Scales of Infant Development. The Psychological Corporation, New York, 1969.
71. Stillman RD: The Callier-Azusa Scale. Dallas, Regional Center for Services to Deaf-Blind Children, 1973.
72. Bruininks RH: Examiners Manual for Bruininks-Oseretsky Test of Motor Proficiency. American Guidance Service, Circle Pines, MN, 1978.
73. Vlach V: Some exteroceptive skin reflexes in the limbs and trunk in newborns. In MacKeith R, Bax M (eds): Studies in Infancy. Clinics in Developmental Medicine, No 27. Spastics International Medical Publications, Lavenham, England, 1966.
74. Kopits SE: Orthopedic Aspects of Meningomyeloceles. In Freeman JM (ed): Practical Management of Meningomyelocele. University Park Press, Baltimore, 1974.
75. Townsend PF, Cowell HR, Steg NL: Lower extremity fractures simulating infection in myelomeningocele. Clin Orthop 144:255, 1979.
76. Hensinger RN: Orthopedic problems of the shoulder and neck. Ped Clin North Am 24:889, 1977.
77. Drennan JC: Orthotic management of the myelomeningocele spine. Dev Med Child Neurol, suppl 18 37:97, 1976.
78. McKibbon B: The use of splintage in the management of paralytic dislocation of the hip in spina bifida cystica. J Bone Jt Surg 55B:163, 1973.
79. Jaeger DL: Splint for infant with myelomeningocele. Phys Ther 61:913, 1981.
80. Redford JB: Principles of orthotic devices. In Redford JB (ed): Orthotics Etcetera. 2nd Ed. Williams and Wilkins, Baltimore, 1980.
81. Fischer BH: Topical hyperbaric oxygen treatment of pressure sores and skin ulcers. Lancet 2:405, 1969.
82. McFadyen GM, Stoner DL: Polyurethane foam wheelchair cushions: Retention of supportive properties. Arch Phys Med Rehabil 61:234, 1970.
83. Stewart SFC, Eng M, Palmieri V, et al: Wheelchair cushion effect on skin temperature, heat flux and relative humidity. Arch Phys Med Rehabil 61:229, 1980.
84. Carpendale MFT, Redford JB: Beds for patients. In Redford JB (ed): Orthotics Etcetera. 2nd Ed. Williams and Wilkins, Baltimore, 1980.
85. De Souza LJ, Carroll N: Ambulation of the braced myelomeningocele patient. J Bone Jt Surg 58A:1112, 1976.
86. Oppenheimer S: Comparative statistics—Treatment vs non-treatment. In McLaurin RL (ed): Myelomeningocele. Grune and Stratton, New York, 1977.
87. Hoffer MM, Feiwell E, Perry R, et al: Functional ambulation in patients with myelomeningocele. J Bone Jt Surg 55A:137, 1973.
88. Streissguth AP, Streissguth DM: Planning for the psychological needs of a young child in a double spica cast. Clin Pediatr 17:277, 1978.
89. Molnar G: Orthotic management of children. In Redford JB (ed): Orthotics Etcetera. 2nd Ed. Williams and Wilkins, Baltimore, 1980.
90. Main BJ: Effects of immobilization on the skeleton. In Owen R, Goodfellow J, Bullough P (eds): Scientific Foundations of Orthopaedics and Traumatology. Saunders, Philadelphia, 1980.

91. Lehmann JF: Lower limb orthotics. In Redford JB (ed): Orthotics Etcetera. 2nd Ed. Williams and Wilkins, Baltimore, 1980.
92. Fulford GE, Cairns TP: The problems associated with flail feet in children and their treatment with orthoses. J Bone Jt Surg 60B:93, 1978.
93. Rose GK: Principles of splints and orthotics. In Owen R, Goodfellow J, Bullough P (eds): Scientific Foundations of Orthopaedics and Traumatology. Saunders, Philadelphia, 1980.
94. Smith EM, Juvinall RC: Mechanics of orthotics. In Redford JB (ed): Orthotics Etcetera. 2nd Ed. Williams and Wilkins, Baltimore, 1980.
95. Taylor N, Sand P: Verlo brace use in children with myelomeningocele and spinal cord injury. Arch Phys Med Rehabil 55:231, 1974.
96. Rose GK, Stallard J, Sankarankutty M: Clinical evaluation of spina bifida patients using hip guidance orthosis. Dev Med Child Neurol 23:30, 1981.
97. Lindseth RE, Glancy J: Polypropylene lower-extremity braces for paraplegia due to myelomeningocele. J Bone Jt Surg 56A:556, 1974.
98. Nuzzo RM: Dynamic bracing: Elastics for patients with cerebral palsy, muscular dystrophy and myelodysplasia. Clin Orthop 148:263, 1980.
99. Taylor N, Sand PL: Verlo orthosis: Experience with different developmental levels in normal children. Arch Phys Med Rehabil 56:120, 1975.
100. Hester SB: Effects of behavioral modification on the standing and walking deficiencies of a profoundly retarded child: A case report. Phys Ther 61:907, 1981.
101. Manella KJ, Varni JW: Behavior therapy in a gait-training program for a child with myelomeningocele. Phys Ther 61:1284, 1981.
102. Kamenetz HL: Wheelchairs and other indoor vehicles for the disabled. In Redford JB (ed): Orthotics Etcetera. 2nd Ed. Williams and Wilkins, Baltimore, 1980.
103. Spiegler JH, Goldberg MJ: The wheelchair as a permanent mode of mobility: a detailed guide to prescription. Am J Phys Med 47:315, 1968.
104. Ford JR, Duckworth B: Physical Management for the Quadriplegic Patient. Davis, Philadelphia, 1974.
105. Palmer ML, Toms JE: Manual for Functional Training. Davis, Philadelphia, 1980.
106. Glaser RM, Sawka MN, Wilde SW, et al: Energy cost and cardiopulmonary responses for wheelchair locomotion and walking on tile and on carpet. Paraplegia 19:220, 1981.
107. Hildebrandt G, Voigt ED, Bahn D, et al: Energy costs of propelling wheelchair at various speeds: Cardiac response and effect on steering accuracy. Arch Phys Med Rehabil 51:131, 1970.
108. Glaser RM, Sawka MN, Durbin RJ, et al: Exercise program for wheelchair activity. Am J Phys Med 60:67, 1981.
109. Cohen MA, Gross PJ: The development of self-help skills. In Cohen MA, Gross PJ (eds): The Developmental Resource. Vol 1. Grune and Stratton, New York, 1979.
110. Nakos E, Taylor S: Myelomeningocele infant mat program. In McLaurin RL (ed): Myelomeningocele. Grune and Stratton, New York, 1977.
111. Gluckman S, Barling J: Effects of a remedial program on visual-motor perception in spina bifida children. J Genet Psychol 136:195, 1980.

8 | Head Trauma

Jocelyn Blaskey

Of the five million children who suffer a head trauma each year,[1,2] Raphaely and coworkers[1] estimate that 200,000 require hospitalization. Statistics describing mortality from severe head injury vary from 6 to 45 percent.[3-6] The cause of death is seldom the primary brain damage but rather intracranial or extracranial secondary complications of the brain damage or concomitant injuries.[3,7-9]

The majority (70 to 98 percent) of severe head injuries result from motor vehicle accidents.[3-7,9] These types of accidents, more prevalent in older children, often result in severe cranial injuries with focal deficits and long-lasting neurologic problems.[4,10] Blunt trauma due to falls from trees, swings, or jungle gyms to grass or concrete, typical of midchildhood, often result in skull fractures and more generalized cerebral injury.[2,4,10-13] Falls or battering resulting in fractures along the cranial sutures are most frequent in children less than 1 year of age.[4,12]

PATHOLOGY

Trauma resulting from head injuries includes scalp and cranium injuries, contusions, concussions, extraparenchymal or intracranial hematomas, cranial nerve injuries, and herniations caused by edema.[14-21] Head injuries can be classified according to how they are inflicted, including acceleration/deceleration injuries, crush injuries, and penetration injuries. Acceleration/deceleration injuries, the most common head injuries, result when the head hits an immobile object or a mobile object hits an immobile head. The cerebral injury is dependent on the acceleration/deceleration forces on the cranium and brain, the force, direction, and point of impact on the head, as well as the motion of the head preceding the impact.[14] Hardman,[11] Morley,[14] and Ommaya[15] discuss the forces involved and their effect on the cerebral tissue.

The cerebral damage resulting from these forces does not account for the loss of consciousness typically seen in traumatic head injuries. Loss of consciousness and death can be explained by a series of secondary complications resulting from traumatic damage to the cerebral tissues. Cerebral edema occurs as a normal reaction to trauma, but is restricted by the amount of room available in the cranium. The intracranial pressure increases as the cerebral tissues swell, eventually resulting in diffuse compression and ischemia of brain tissue. As the intracranial pressure rises, the hippocampus herniates through the foramen magnum, compressing the brainstem and causing unconsciousness when the reticular system is affected. Rapid increases in intracranial pressure and hippocampal herniation may result in hemorrhages in the midbrain and pons leading to death.[11,14]

In children and adolescents, cerebral edema may evolve after a trivial head injury and is not associated with a hematoma, hemorrhage, or contusions as is commonly seen in adults. Cerebral blood flow studies and computed tomogram densities suggest that the brain contains more blood than normally.[11,20] Further discussion of mechanisms responsible for loss of consciousness are offered by Lewin[16] and Shetter and Demakas.[17]

MEDICAL MANAGEMENT

Acute medical management primarily prevents and treats the secondary complications of head injury in order to provide optimal conditions for neurologic recovery. Current medical research is evaluating diagnostic tests used to predict and define changes in the patient's neurologic status. Improved diagnostic testing may increase the accuracy of outcome prediction and permit closer evaluation of present medical regimens. Orthopedic intervention includes acute fracture stabilization and management of spasticity through the rehabilitation process, reserving surgical intervention to improve function for 18 months after injury.

Neurologic Evaluation

The neurologic evaluation assesses the disruption and evolution of consciousness after trauma in order to diagnose and thereafter manage primary and secondary traumatic brain lesions. Raphaely[1] and Greenberg and colleagues[22] discuss the significance of neurologic findings.

Documentation of level of consciousness permits ongoing assessment of progressive changes in consciousness. The Glasgow Coma Scale, devised by Jennett and Teasdale,[23] has been used internationally as an assessment of the depth and duration of impaired consciousness and coma during the acute stage. The Glasgow Coma Scale was conceived as a graded measurement of three aspects of behavior: motor responsiveness, verbal performance, and eye opening. The best response for each behavior is recorded. The sum of the grades for each response is an indication of the depth of coma ranging from 3 to 15.[23]

Brink and associates[2,13] and Cartlidge and Shaw[4] adapted Ommaya's original classifications of five levels of consciousness[15] to evaluate depth and duration of coma and return to consciousness.

At Level V, no response to stimuli can be elicited. A generalized response to sensory stimuli indicates Level IV. At Level III a consistent localized response to a stimulus is evident. By Level II, the child has become responsive to the environment. Level I is attained when the child is oriented to time and place, and is recording ongoing events. Brink[2,13] designed three tables to further define behaviors appropriate to each age group in determining level of consciousness. The age groups are as follows: infants 6 months to 2 years of age; preschool children aged 2 to 5 years; and school-age children 5 years and older.

Further diagnostic tests include x-rays of skull and neck to identify fractures, angiography to assess blood flow patterns, echoencephalography to detect lateral displacement of the cerebral midline suggesting mass lesion or brain shift, and, at a later point, electroencephalogram as a tool to monitor the patient's course. Computed tomography (CT) and multimodality evoked potential studies assist with diagnosis of brain lesions and evaluating severity of involvement. Recent articles review the use of a multimodality evoked potential study for the localization and evaluation of brain dysfunction and the implications for management and prognostication in the severely head-injured patient.[22,24-29]

Acute Medical Management

The goal of initial medical management is maintenance of vital functions. Because the child's reaction to cerebral damage is labile, clinical signs can change rapidly. Serial monitoring of respiratory rate, blood pressure, pulse rate and rhythm, temperature, and level of consciousness will indicate the child's change in status. A tracheostomy and artificial ventilation control obstruction and prevent repeated episodes of hypoxia and cyanosis. Close monitoring of increased intracranial pressure permits appropriate management, including hyperventilation, hypertonic mannitol or dexamethasone, barbiturate coma, or hypothermia.[3,21,30] In prolonged coma, nasoesophageal tube feeding provides fluid and nutrient requirements.

Seizures occur most frequently within the first week after injury. Anticonvulsant therapy depends on the risk of recurrence, which increases to 70 percent after the first week post injury. Generally seizure prophylaxis is provided with phenobarbitol for one year. Discontinuance is dependent on electroencephalography (EEG) results.[18]

Hypertension with systolic pressures between 160 and 180 mmHg and diastolic pressures between 100 and 140 mmHg are not uncommon. Systolic blood pressure greater than 130 mmHg and diastolic pressure greater than 100 mmHg, persisting for more than 6 weeks after injury, decreases the chance of significant neurologic recovery.[13] Return of blood pressure to normal levels coincides with neurologic improvement.[18]

Orthopedic Management

Orthopedic problems associated with traumatic head injury include spinal cord injury, brachial plexus injury, fractures and dislocations resulting from concomitant trauma to limbs and spine, and spasticity, contractures, pressure sores, ectopic ossification, scoliosis, and limb length discrepancies associated with the brain damage.[30-33] Injuries are difficult to diagnose in the unconscious child.

Heterotopic ossification of soft tissues occurs in some patients with prolonged unconsciousness, typically 2 to 4 months after head injury. The most common sites are the shoulder, elbow, hip, and knee. Whether mobilization is beneficial during the acute phase is controversial. In children, ectopic bone is often spontaneously resorbed, therefore surgical excision of bone to improve function is delayed. However, recurrence of bone growth may follow surgery.[16,18,31]

Spasticity, a common sequela of head injury increases during the first few months after injury, peaking at 2 to 3 months, then gradually decreases, sometimes for over 2 years.[8] Bilateral moderate to severe spasticity is most common in patients comatose for more than 4 weeks.[2] Conservative management, including passive range of motion, static stretching, serial plaster casts, dropout casts, and positional splints, attain full range of motion before function returns.[18] Surgical management of spasticity is delayed until 12 to 18 months post injury, permitting the unpredictable neurologic recovery to take its course.[18,31] Refer to Hoffer and associates,[18,33] Brink and Hoffer,[31] and Meyler and associates[32] for further discussion of acute and long-term orthopedic management.

Prognosis

Although recovery of consciousness and preinjury functional status is usually complete within 3 weeks, behavioral difficulties, shortened attention span, and irritability persist longer.[1] It is estimated that 5 to 10 percent of those hospitalized will manifest neurologic and/or psychologic sequelae 6 months or more after injury. The severity of neurologic sequelae correlates with the severity of trauma; however, the psychologic sequelae do not demonstrate this relationship.[8] The interplay between the neurologic and psychologic sequelae, as well as the effect of the child's preinjury developmental and mental status, family support and interaction, and availability of appropriate professional and nonprofessional intervention support systems, combine to determine the ultimate reintegration of the child into society.[6,7,34] Much research attempts to expand the confidence with which physicians can predict the ultimate outcome from the patient's status within the first few hours. Physical and mental improvement is evident 2, 3, and even 7 years after the injury;[2] however, it is generally agreed that the maximum gains occur by the first 6 to 12 months after injury.[2] Assessing the outcome of a child is more complex than assessing that of an adult, as the child is not expected to regain his former status, but to continue to mature developmentally and mentally, sequentially achieving "age-appropriate" milestones in all aspects of behavior. Established outcome categories, recently reviewed by Jennet and associates[34,35] and referred to in many reports[3,27,34,36] are as follows: (1) death, (2) persistent vegetative state, (3) severe disability, (4) moderate disability, and (5) good recovery. An initial Glasgow Coma Score ≤4 portends a poor outcome, often death.[1,24,36] Young and associates[36] report outcomes equally distributed with Glasgow Coma Scores 5 to 7 and 95 percent good to moderate recovery with scores greater than 7. Changes in the Glasgow Coma Score during the first 24 hours improve the precision of prediction of outcome.[36] Slow response time and difficulties with short-term memory are major residual abnormalities with intial Glasgow Coma Scores 5 to 8. Refer to studies by Jennett and associates,[34,35] Bruce and associates,[3] Greenberg and associates,[27] Gilchrist and Wilkinson,[6] Cartlidge and Shaw,[4] and Mayer and associates[5,30,37] for detailed reviews of outcome.

Brink[13,33] reports that the length of time unconscious, specifically the amount of time elapsed from injury until the child can follow commands or imitate gestures (Level II), reflects the severity of trauma. A good or moderate outcome is expected if coma does not exceed 6 weeks. Coma persisting longer than 3 months portends poor return of motor function.[13,31,33] The frequency and severity of spasticity and ataxia increases as the length of coma increases.[13] The incidence of spasticity and ataxia in severely head-injured children is high, about 65 and 50 percent, respectively, with 35 percent incidence of ataxia and spasticity combined.[2,13,31,33] Around 75 to 80 percent of all children with severe head injuries achieve independence in ambulation and self-care.[6,13,18,31]

Psychologic sequelae, including cognitive and behavioral problems, do not correlate with severity of trauma and may reflect diffuse injury.[8,35] Improvement in cognition parallels that of level of consciousness. Initial agitated behavior in response to cerebral irritation resolves as the level of consciousness improves, and the child is able to respond to the environment. Confused behaviors resolve as memory and cognition improve. Persistent deficits in learning and memory may be severe; the younger the age of onset, the more pronounced the effect on intellectual performance. IQ at one year after injury relates directly to length of coma.[2,18] Changes in personality and behavior include hyperactivity, distractibility, low tolerance for frustration, poor social judgment, lack of impulse control, and aggressiveness.[4,8,18] The intellectual deficits and personality changes that persist require special school placement and are more difficult for the family to manage.[35]

PHYSICAL THERAPY EVALUATION

Evaluation of the head-injured child is a continuous process. The unpredictable and varied rate of recovery and the complex mechanisms of recovery necessitate constant evaluation and modification of therapeutic intervention to appropriately enhance the recovery that is occurring. The simultaneous but varied rates of recovery in all aspects of behavior requires close communication between professional team members. Each therapist affects the whole child with each intervention. Understanding the deficits and abilities of the patient in all behaviors assists each discipline to employ strategies to best achieve their goals while reinforcing recovery in all aspects of performance.

A head-injured patient's loss of consciousness and diminished cognitive abilities require modification of the traditional evaluation. Evoking the response appropriate to the area of assessment is a challenge to the therapist. Careful observation of the timing, force, duration, direction, and location of movement in response to controlled stimulation provides information as to the status of sensory, motor, and sensorimotor integrative aspects of movement. Conscious manipulation of intervention determines the precise amount and timing necessary to elicit the desired response. Intervention may be modified as to amount or intensity of stimulation, duration, complexity, and rate of input. When evoking a response to sensory stimulation, allow for a delay for processing. After sufficient delay, the stimulus may have to be repeated a few times to evoke the desired response. Note the best response observed, as this indicates the potential of the patient. Information concerning the injury, the child's preinjury status, and rate of progress is available from a chart review and/or family interview. Physical assessment requires multiple short sessions to assure accurate evaluation.[38,39]

Behavioral Considerations

The challenge of evaluating a head-injured patient is in eliciting the appropriate response. Decreased consciousness, maladaptive behaviors, and impaired cognition interfere with the child's ability to participate in the evaluation. Evaluation techniques are modified according to the child's level of consciousness and cognitive function. A child at Levels V, IV, or III, according to Ommaya's scale, is unable to follow commands; assessment, therefore, employs passive manipulation. A child at Level II can follow simple one-step commands; however, distractibility, limited attention span, and memory impairments may preclude following commands with more than one step, attending to a task for more than a few seconds, or attending to your stimulus at all. Elicitation of automatic activities provide purposeful motion for evaluation of motor control. A child at Levels IV, III, and II may appear to change level of consciousness several times during the day. When the child is most alert, the best responses will be evinced. Fatigue may occur after 15 minutes, at which time earlier responses cannot be reproduced.

By Level I, the child is oriented to self, time, and place. Although distractibility, limited attention span, and memory impairments remain, their severity has decreased sufficiently to permit use of traditional evaluation tools for short testing periods. Behaviors such as aggression, lack of self-initiation, low frustration tolerance, emotional lability, or withdrawal require short sessions and a structured environment. At Levels II and I, a quiet environment facilitates accurate evaluation of motor control; however, the child's ability to perform activities with the usual distractions may elucidate functional impairments limited by cognitive status.

The agitated patient presents the greatest challenge for evaluation and treatment. One must remember that the child is responding to cerebral irritation and internal confusion as he or she tries to come to grips with the environment. Finding a means to calm the child facilitates assessment. In a calm environment with structured stimuli, the child may follow commands for short periods of time. Touching the child, or demanding a motion too difficult or complex, will quickly cause frustration and agitation. Purposeful movements, observed with a critical eye, provide range of motion, sensation, motor control, equilibrium, and strength information. Children often demonstrate their best developmental or functional level when most agitated.

Chart Review

The patient's age and preinjury developmental status provide a baseline for assessing motor ability and identifying preinjury problem areas. Preinjury behavior and cognitive abilities are apparent in school performance records and through family interview. Knowledge of favorite play activities aids in establishing a baseline as well as goals in determining treatment.

The etiology of head injury and neurosurgical reports suggest the location and extent of cerebral injury. The circumstances of the injury alert the therapist to suspect concomitant injuries that may not be apparent until the patient gains consciousness. Peripheral nerve injuries and fractures may be missed during the acute stages.

The status of concomitant injuries and necessary precautions must be known before beginning the physical evaluation. Peripheral nerve injuries should be suspected if traction or external immobilization has been used.

Medical complications and present status alert the therapist to precautions necessary during evaluation and treatment. During the acute stage, aggressive chest physical therapy may increase intracranial pressure. Elevation of the head 30 to 45 degrees and preventing neck rotation assist in preventing increased intracranial pressure. Coordination with nursing, supervision of proper positioning, and modifying chest physical therapy according to the patient's tolerance assures safety for the patient. Labile or hypertensive blood pressures may result from the head injury or medications. Muscle stretching during range of motion or casting and changes in position may cause sudden increases in systolic and diastolic pressure and an associated tachycardia. Monitoring during treatment is recommended. Familiarity with nasogastric tube and tracheostomy precautions prepare the therapist for unexpected problems such as coughing out the inner cannula or regurgitation through the tube. Some centers do not recommend activities that lower the head below the stomach when the patient has a nasogastric tube in place, as the cardiac sphincter of the stomach is relaxed and open, and regurgitation and aspiration may take place.[38] Changes in position and chest physical therapy will loosen tracheal secretions, requiring suctioning. Careful review of the patient's medical record will alert the therapist as to which of these precautions may be necessary during evaluation and therapy.

Level of consciousness or coma score at onset and changes during the first 24 to 48 hours are key prognosticators. The present level of consciousness, the time since the injury, and the duration of coma provide greater indication of the severity of injury and the expected outcome.

A history of decerebrate or decorticate posturing alerts the therapist to expect contractures and possible pressure areas. Prolonged posturing may result in unrelieved pressure, causing damage to superficial nerves, especially the ulnar or peroneal nerves. Heterotopic ossification, associated with trauma or spasticity, causes painful and limited joint range of motion.

Family involvement since hospitalization gives an indication of involvement expected after discharge. A supportive and involved family facilitates the rehabilitation and guarantees continuation of the process after discharge. In-hospital care only initiates the prolonged process of recovery and reintegration into society. The functional achievements must become part of the child's and family's daily routine. Goals and methods must be modified to meet the family's needs, as they will be the full-time therapists once the child leaves the hospital.

Previous therapeutic evaluation and progress reports indicate the child's progression thus far. The child may appear totally different from the most recent evaluation as neurologic improvement may occur rapidly. At times the new environment and transition may totally confuse the patient or result in an apparent decrease in level of consciousness until he or she adapts to the new surroundings.

Sensory Testing

The child's response to a specific sensory stimulus changes as level of consciousness changes. Stimuli through intact auditory, visual, olfactory, gustatory, and pain pathways evoke a response at all levels of consciousness, except Level V.

A Level IV child demonstrates a generalized response to any sensory input. The response is the same regardless of the type of stimulus presented. Increased respiratory rate, sweating, increased pulse rate, change in tone throughout the body, grimace, or total body movements are frequently noted.

At Level III, the child's response is specific to the stimulus presented. Often a delay occurs before the response and the stimulus may need to be repeated. Examples of localized responses to selected stimuli are listed in Table 8-1.

Proprioception can be grossly assessed once the child initiates purposeful movements (Level II). Specific testing is limited by cognition and the child's age. Sharp-dull and two-point discrimination testing require memory, the ability to process information, and the ability to follow complex commands.

Hypersensitivity to touch must be assessed. Total body, perioral, and oral hypersensitivity most often result from prolonged lack of stimulation and resolve nicely in response to desensitization therapy.

Table 8-1. Localized Response to Sensory Stimuli

Sensory Tract	Stimulus Examples	Response
Auditory	Voice	Eye opening
	Bell	Looking toward stimulus
	Hand clapping	Turning head toward/away from stimulus
Visual	Threat near eyes	Blinking
	Bright object	Focusing and tracking
	Familiar toy	
	Familiar person	
Olfactory	Ammonia	Grimace or turn away
Gustatory	Sugar	Smile
	Lemon	Grimace
Pain	Squeeze muscle belly	Pull extremity away
	Squeeze nail bed	Look toward pain
	Pin prick	

Range of Motion

Assessment of which factors are interfering with full range of motion determines whether full range can be gained or the child must learn to compensate. Heterotopic ossification is often associated with a warm joint and painful range. A bony end point is noted if one can range through the child's resistance. Range may become more limited and the pain of movement through the range may interfere with functional activities. While heterotopic bone often is reabsorbed in children, short-term and potentially long-term compensation for lack of range is necessary. Hypertonus may favor prolonged habitual posturing and the potential development of soft tissue and joint capsule contractures. Positioning the patient to minimize tone aids in determining passive joint range of motion. Appropriate conservative or surgical methods gain range of motion to permit functional use of the extremity.

A child who is agitated, confused, or unable to follow commands may appear to resist ranging and cry as if in pain. Observing joint range of motion used in spontaneous movements and functional activities confirms that full range of motion is present, or further challenges the therapist to determine what is truly limiting range.

Tone

Assessment of muscle tone, the amount of resistance to passive movement, may reveal varying degrees of increased or decreased tone. Hypotonicity may result from muscle weakness, impaired sensorimotor integration, impairment in excitatory centers of postural tonic control, and possibly damage to reticular activating centers. Hypertonicity may result from release of spinal level excitatory influences from the descending inhibitory influence of the reticular system, or as an exaggeration of the normal tendency to revert to tonic reflex influence in difficult activities. The pattern of relative hyper- or hypotonicity reveals the balance of excitatory and inhibitory influences on the motoneurons. Changes in interoceptive and exteroceptive input will affect this balance, resulting in changes in muscle tone. The child's alertness, difficulty of the task, tonic neck, tonic labyrinthine, positive supporting reflexes, and modified vestibular, tactile, and proprioceptive input affect the muscle tone and ability to move. Assessing the muscle tone relative to modifications in sensory input assists in program planning.

A transition from decerebrate or decorticate posturing to hypotonicity often follows neurologic recovery. Hypotonus eventually changes to hypertonus or alternating hypo- and hypertonus. Prolonged hypotonus is often associated with ataxia; however, ataxia may not be apparent until the child initiates purposeful movements.

Motor Control

Movement reflects the status of level of consciousness, behavior, cognition, sensation, sensorimotor integration, and neuromuscular status. The quality of movement is the product of the interaction of the uninvolved centers of control. Apparent deficits represent the inability of remaining centers to compensate for actual deficits caused by damage to or suppressed functioning of major motor control centers.

Initially, the quality of movement is assessed in general terms. Whether movement occurs spontaneously or only in response to stimulation reflects the level of consciousness or the presence of limb neglect as a result of sensory deficits. Level of consciousness determines whether motion is purposeful or nonpurposeful (random movement). Structure and the child's level of alertness may influence the type of motion noted. Determining whether movement is patterned or selective is especially difficult in the infant. Patterned movements are often most prevalent. Careful observation of spontaneous movements and manipulating positioning, and type and location of stimulus to encourage a selective response, determines if selectivity is present. Often selective movements and normal movement patterns replace the abnormal flexion and extension patterns as the child's level of consciousness and cognition improves and motor learning progresses; however, if moderate-severe spasticity combines with abnormal patterned motion, resolution to selective control is less likely. Assessment of movement in gravity-eliminated positions and against gravity determines the relative strength of muscle groups and assists in identifying peripheral nerve injuries. Determining good and normal strengths of individual muscles is difficult. Often a child will not maintain a joint position against resistance. Lifting body weight or weighted items and the way in which a child moves between postures and maintains postures may suggest weaknesses. Muscle endurance may be impaired from prolonged inactivity, especially if hypotonus is present. It has been argued that brain-damaged patients "suffer from lack of central control over movement and not actual muscle weakness."[40] In my experience, some children suffering severe head injuries and prolonged unconsciousness demonstrate muscle weakness and limited endurance contribution to impaired motor control, especially of the neck and trunk. Areas of weakness then demand consideration in planning treatment.

The influence of muscle tone, sensation, and muscle strength and endurance on the selective or patterned control available determines the achievable motor control of each extremity, neck, and trunk in isolation. Observation of function identifies the child's ability to use the motor control available. Deficits in sensorimotor integration (e.g., apraxia, impaired motor planning, or visual discrimination), impaired cognition (limited attention to task, impaired memory or sequencing, inability to imitate), and decreased level of consciousness affect the functional use of motor patterns available.

Observing the developmental sequence of postures and movement in and out of various positions assists in identifying the influence of muscle tone, sensation, muscle strength and endurance, sensorimotor integration, and cognition on motor control. Testing equilibrium and righting reactions usually demonstrates delayed and exaggerated responses, which resolve as level of consciousness improves. Tone interfering to prevent a protective or equilibrium response portends residual impairment, although improvement occurs. The reintegration of the influence of tonic reflexes into normal postural reactions most often follows a pattern similar to the developmental sequence on an accelerated time line. Although righting and equilibrium reactions are apparent in supine, prone, and four-point positions, sitting and standing may prove too difficult or stressful, resulting in tonic reflex influences dominating motor responses; however, the quality of righting and equilibrium reactions in lower level developmental activities portends the eventual quality of these reactions in higher level postures.

Observations of purposeful movement in response to a command may indicate cognitive or sensorimotor integration deficits in addition to motor control impairments already identified. A classic case is the child's apparent inability to move the arms when asked to lift the arm as high as he or she can and to touch your hand or reach for a toy. However, if you throw a ball the child will automatically catch it with perfect control! Whether the child is unable to attend, to initiate movement, or to sequence the activity, or has sensorimotor integration deficits is difficult to determine. Team members specializing in these areas of evaluation identify specific deficits and suggest intervention strategies for improvement of function or compensation for deficits. Developmental tests have not been standardized for the head-injured population. With the complexity of deficits in each child, the validity of these tests is questionable; however, selection of testable items provides an index of the abilities of the child at a point in time and a baseline for comparison as recovery occurs. The validity of standardized tests in defining outcome or confirming total recovery has not been evaluated.

Cardiopulmonary Status

In the acute setting, cardiac and respiratory impairments may result from trauma to the chest, pharyngeal spasm, respiratory center depression from brainstem damage, and labile reactions to trauma. Endotracheal intubation or tracheostomy permit maintenance of an airway for provision of mechanical ventilation and suctioning.

Laboratory study results and chest radiographs assist in identifying the respiratory problem. In the acutely ill patient mechanical devices such as arterial, central venous, and Swan-Ganz catheters, electrocardiograms, intracranial pressure transducers, and respiratory gas analyzers provide baseline data, as well as indication of tolerance for treatment. Observation of breathing rate, rhythm, and pattern, chest expansion measurements and palpation, percussion, and auscultation complete the clinical evaluation.[40–43]

The child no longer needing mechanical monitors may continue demonstrating labile physiologic responses to change in position or stretch. Baseline heart rate, rhythm, and blood pressure are determined at rest and in response to exercise.

Orofacial Control

Children suffering severe head injuries frequently require nasogastric tube feeding, as brainstem involvement has impaired the swallow, gag, and cough reflexes. Prolonged nasogastric tube feeding often results in deprivation of oral sensation and therefore delay in return of normal reflex responses for swallowing and preventing aspiration.

Sensory evaluation of the face, lips, gums and tongue, soft palate, and posterior pharyngeal wall may identify hypo- or hypersensitivity to touch. Children with a history of decorticate posturing often demonstrate abnormal reflex responses to stimulation, including the following: rooting reflex, pursing reflex, reflex chewing followed by a reflex suck-swallow. The reflex swallow, gag, and cough are evaluated in all patients. A reflex gag, normally elicited on the posterior third of the tongue, may be hypersensitive (elicited in middle to anterior third) or diminished (elicited only on soft palate or posterior pharyngeal wall). Voluntary initiation of a swallow and cough is requested if the child can follow commands. If unable to follow commands, a small amount of water placed in the side of the mouth with a straw will usually elicit a swallow. An audible swallow, multiple attempts, delayed initiation, or inadequate laryngeal excursion indicate incoordination and possible aspiration. If a reflex cough is not elicited, and the status of the swallow suggests possible aspiration, further evaluation is necessary before initiating feeding. If a child has a tracheostomy, feeding the child a small amount of pureed food with blue food coloring added followed by suctioning will reveal if aspiration has occurred. A swallowing fluoroscopy may be necessary to confirm the absence of aspiration when a tracheostomy is not present.

Selective and voluntary control of the lips, tongue, and jaw can be observed in response to stimulation with a tooth swab, gloved finger, or tongue blade to the gums and tongue. Expected motor control for the child's age must be considered. Adequate ability to maneuver food to the sides and back of the mouth and presence of a reflex swallow, reflex gag, and reflex cough are indications for a feeding trial.

Determining Realistic Functional Goals

Ideal long-term goals include attainment of age-appropriate gross motor activities, functional abilities, and diet. Reasonable outcomes considering length of coma have been discussed. Ataxia and spasticity are the most common factors interfering with functional activities and, if severe, may prevent ambulation. Mental and cognitive deficits are often more disabling than physical deficits in determining overall outcome. The need for constant supervision and residual aggressive, impulsive, and destructive behavior require an involved caretaker for successful postdischarge management. Intellectual deficits, common when a severe head injury is sustained in childhood, may limit potential vocational abilities. Adolescents commonly demonstrate poor judgment and difficulty with problem solving, which seriously hinder vocational potential and financial independence.[16]

Considering developmental and functional abilities appropriate to the child's age, the length of time in coma, and the physical findings and cognitive status in light of the length of time from onset, a potential functional status can be estimated. To determine if the predicted status is achievable and realistic for the patient, consider preinjury development, setting after discharge, and involvement of caretakers. Realistic goals can thereby be determined. Family may not be available for constant supervision, and household barriers (and monetary constraints) may prevent use of assistive devices for independence, limiting function in transfers to those requiring assistance. The availability of therapy through school or infant stimulation groups permits discharge at lower levels of function with the knowledge that therapy will be continued on an outpatient basis. Unrealistic family expectations for recovery require immediate and continuing family involvement and education. If alternative placement is necessary, realistic goals and equipment are chosen appropriate to the discharge setting, where time restraints and staffing may limit supervision and follow-through on programs.

Level of consciousness and cognitive function may limit achievement of goals expected, based only on physical findings. Children at Levels IV and III demonstrate generalized or localized responses when stimulated, but do not initiate interaction with the environment. Wheelchair positioning to prevent contractures and assist respiratory status is realistic. Bed positioning, range of motion, and possibly a respiratory-postural drainage-vibration program may be carried out by an involved family. Feeding reflexes may permit the child to be fed a pureed or soft diet. Mobility in bed is dependent, but instructions for caretakers on body mechanics and facilitation of rolling may assist the care of the adolescent. Transfers are dependent. A lift is recommended.

A child at Level II is able to follow commands and initiate purposeful activity. The child may be able to relearn automatic activities such as rolling, coming to sit, crawling, standing, ambulation, and self-feeding, if physical deficits are minimal. The absence of judgment and problem-solving abilities requires constant supervision and often assistance to prevent injury to the child. Carryover of the same activity in new environments will require assistance and much repetition until the pattern is relearned in the new situation. A child with moderate-severe motor deficits has difficulty learning to compensate due to poor memory and sequencing abilities. Learning mobility with equipment may not be possible. Bed mobility and transfers may require minimal to moderate assistance.

A child reaching Level I is oriented to time, place, and self and is recording ongoing events. Independence in mobility at home, self-care and feeding are realistic goals. Proper use of adaptive equipment can be learned. A child normally requires supervision in the community, however. This must be emphasized with caretakers as poor frustration tolerance, lack of problem solving, impaired judgment, and poor impulse control demand closer supervision than preinjury. The adolescent will also require supervision in the community where the multitude of stimuli may be confusing, and residual judgment and problem-solving deficits may make new situations difficult to manage.

PHYSICAL THERAPY

General Treatment Principles

The therapist does not cause neurologic recovery, but rather channels the spontaneous recovery that is occurring. Whether recovery is the result of diaschisis, equipotentiality, compensation, vicariation and/or collateral regeneration and hypersensitivity remains controversial.[44–49] The timing, frequency, and type of therapeutic intervention to effect a given outcome has not been objectively ascertained. Valid tools to define deficits, and methods of differentiating recovery due to neurophysiologic mechanisms from that resulting from learning compensatory behaviors are yet to be developed.

A systematic evaluation permits determination of the major problems interfering with function, the abilities retained, and intact exteroceptive and proprioceptive systems through which proper adaptive behaviors can be stimulated. Treatment is an extension of the evaluation process. With the complexity of deficits, uniqueness of each child and spontaneous recovery occurring, no single method of treatment is appropriate in every situation. The patient's adaptive response to a specific intervention may change within a treatment period as well as between treatment periods. The therapist must know the adaptive response he or she is trying to evoke. Then the therapist, considering evaluation findings and responses to this point, must provide the appropriate cues. Immediate evaluation of the child's response, both subtle tone changes as well as gross movements, provides feedback as to modifications needed in the handling provided.

The normal learning process may account for apparent recovery. Carr and Shepherd[40] identified key factors in the process of relearning of movement. The goal must be identified and relevant to the child. The therapist must guide the child through the proper sequence of movement providing cues as needed. The therapist assists with the inhibition of unnecessary activity that normally occurs as the movement is refined, thus reducing the energy cost of movement.

Normal postural reactions necessary to maintain balance and position against gravity permit progression from stability to controlled mobility and enhancement of sensorimotor integration. The proper body alignment and mental set in preparation for and throughout the movement are provided by the therapist through handling. Guided and controlled practice, motivation and knowledge of results, and feedback further enhance learning.[40] Temporary regression to less selective and more primitive motor activity when former well-coordinated movements are used in different combinations of patterns in more difficult tasks is apparent in normal acquisition of new skills. The therapist is intimately involved in intricate modifications of handling to provide a relevant and normal sensorimotor experience. Designing play activities, appropriate to the child's cognitive abilities, which are goal directed, provide success, encourage movement, and yet permit adequate handling by the therapist to ensure a normal sensorimotor experience, is a skill developed through practice.

Treatment is most effective with a well-coordinated team approach.[50] This requires a basic knowledge of each professional's expertise in the child's rehabilitation. Common definitions of terms describing deficits and abilities permit accurate communication. Stichbury and colleagues,[51] in reviewing the importance of an interdisciplinary approach to treatment, beautifully demonstrate the process of identifying the primary deficit and then structuring the treatment environment to facilitate an appropriate adaptive response by the patient.

A coordinated team effort enhances learning through additional reinforcement of appropriate skills incorporated into the treatment sessions of each team member. For example, a child now able to sequence three items, but requiring upper extremity stabilization for fine motor control, may work on sequencing with appropriate-size toys while standing on the tilt table. Generally each team member contributes to orienting the child, beginning and ending each session by telling the child his or her name, where he or she is, what he or she is going to do, and the therapist's name.

As discussed under goals, the child's cognitive abilities and behaviors influence the therapist's goals and likewise the approach to treatment. At Levels IV and III the child cannot actively initiate participation in the therapeutic program. Emphasis at this time is to increase the time the child will attend to the stimuli, and decrease the delay to respond. Maintaining or improving range of motion and stimulating equilibrium and righting reactions prepares the musculoskeletal system for the time when the child can participate. Decreasing hypersensitivity and facilitating normal reflex responses of gag, swallow, and cough prepare the child for feeding. An active respiratory program prepares the physiologic response.

When the child reaches Level II he or she can initiate interaction with the environment. Structuring the environment controls the sensory input and therefore assists to organize the input in evoking an appropriate response. The child may be able to "learn" a previously learned activity with much repetition. Generally providing simple verbal directions, demonstrating your command and assisting the child through the activity provides appropriate cues and structures. However, if the child responds only verbally to verbal cues, but will roll when the command is gestured, and is facilitated, these cues are then repeated without speaking. Gradually assistance through the activity is decreased so that the therapist initiates the activity but expects the child to complete the roll. Success is always made possible and reinforced when achieved. Eventually, with only a gesture or command, the child can initiate the activity and have the components in the proper sequence to achieve the goal. Carryover from session to session requires memory. Independent carryover in a different environment is not expected until the child can solve problems; therefore, although physically able to perform an activity, the child may require assistance to repeat the same activity in a different environment.

As the child's memory improves he or she can carry over activities in new environments and remember them from day to day. Lability and distractibility tend to decrease; however, often irritability and difficulties with judgment and problem solving persist at Level I. Expecting the child to take responsibility for getting to classes on time, choosing clothes, and other age-appropriate expectations of independence are gradually encouraged. Community outings challenge the child's judgment and problem solving. Exercising safety in street crossings at busy corners and running errands to small stores or fast food restaurants test the child's cognitive, emotional, social, and physical abilities in the community.

Inadequate Range of Motion

Management of inadequate range of motion depends on the factors limiting range and the severity of the factors. Heterotopic ossification is the most difficult to manage. The child splints against passive range of motion and will not move the joint through full range actively. If the pain interferes with functional activities, immobilization in plaster may relieve the pain sufficiently to permit rehabilitation to continue. The child must compensate for the limited range until the bone is reabsorbed or possible surgical resection is complete after 18 months.

Hypertonicity, hypotonicity, or peripheral nerve injury prevent spontaneous movement of each joint through its normal range of motion and encourage prolonged posturing, resulting in myostatic or capsular contracture. A range of motion program incorporating positioning, static stretching, casts, splints, orthoses, and/or electrical stimulation is designed considering the apparent soft tissue contracture and factors affecting its development. Static stretch or serial casting may decrease soft tissue contracture followed by splints and positioning to maintain range.

The effect of tone on postures may be relieved through proper positioning. Positioning is difficult to maintain in an active patient. Most applicable in early management, positioning serves to maintain range of motion by preventing prolonged postures in abnormal positions. Bed positioning with pillows and rolls should encourage slight neck and trunk flexion, shoulder protraction, slight elbow flexion and forearm pronation, and wrist extension. Pelvic anterior tilt and slight flexion of the hip, knee, and ankle may relax lower extremity tone.

Extremity positioning is alternated between flexion and extension as long as tone is relaxed. Placement in the prone position is encouraged when medically cleared. Moderate-severe tone not decreased with positioning may respond with the addition of casts and splints.

Wheelchair positioning to control tone must consider the influence of the head position on tone and the key points where control affects the tone of the rest of the body. Generally, a slightly reclined position prevents fatigue and provides support when tone is diminished, as well as preventing increased tone from increased stress. Travel chairs may be modified to normalize tone and provide adequate support. Shoulder protraction, support of upper extremities on lap board or bolsters, lateral trunk support, pelvis upright or slightly anteriorly tilted, hips flexed and abducted with wedge cushion and abduction bolster, and feet supported encourages symmetrical weight bearing on buttocks, normalized tone, and stability. Posterior splints may position ankles with slight spasticity or protect weak muscles from being stretched.

Shoulder and hip range of motion limitations are best managed with traditional static stretching and passive range of motion methods combined with positioning to maintain the range available. If the child has lower extremity casts, simple modifications will assist with hip positioning. An abductor bar attached to short leg or long leg casts or splints maintain hip abduction in the supine and prone positions. A single bar attached to the lateral side of lower extremity casts or splints prevents posturing in external rotation. Depending on the child's therapy program, abductor bars and outriggers are attached permanently to present casts or splints, or are attached to plaster cups which fit on the heel of a short leg cast or at the knee of a long leg cast, permitting removal for dressing or sidelying positioning.

Cylinder casts do not decrease central spasticity, rather they serve to maintain muscle length and minimize the sensory input eliciting the stretch responses. Casting and orthoses provide temporary management while neurologic recovery is occurring, with the expectation that spasticity will decrease as recovery progresses. Casts are preferred in severe spasticity as anterior/posterior splints permit motion that encourages stretch responses and may result in pressure sore development.

Ankles and knees often respond well to serial casting. Well-padded cylinder casts applied with the joint positioned just short of its maximum passive range are changed every 8 to 10 days. At each cast change the joint is put through full range and a new cast applied at maximum available range. Generally two to three cast changes are necessary to achieve full range. Once the desired range is achieved, a "holding cast" maintains the corrected range for 1 to 3 weeks. This cast may be bivalved and converted to an anterior-posterior splint. Gradual weaning to using splints at night, and positioning orthoses and range of motion during the day, proceeds as long as range is maintained. Splinting continues until neurologic recovery results in decreased spasticity and improved motor control. Dropout casts combined with positioning for gravity-assisted range of motion hasten decreasing elbow flexion contractures and knee flexion contractures of less than 60 degrees.[106] Dropout casts may need to be changed every 3 to 5 days as range will increase quickly. Serial casting is most often incorporated in early management to achieve functional range by the time coma has decreased, permitting the child's participation in therapy. During this time children may demonstrate physiologic lability to pain and stretch and cannot communicate location or intensity of pain. Labile vital signs or other indications of pain necessitate changing casts to decrease stretch and or relieve localized skin pressure.[16,33,38,50,52,53]

Tone-inhibiting casts encouraging hyperextension of the toes, pressure under the metatarsal heads, a stable ankle position, and deep tendon pressure along the tendocalcaneous may normalize dynamic hypertonicity when functional activities in the upright position are initiated.[50,54] Traditional ankle-foot orthoses or specially modified tone-inhibiting orthoses may maintain ankle range of motion and modify persistent hypertonicity during functional activities until neurologic recovery permits adequate motor control or surgical procedures are considered at 18 months to 2 years post injury.[16,33,52] Clinical evaluation of function with traditional short leg casts and function with tone-inhibiting short leg casts may assist in determining the most effective orthotic management.

Electrical cycling of muscle groups antagonistic to spastic muscles may be incorporated with use of casts or separately to increase range of motion at the knee, ankle, elbow, and wrist.[50,55] Cycling in a functional position, such as standing, increases joint range while assisting to reeducate normal muscular control. A child with knee flexor contractures and/or hamstring spasticity interfering with extension control in the upright position may benefit from functional electrical stimulation of the quadriceps muscle in standing combined with weight shift to the involved side during stimulation. Electric stimulation of the peroneal nerve may facilitate a decrease in extensor tone and positive support in weight bearing. Tolerance for electrical stimulation and the effect of stimulation on spastic musculature elsewhere in the body is variable; therfore judicious use of this modality as an adjunct to the therapeutic regimen is recommended.[55]

Children discharged nonambulatory require special consideration of wheelchair positioning and a home program to maintain joint range of motion and muscle length. Choice of wheelchair and modifications that normalize tone may assist in preventing postures resulting in dislocation or bony deformities. Orthotic management with ankle-foot orthosis, hip abduction braces, and body jackets may assist positioning in the presence of moderate tone but are rarely tolerated if tone is severe. A body jacket as an adjunct to positioning may assist in preventing spinal deformity in a child with trunk weakness or hypotonicity. Aggressive management to maintain range of motion during the growing years may prevent severe deformities leading to pain, pressure areas, and difficult wheelchair positioning, which will diminish sitting tolerance in later years.

Inadequate Motor Control

Evaluation of muscle strength, endurance, joint range of motion and the influence of tone on postural control, and mobility of the head, trunk, and extremities identifies the major problems potentially interfering with normal motor control. The ability of the child to perform a functional activity includes factors beyond use of the separate parts; for example, the influence of trunk control, visual perceptual deficits, cognition, and the difficulty of the task affect ability to control the extremities. Observation of the child's difficulty in performing a function challenges the therapist to identify various components of the task that are difficult for the child. Providing additional cues, inhibiting excessive motion, and improving deficits through varied treatment situations will eventually result in independence in the function. Treatment evolves from appropriate integration of principles of Bobath, Rood, Ayres, Brunnstrom, and proprioceptive neuromuscular facilitation. Appropriate strategies are suggested through evaluation findings and observation of adaptive responses to handling, providing various types and amounts of sensory cues. The child's adaptive responses provide feedback and therefore indicate modifications of intervention necessary to refine the response.

Ommaya describes the reintegrative phenomena displayed by patients as they slowly struggle toward full consciousness in a distorted and irregularly accelerated reproduction of ontogenetic development. The patient retraces general behavioral development as well as the neurologic pattern of his or her own growth and maturity.[15] It is fascinating to watch the recovery of young children. They often cry or refuse to progress too quickly. Tonic influences in difficult postures and reintegration of normal postural reactions are dramatic. Often the child spontaneously progresses to the next developmental level. Facilitating normal tone, movement, and increased sensory awareness, and providing a structured environment to reinforce normal postural reactions and mobility, while preventing repetition of abnormal movement, affects internalization and independent imitation of normal postural reactions and movement patterns. Whether the therapist is assisting with or permitting the learning process, enhancing access to intact control centers through amplification of previously less-developed proprioceptive access systems or whether recovery is independent of outside intervention defies determination; however, maintaining the musculoskeletal status, channeling the functional use of recovery that occurs, and teaching compensation for residual deficits are minimal roles of the therapist.

Motor control of the extremities is influenced by head and trunk control and head position. Posturing of the trunk is influenced by extremity tone and head position. Head control is influenced by trunk control. In short, the movement of any part of the body is influenced by and influences the postural control of other parts of the body. Therefore treatment planning must include consideration of the whole body (and cognitive status).

Motor control at Levels III and IV is facilitated through stimulation of exteroceptors eliciting reflex responses and proprioceptors effecting tonic and postural responses. Wheelchair and bed positioning programs aim to provide appropriate proprioceptive input to encourage normalization of tone, as well as maintaining range. Positioning on the tilt table and supported sitting on a mat provide varying proprioceptive input. Assisted rolling and coming to sit facilitate righting and equilibrium reactions to somatic proprioceptive and vestibular input. Handling encourages appropriate adaptive responses while inhibiting abnormal tonic influences.

Wheelchair positioning for hypotonic patients is similar to the wheelchair positioning described earlier. Hip flexion, slight anterior pelvic tilt, and feet supported encourages equal weight bearing on the buttocks and provides a stable base to enhance head and trunk control. A wedged cushion with depth and thickness appropriate for thigh and tibial length adapts a junior chair to a small child. Feet are supported on the wheelchair seat. Travel chairs accommodate the larger child. Lateral trunk supports, a somewhat reclined wheelchair back and chest rests, H-straps or soft ties provide lateral and anterior support preventing kyphosis and lateral lean. Upper extremity support on a lap board or bolsters assists to provide lateral support and prevent forward lean of the upper trunk.

A stable pelvis and trunk are prerequisites for controlling head position. Maintaining slight cervical extension and capital flexion with neutral rotation and lateral flexion provides a normal sensorimotor experience through visual orientation, and vestibular and somatic proprioceptive systems. Lateral head supports control rotation and lateral flexion as long as the wheelchair back is well reclined. Medium density 6-inch-thick cushions may be carved to provide appropriate cervical extension, preventing lateral flexion and rotation. Carving a cap within the foam to cover part of the forehead assists in controlling capital positioning. A sayer sling setup permits neck rotation while controlling lateral flexion and flexion/extension in a more upright position.

As the child reaches Level II, play activities encourage purposeful goal-directed responses initiated by the child. Inhibition of abnormal postures and movement and facilitation of the greatest possible variety of innate and potentially normal basic motor patterns is the goal of each treatment. Head control, head and trunk righting, extremity control for support and mobility, rotation, and equilibrium reactions are considered in choosing activities and treatment techniques. Tactile stimulation and techniques of proprioceptive neuromuscular facilitation, such as use of maximal resistance and rhythmical stabilization, as well as tapping, approximation, and weight bearing provide increased sensory input in the presence of apparent or real weakness of muscles after decreasing abnormal tone or hypotonicity.[56]

Play activities are designed with combinations of postural demands of head and trunk and gross and fine motor demands of extremities in different postures. Progression of treatment includes decreasing the amount of postural assistance provided through handling or increasing the difficulty of movement expected. Providing sufficient handling for postural control while using an activity to facilitate or challenge postural control may require two people. The therapist handling the child receives constant feedback as to the child's postural tone. The therapist then directs the assistant or designs the play to encourage mobility, which challenges the postural control to the point just short of where the child reverts to abnormal reflex responses. A child straddling a bolster with hips and knees flexed to 90 degrees, feet flat on the floor, may require approximation through the pelvis to encourage equal weight bearing through the buttocks and feet. Reaching above the head in midline for a "nerf ball" and placing it in a box at eye level may encourage adequate extensor tone to provide sufficient postural control for this simple task. Asking the child to throw the object, to place the object in a box by the feet or to reach for the object so that he or she must rotate the trunk and shift weight to one side may be too difficult. The therapist providing stability will feel a decrease in postural tone or a reversion to primitive tonic reflexes to provide the tone needed. Dynamic modification of handling will guarantee successful completion of the task and a normal sensorimotor experience. This same child may be able to rotate within the body axis in supine or when well supported in a standing table. Weight shifting for single limb support and performing a one-handed fine motor activity may be tolerated when prone on elbows.

Goldberger[57] suggests that spontaneous recovery from cerebellar ataxia is dependent on peripheral feedback and is not dependent on training or enhanced by training. Inaccuracy in timing and movement is compensated for by greater accuracy in position (mediated in part through the cerebral cortex). Initial ataxia is replaced by tremor as the oscillation amplitude decreases, frequency increases and rhythm becomes more regular. The dorsal roots, dorsal columns, pre- and postcentral gyrus, and pyramidal tract are implicated in compensating for cerebellar dyskinesia resulting from dentate-interpositus lesions.[57]

Ataxia becomes apparent once the child initiates purposeful movements. The oscillations decrease in amplitude as each developmental level is mastered; however, progression to a less stable posture or demanding a fine motor activity with the hand at a distance away from the body exacerbates the oscillations. The child stabilizes against a hard object, with upper extremities against the body or a table when performing fine motor activities. Moving from one position to another, the child will maintain as many points of contact with a steady surface as possible. Postural stability, rotation within the body axis and equilibrium reactions are facilitated through proprioceptive input. Studies on long-term follow-up of resolution of ataxia and long-term interference with ambulation as an adult are not available.

Nelson,[58] in reviewing neuro-otologic aspects of head injury, presents evidence of cervical vertigo produced in animal studies and apparent in clinical experience but without a pathophysiologic explanation. Ataxia can be produced in rabbits, monkeys, and humans by local anesthetic injected into the neck muscles. Humans report a sense of falling or tilting. Nystagmus cannot be demonstrated. Unilateral injection results in a clinical picture of ipsilateral ataxia, past pointing, and hypotonia. A cervical collar relieves the ataxia. Clinically symptoms arise ½ to 1 day after a whiplash injury and may persist weeks or months even when near-normal neck range of motion is attained.

Clinically, the comatose head-injured patient demonstrates vestibulo-ocular reflex impairment to head-turning or caloric irrigation of the ears. As the patient regains consciousness, a strong direction-fixed nystagmus, most suggestive of a unilateral vestibular lesion, is demonstrated. Nystagmus and vertigo largely subside over a 2- to 3-week period because of central compensatory mechanisms. Ambulatory patients complain of ataxia in the absence of paresis or cerebellar tremors with a tendency to list toward one side or difficulty changing directions when sudden head turns are required. Residual ataxia is apparent for up to several weeks and symptomatic treatment is suggested.[58]

Generally, as cognition and level of consciousness improve, motor control improves. Refinement of sensorimotor integration, and therefore motor control in upright postures, often occurs spontaneously in preschool children or is enhanced by intervention through school therapy units. Once the children are mobile, they are in constant motion, thereby naturally refining and adapting present motor patterns to perform more difficult activities. Treatment activities should be designed considering muscle strength and endurance and physiologic responses to exercise to decrease the demand of functional activities. Auditory rhythm[59] and dance therapy[60] provide further enhancement of postural control.

Neuromuscular electrical stimulation may assist in increasing sensory input for muscle reeducation in a child with low tone. Paraspinal stimulation to encourage head control and lower extremity stimulation during standing and ambulation are generally preceded by a period of increasing tolerance to stimulation and strength and endurance of muscle contraction. Specific muscle strengthening may also be a goal of electrical stimulation.[55]

Pickup walkers with front wheels provide balance assistance for household mobility. The addition of weight (lead BB's in the walker legs) provides additional stability for ataxic children. Helmets are generally recommended for all ambulatory children lacking protective balance reactions sufficient for safety. Ankle-foot orthoses, besides controlling hypertonicity, may provide additional stability for ataxic children. Weights added to shoes may also improve control and stability. Bathroom equipment may include strategically placed grab bars to assist balance during transfers. A towel or nonskid stickers on the floor of the tub may assist with safety in sitting and transfers; bath loungers may be necessary if balance reactions in sitting are poor.

Reintegration of the child into the school setting requires ongoing coordination with teachers and school therapists. Sensorimotor integration deficits not apparent initially may manifest later when the child appears clumsy in certain playground activities. Observing the child performing the activity and determining the motor and sensorimotor integration skills necessary for smooth completion of the task permits identification of the residual deficits. Baum, finding a significant relationship between dressing ability scores and three constructional praxis scores, concluded that a portion of the patient's inability to dress was perceptual rather than motor in nature.[61] Activities to encourage development of missing skills and suggestions for modifying activities to compensate for deficits permit continued motor control improvement while promoting good self-esteem through peer interaction.

Inefficient Cardiopulmonary System

In the acutely ill patient, chest physical therapy assists in preventing the complications of atelectasis and pneumonia. Positioning, bronchial drainage, and manual techniques of percussion and vibration assist in mobilizing secretions and increase airflow to the dependent lung.[40,43] Becker and colleagues[62] report reduced values for vital capacity, inspiratory capacity, total lung capacity, and forced expiratory volume at 1 second in young adult head-injured patients when compared to normals. Less efficient circulatory and ventilatory responses to exercise among the head-injured group were identified. They suggest the inefficiencies may be inherent to brainstem disturbances, resulting in deficient automatic motor performances, which contribute to development of secondary deconditioning.

Inadequate Orofacial Control

The major problems interfering with feeding are cognition, hypo- and/or hypersensitivity to stimulation, level of consciousness, and poor head and trunk control. Although voluntary initiation and modification of orofacial motor control is lacking, most children, even at Levels III and IV, demonstrate the rhythmical transient or phasic jaw closing and opening reflexes, the tonic opening reflex, and the repeating-tongue-movement reflex followed by reflex swallow described by Campbell.[63] These rhythmic oral motor patterns follow a yawn, oral stimulation, and at times noxious tactile stimulation as a generalized response to stimulation. Although the rooting reflex and pursing reflex may be elicited, generally these do not interfere with feeding and tend to be inhibited after three or four repetitions of stimulation.

Perioral and intraoral hypersensitivity resulting in a tonic bite and a gag will interfere with jaw opening to get food into the mouth and the swallow reflex, respectively. Techniques of desensitization, such as firm pressure on the lips, firm stroking of the gums, and firm stroking and pressure with a toothette or tongue blade intraorally and on the tongue assist inhibiting these responses. Desensitization may be necessary preceding each feeding session.

Hyposensitivity, often seen with prolonged nasogastric tube feeding, will modify the rhythmic oral motor patterns such that the rhythmic tongue movement may cease before the bolus reaches the pharynx, the reflex swallow may be delayed, and laryngeal excursion may be incomplete. Considering that the central pattern generator may exist in the brainstem reticular formation,[63] sensitization techniques such as quick stroking periorally and intraorally prior to feeding, which also tend to increase the alertness of the patient, may be affecting the rhythmic motor reflexes through affecting the general excitatory status of the reticular activating system.

The brief alert periods and short attention span of the patient are most limiting to actual feeding as the motor reflexes are elicited for only short periods of time. Generally, the amount of time the child is alert is insufficient to maintain nutritional status through oral feeding. The lack of fine motor control necessary to swallow liquids without aspiration (possibly due to hyposensitivity) precludes safe and sufficient oral liquid intake.

Head and trunk control affect orofacial control in three ways. The alignment of the structures of the oropharynx and larynx affect the speed and ease of the flow of liquids and food and therefore the needed motor control to facilitate or control the food. The strength and endurance of neck and trunk musculature, as well as oral musculature, affect the energy cost of this simple activity and therefore the length of time the child can sustain it. The status of the central nervous system which accounts for hypertonicity or hypotonicity of the musculature may influence the central control mechanism if one accepts the hypotheses that the central pattern generator can be influenced by voluntary commands from higher centers, by sensory information from the oral cavity and from the muscles, and by the state of the central nervous system.[63] Techniques of facilitation and inhibition, such as positioning of head, trunk and extremities, manual jaw and lip control, and quick stretch, ice and resistive exercises to lips, larynx, orofacial and neck musculature, appear to improve motor control in response to sensory input. Whether voluntary control, increased muscular strength and endurance, a change in acuity or threshold of peripheral sensory endings, or the neurophysiologic changes of the state of the central nervous system account for improved motor control, few children lack sufficient recovery for oral feeding.

Initiation of feeding may occur earlier than one might expect. Winstein and colleagues[52] list six indications for initiation of feeding: (1) adequate cognition, (2) adequate intraoral manipulation, (3) adequate laryngeal elevation observed with reflex swallow after administration of small amount of water, (4) presence of gag or weak posterior pharyngeal wall motion, (5) no active respiratory problem, and (6) no evidence of aspiration.

Active respiratory problems or a nonfunctional cough after or during swallowing may indicate aspiration. In the presence of a tracheostomy, suctioning after feeding with a small amount of dye-containing substance will verify the presence or absence of aspiration. If there is no tracheostomy, a functional reflex cough cannot be elicited, and laryngeal control is questionable, a swallowing fluoroscopy is recommended to determine if aspiration is occurring. (*Note:* If a swallowing fluoroscopy is necessary, the therapist must consider positioning, facilitation, and inhibition techniques, and the consistency of the substance swallowed for a true assessment of aspiration to be expected during therapeutic feeding. A fluoroscopy of a low level patient, in supine with hyperextended neck, swallowing a liquid substance will most likely demonstrate aspiration, but is not a true representation of control expected in the therapeutic setting.)

When initiating a feeding trial, head and trunk positioning and handling techniques will modify the motor control. The consistency of food and viscosity of liquids are modified according to the motor control and endurance of the musculature. Pureed foods over the middle part of the tongue will elicit the reflex repeating-tongue-movement, which leads to a swallow. Soft foods of a thicker consistency require greater endurance of intraoral musculature. Ground foods provide a greater variety of sensory input and require a greater variety of tongue control to gather the pieces into a bolus, but they often stimulate this activity and may be handled better. A regular diet requires tongue lateralization and control of jaw motion for chewing. Progression of diet follows evaluation of motor control and muscular endurance and must consider age expectations. Considerations in choice of foods include hypersensitivity to taste, often present initially, cultural preferences (even a taco can be pureed in a blender), and the tendency of dairy products to increase secretions.

Liquids are the most difficult to swallow as they may pass quickly through the oropharyngeal passages providing little sensory stimulation to elicit adequate motor control. Thickening liquids with gelatin or cereal may increase the viscosity sufficiently to permit adequate motor control. Proper hydration often requires continued nasogastric tube feedings. The increased sensory stimulation of carbonated beverages may facilitate adequate motor control to prevent aspiration. (The advisability of hydration through carbonated beverages must be discussed with the physician, but do not be surprised to find Johnny easily downing Coca Cola during a visit with Mom and Dad and yet aspirating on milk for dinner.) Once a child can complete a meal in 30 minutes without aspiration, family members and/or nursing staff are instructed on proper positioning and simple facilitation techniques. Progressing the child to completing three meals a day orally may initially require supplemental feedings through a nasogastric tube.

Cognition and behavior often interfere with self-feeding even after adequate orofacial motor control and endurance are achieved. A short attention span and absent memory result in distractibility and confusion. The child may forget to swallow and be attending to other stimuli, but when reminded to swallow and redirected to the eating activity, can complete a meal. The confused child does not know that you drink from a cup and may put it on his head. The child may continually stuff food into the mouth, apparently forgetting that food has just been put into the mouth, and also forgetting to swallow. (A more highly textured diet may facilitate automatic reactions.) Supervision and structure initiated by the therapist may be carried through by the family or nurses to remind the child to swallow after each bite, not allow scooping more food from the plate before swallowing, and to structure him or her not to use the spoon when "eating" the milk or try to drink from the plate. If initiation and sequencing are a problem, appropriate assistance and supervision are provided. If upper extremity motor control does not preclude self-feeding, once a child reaches Level II, initiating purposeful activities, necessary supervision, and assistance to permit successful self-feeding are preferred over passive feeding of the patient. Although one meal may take an hour to complete, self-feeding for at least one and preferably two meals is encouraged.

PARENT/CLIENT EDUCATION

Education of the parents during the acute and inhospital rehabilitation phases of recovery involves the whole team. By the time of discharge, the parents must have accepted the role of primary therapist in all aspects of the child's behavior. The parents must implement the child's reintegration into society, the ultimate goal of rehabilitation. They must recognize the child's abilities and understand his or her disabilities, structuring the day and activities to meet the child's needs and eventually to nurture independence. They must accommodate this child while continuing their own lives and caring for other family members.

Education of the family during the acute stage includes understanding the significance of the trauma and the prognosis expected. The inability of the neurosurgeon to accurately predict outcome 100 percent of the time adds to the confusion. The stages of grieving the family experiences often preclude actual hearing and understanding of explanations. Education of the need for intensive care of the child is ongoing.

As the level of consciousness improves, hope is nurtured. Unrealistic expectations of recovery may interfere with understanding the need for therapeutic intervention and family education. Following evaluation of the child by each team member, a conference is held for team members and the child's parents. Each team member identifies his or her role in rehabilitation, the abilities and problems the child has at present, and the expected abilities at discharge from the hospital. Team members must explain the child's problems and reasons for expected discharge abilities (which are less than normal function) so that the family can begin to understand problems that will remain and become involved in the rehabilitation program.

Family educational programs involving a few families, mediated by a social worker or psychologist, provide education and interaction with the child's therapists as well as supportive therapy from other families experiencing similar feelings and problems. Minislide presentations and discussions by each team member convey the role of that discipline in the child's rehabilitation, demonstrate the usual progression of improvement, and therapeutic activities the child will experience, as well as defining terms commonly used to identify cognitive problems and behaviors.

Although most families of young children have working parents, they are encouraged to spend an occasional day attending the child's therapy sessions. Nursing staff provide most of the ongoing education when the parents visit in the evenings. Assistance and supervision in play, self-care, and transfers is encouraged early in preparation for home therapeutic passes.

Home therapeutic passes usually begin when the child is eating, although training parents in nasogastric tube or gastric tube feeding would permit earlier passes. Assistance and supervision in play, feeding, self-care, and mobility are practiced at home and updated weekly. Structural barriers and safety hazards are identified and solutions explored immediately to facilitate the discharge process.

As discharge approaches and adaptive equipment needs are identified, the family participates in choosing adaptive equipment and determining acceptable methods of mobility in order to assure carryover. By the time of discharge the family understands the child's needs and is able to assist and progress his or her activities.

Follow-up as an outpatient usually is through clinic visits. Evaluation of neurologic recovery and improvement in play, socialization, speech, feeding, and mobility provides team members with information for further intervention and appropriate referrals to outside agencies or staff team members. As the child matures into an adult, needs change and residual problems affect him or her in different ways. Continued follow-up assures continued family and child education to facilitate reintegration into society. Referral to appropriate community resources such as special schools, school therapy units, vocational training centers, driver's training centers, health professionals, the National Head Injury Foundation (18A Vernon St., Framingham, MA 0l707) and other nonprofit organizations assists in meeting the needs of the family and client.

OTHER MANAGEMENT

The members of the rehabilitation team include a pediatrician, psychologist, social worker, nurses, occupational therapist, and speech therapist, with consultation by orthopedic surgeons, neurologists, and neurosurgeons. The roles of the health team members vary according to the centers, the team members available, and the strengths of the staff. I will briefly highlight the management characteristic of each professional at our center.

The speech pathologist assesses and treats the cognitive and language deficits; controlling the amount and complexity of stimuli and the rate and duration of presentation, the speech pathologist assists the child to relearn the process of organizing, integrating, and expressing thoughts. Increasing attention, concentration, visual discrimination, sequencing, categorization, memory, and orientation to time, self, and place are emphasized at Level II. At Level I therapeutic activities encourage the development of skills in analysis and synthesis, judgment, problem solving, reasoning, and abstract thinking. Specific speech production problems are evaluated and treated.[10] The higher cognitive functions of decision-making, judgment, and problem solving are usually not expected to recover by discharge and require constant supervision to assure the child's safety. Review of what the child should do if he or she wants to cross a street and observation of performance in actual community situations assess the child's ability and identify deficits.

Linguistic function, auditory and visual reception and retention, language formulation, and expression are tested. Relearning of reading, spelling, writing, and gestural communication skills are initiated in the rehabilitation hospital and continued in the school setting.

The child's common behaviors during recovery, such as lack of cooperativeness, poor self-initiation, low frustration tolerance, exaggerated response to stress, emotional lability, and tendency to aggressiveness may result from cognitive deficits in memory and concentration. Social workers, psychologists, and psychiatrists may provide family counseling to deal with residual hyperactivity, lack of impulse control, low tolerance for frustration, aggressiveness, and poor social judgment.[18] Enuresis may signify a return to dependence.[64] Psychologic testing identifies significant slowing of response, reduction in performance IQ compared to the preinjury state, and difficulty with auditory and visual perception, all of which markedly limit school performance.[1] Only 30 percent in a series of 300 severely head-injured children had normal intelligence, however 64 percent can benefit from an educational program. Psychologic testing prior to discharge assists with school placement.[2,18]

Social worker intervention with the families varies with the child's level of consciousness. Assessment of the family support system facilitates assisting family adjustment. Through individual and group mediums, initial intervention assists the family to cope with the devastating disruption to their lifestyle and the issue of life or death. Education on the rehabilitation process and the family's coping strategies attempts to shift them to coping day to day rather than trying to prepare for the long term. As the child recovers, the family responds on an emotional roller coaster of highs as the child lives, wakes up, and progresses—and lows as progress hits plateaus and residual physical, cognitive, and psychologic deficits, and behavioral changes are compared with preinjury identity. The social worker assists the families to deal with their feelings, anxieties, frustrations, and depression in considering the child's reentry to home and the resultant threat to their lifestyle and marriage. As discharge approaches, families are informed of financial, school, mental health, regional center, and voluntary agency resources. The social worker and psychologist also assist other team members in coping with the family's and child's behaviors.[65] Outpatient intervention assists the family and child in dealing with the child's inappropriate social behavior, social isolation, peer rejection, and low self-esteem to assist reintegration into society.

A nurse specializing in assisting the return to school coordinates the necessary testing and referrals to smooth the transition. As a liaison to the community, the nurse confers with the team members to identify proper school placement where appropriate therapy and educational needs can be met.

Occupational therapists and physical therapists work closely together. The occupational therapist emphasizes fine motor, self-care, and perceptual skills. Age-appropriate socialization and play skills are encouraged within the child's physical abilities. Social and play development, perceptual motor development, and daily living skills at home and in the community are delayed after a head injury. Activities and intervention to develop these skills to age-appropriate levels are continued in outpatient follow-up and therapy at school. Disabilities in these areas contribute to peer rejection, isolation, and poor self-esteem.

REFERENCES

1. Raphaely RC, Swedlow DB, Downes JJ, et al: Management of severe pediatric head trauma. Pediatr Clin North Am 27:715, 1980.
2. Brink JD, Garrett AL, Hale WR, et al: Recovery of motor and intellectual functions in children sustaining severe head injuries. Dev Med Child Neurol 12:565, 1972.
3. Bruce DA, Schut L, et al: Outcome following severe head injuries in children. J Neurosurg 48:679, 1978.
4. Cartlidge NEF, Shaw DA: Head Injury. In Walton Sir JN (ed): Major Problems in Neurology, Vol 10. Saunders, Philadelphia, 1981.
5. Mayer T, Walker ML, Johnson DG, et al: Causes of morbidity and mortality in severe pediatric trauma. JAMA 245:719, 1981.

6. Gilchrist E, Wilkinson M: Some factors determining prognosis in young people with severe head injuries. Arch Neurol 36:355, 1979.
7. Jennett B: Head injuries in children. Dev Med Child Neurol 14:137, 1972.
8. Ommaya AK: Head injuries: aspects and problems. Med Ann DC 32:18, 1963.
9. Carlsson C-A, von Essen C, Löfgren J: Factors affecting the clinical course of patients with severe head injuries. J. Neurosurg 29:242, 1968.
10. St. James-Roberts J: Neurological plasticity, recovery from brain insult, and child development. Adv Child Dev Behav 14:253, 1979.
11. Hardman JM: The pathology of traumatic brain injuries. Adv Neurol 22:15, 1979.
12. Bruce DA, Schut L: The value of CAT scanning following pediatric head injury. Clin Pediatr (Phila) 19:719, 1980.
13. Brink JD, Imbus C, Woo-Sam J: Physical recovery after severe closed head trauma in children and adolescents. J Pediatr 97:721, 1980.
14. Morley TP: Some considerations of head injury. Postgrad Med 22:53, 1957.
15. Ommaya AK: Trauma to the nervous system. Ann R Coll Surg Engl 39:317, 1966.
16. Lewin W: Head injuries in children. In The Management of Head Injuries. Williams and Wilkins, Baltimore, 1966.
17. Shetter AG, Demakas JJ: The pathophysiology of concussion: A review. Adv Neurol 22:5, 1979.
18. Hoffer M, Brink J, Marsh JS, et al: Head injuries. In: Lovell WW, Winter RB (eds): Pediatric Orthopaedics. Lippincott, Philadelphia, 1978.
19. Clifton GL, McCormick WF, Grossman RG: Neuropathology of early and late deaths after head injury. Neurosurgery 8:309, 1981.
20. Bruce DA, Alavi A, Bilaniuk L, et al: Diffuse cerebral swelling following head injuries in children: The syndrome of "malignant brain edema." J Neurosurg 54:170, 1981.
21. Miller JD, Butterworth JF, Gudeman SK, et al: Further experience in the management of severe head injury. J Neurosurg 54:289, 1981.
22. Greenberg RP, Stablein DM, Becker DP: Noninvasive localization of brain-stem lesions in the cat with multimodality evoked potentials, J Neurosurg 54:740, 1981.
23. Teasdale G, Jennett B: Assessment of coma and impaired consciousness. Lancet 2:81, 1974.
24. Narayan RK, Greenberg RP, Miller JD, et al: Improved confidence of outcome prediction in severe head injury. A comparative analysis of the clinical examination, multimodality evoked potentials, CT scanning and intracranial pressure. J Neurosurg 54:751, 1981.
25. Greenberg RP, Becker DP, Miller JD, et al: Evaluation of brain function in severe human head trauma with multi-modality evoked potentials. Part 2: Localization of brain dysfunction and correlation with posttraumatic neurological conditions. J Neurosurg 47:163, 1977.
26. Greenberg RP, Mayer DJ, Becker DP, et al: Evaluation of brain function in severe human head trauma with multimodality evoked potentials. Part I: Evoked brain injury potentials, methods, and analysis. J Neurosurg 47:150, 1977.
27. Greenberg RP, Newlon PG, Hyatt MS, et al: Prognostic implications of early multimodality evoked potentials in severely head-injured patients: A prospective study. J Neurosurg 55:227, 1981.
28. Tsubokawa T, et al: Assessment of brainstem damage by the auditory brainstem response in acute severe head injury. J Neurol Neurosurg Psychiatry 43:1005, 1980.
29. Chiappa KH, Gladstone KJ, Young RR: Brain stem auditory evoked responses. Arch Neurol 36:81, 1979.

30. Mayer T, Walker ML, Shasha I, et al: Effect of multiple trauma on outcome of pediatric patients with neurologic injuries. Child Brain 8(3):189, 1981.

31. Brink JD, Hoffer MM: Rehabilitation of brain injured children. Orthop Clin North Am 9(2):451, 1978.

32. Meyler WJ, Bakker H, Kok JJ, et al: The effect of dantrolene sodium in relation to blood levels in spastic patients after prolonged administration. J Neurol Neurosurg Psychiatry 44:334, 1981.

33. Hoffer MM, Brink JD: Orthopedic management of acquired cerebral spasticity in childhood. Clin Orthop 110:244, 1975.

34. Jennett B, Snoek J, Bond MR, et al: Disability after severe head injury: observations on the use of Glasgow Outcome Scale. J Neurol Neurosurg Psychiatry 44:285, 1981.

35. Jennett B, Bond M: Assessment of outcome after severe brain damage. A practical scale. Lancet 1:480, 1975.

36. Young B, Rapp RP, Norton JA, et al: Early prediction of outcome in head-injured patients. J Neurosurg 54:300, 1981.

37. Mayer T, Matlak ME, Johnson DG, Walker ML: The modified injury severity scale in pediatric multiple trauma patients. J Pediatr Surg 15:719, 1980.

38. Guentz S: Rehabilitation nursing techniques. In Professional Staff Associates of Rancho Los Amigos Hospital: Rehabilitation of the Head Injured Adult: Comprehensive Physical Management. Downey CA, 1979.

39. Lance JW: The control of muscle tone, reflexes and movement: Robert Wartenberg Lecture. Neurology 30:1303, 1980.

40. Carr JH, Shepherd, RB: Physiotherapy in Disorders of the Brain. Heinemann, London, 1980.

41. Kigin CM: Chest physical therapy for the postoperative or traumatic injury patient. Phys Ther 61:1724, 1981.

42. Ciesla N, Klemic N, Imle PC: Chest physical therapy to the patient with multiple trauma. Phys Ther 61:202, 1981.

43. Hammon WE, Martin RJ: Chest physical therapy for acute atelectasis. Phys Ther 61:217, 1981.

44. Robinson RO: Equal recovery in child and adult brain? Dev Med Child Neurol 23:379, 1981.

45. Bishop DVM: Plasticity and specificity of language localization in the developing brain. Dev Med Child Neurol 23:251, 1981.

46. Robinson RO: Plasticity and specificity of language localization in the developing brain. Dev Med Child Neurol 23:387, 1981.

47. Winstein C: Evaluation and management of swallowing dysfunction. In Professional Staff Associates of Rancho Los Amigos Hospital: Rehabilitation of the Head Injured Adult: Comprehensive Physical Management. Downey CA, 1979.

48. Goldman PM: Plasticity of function in the CNS. In Stein DG, Rosen JJ, Butters N (eds): Plasticity and Recovery of Function in the CNS. Academic Press, New York, 1974.

49. Geschwind N: Late changes in the nervous system: An overview. In Stein DG, Rosen JJ, Butters N (eds): Plasticity and Recovery of Function in the CNS. Academic Press, New York, 1974.

50. Garland D (ed): Head Trauma: Comprehensive Rehabilitation. Butterworth, London, in press.

51. Stichbury JC, Davenport MJ, Middleton FR: Head injured patients: A combined therapeutic approach. Physiotherapy 66:288, 1980.

52. Winstein C, Thompson S, Briggs D, et al: Treatment techniques of gaining motor control. In Professional Staff Association of Rancho Los Amigos Hospital: Re-

habilitation of the Head Injured Adult: Comprehensive Physical Management. Downey CA, 1979.

53. Hoffer MM, Garrett A, Brink JD, et al: The orthopedic management of the brain-injured children. J Bone Joint Surg 53A:567, 1971.
54. Zachazewski JE, Eberle ED, Jefferies M: Effect of tone-inhibiting casts and orthoses on gait. Phys Ther 62:453, 1982.
55. Benton LA, Baker LL, Bowman BR, et al: General uses of electrical stimulation. In Professional Staff Associates of Rancho Los Amigos Hospital: Functional Electrical Stimulation Workshop, Downey CA, 1979.
56. Bobath K, Bobath B: The facilitation of normal postural reactions and movements in the treatment of cerebral palsy. Physiotherapy 50:246, 1964.
57. Goldberger ME: Recovery of movements after CNS lesions in monkeys. In Stein DG, Rosen JJ, Butters N (eds): Plasticity and Recovery of Function in the CNS. Academic Press, New York, 1974.
58. Nelson JR: Neuro-otologic aspects of head injury. Adv Neurol 22:107, 1979.
59. Safranek MG, Koshland GF, Raymond G: Effect of auditory rhythm on muscle activity. Phys Ther 62:161, 1982.
60. Couper, JL: Dance therapy: Effects on motor performance of children with learning disabilities. Phys Ther 61:23, 1981.
61. Baum B, Hall KM: Relationship between constructional praxis and dressing in the head-injured adult. Am J Occup Ther 35:438, 1981.
62. Becker E, Bar-Or O, Mendelson L, et al: Pulmonary functions and responses to exercise of patients following craniocerebral injury. Scand J Rehabil Med 10:47, 1978.
63. Campbell SK: Neural control of oral somatic motor function. Phys Ther 61:16, 1981.
64. Dillon H, Leopold R: Children and the post-concussion syndrome. JAMA 175(2):110, 1961.
65. Oddy M, Humphrey M: Social recovery during the year following severe head injury. J Neurol Neurosurg Psychiatry 43:798, 1980

9 | Severely and Profoundly Retarded Children

Karen Yundt Lunnen

There is increasing recognition that retarded individuals are more like us than they are different; that they need, just as we all do, love, joy, activity, a chance to grow and progress, and a chance, wherever possible, to become independent.[1]   Senator Hubert H. Humphrey

The most widely accepted definition of mental retardation is that adopted by the American Association on Mental Deficiency (AAMD): "... significantly subaverage intellectual functioning existing concurrently with deficits in adaptive behavior and manifested during the developmental period" (usually interpreted as being from birth until the eighteenth birthday).[2] Put in another way, retardation is the result of conditions that prevent, reduce, or delay the development of effective ways of interacting with the environment.

CLASSIFICATION OF MENTAL RETARDATION

There is considerable controversy about the classification of mentally retarded individuals, the validity of the intelligence quotient (IQ), and the effects of labeling. However, despite its difficulties, "classification of exceptional children is essential to get services to them."[3] The definition adopted by AAMD at least dictated that classification be based on intelligence *and* adaptive behavior, thus expanding the concept of mental retardation to include more than just intellectual functioning.

Table 9-1. Intellectual Classification Based on Standardized Test Scores

Level of Retardation	Number of Standard Deviations Below Mean	Quotient Range	
		Stanford-Binet	Wechsler
Mild	2–3	52–68	55–69
Moderate	3–4	36–51	40–54
Severe	4–5	20–35	25–39
Profound	<5	≤19	≤24

Intellectual classification is based on a quotient determined by standardized testing (usually Stanford-Binet, Bayley, or Wechsler Scales). Those scoring below 70 are classified as mentally retarded, with subgroupings of increasing severity established at increments of standard deviation units below the normative mean of 100 (1 standard deviation being 15 or 16 points, depending on the test). Table 9-1 presents the usual classification system.

The AAMD has provided general guidelines for the adaptive behavior classification and many adaptive behavior rating scales are in print. The appropriateness of any behavior, of course, varies with age. Table 9-2 presents a summary of an adaptive behavior classification based on the AAMD's expanded definition of mental retardation.[2]

One could legitimately question the validity of these two systems for categorization of mentally retarded individuals. Roszlowski and Spreat[4] found a "strong degree of relationship" (contingency coefficient of 0.77) between psychometric and clinical classificatory systems. However, for 35 percent of subjects the two classifications were discrepant—most often the clinical classification indicated less impairment than the intelligence quotient.

The distribution of IQ's is basically a normal curve, but with slightly increased frequencies at the lower end, representing a greater number of the very severely retarded.[5] Only 11 percent of the mentally retarded population or 0.3 percent of the total population are in the moderate, severe, and profound ranges.[6] Conley[7] estimates that the percentage of severely impaired infants at birth is as high as 1.3 to 2 percent, but that as many as 9 out of 10 with an IQ less than 25 and 1 in 2 with an IQ between 25 and 50 die within the first 5 years of life, most within the first year.

Table 9-2. Adaptive Behavior Classification[a]

Mild:	Children usually can master basic academic skills. (Educable). Adults, with training, can work in competitive employment and maintain themselves independently or semi-independently in the community.
Moderate:	Such persons usually can learn self-help, communication, social and simple occupational skills, but only limited academic or vocational skills. (Trainable).
Severe:	Such persons require continuing and close supervision, but may perform self-help and simple work tasks under supervision. (Dependent).
Profound:	Such persons require continuing and close supervision for survival, but some may be able to perform simple self-help tasks. Often have associated handicaps.

[a] Summarized from the expanded definition of mental retardation of the American Association of Mental Deficiency. (See Ref. 2.)

The Association for Retarded Citizens published estimates of retardation by age and degree in 1979.[8] The severely and profoundly retarded population totals about 330,000.

ETIOLOGY AND PATHOLOGY OF MENTAL RETARDATION

Known, discrete causes of mental retardation are found in only a small percentage of cases, although significantly more of the children with IQ's less than 50 have an identifiable etiology than those with higher IQ's. Treatment strategies are seldom dependent on etiology, and etiology is notably absent from the AAMD definition of mental retardation, but it can be important for genetic counseling aimed at prevention of future cases.

In a study of severely mentally retarded children, Gustavson and associates[9] reported that mean gestational age and birth weights were lower than in average newborns. They also determined that at this level of mental retardation, the insult occurred prenatally in 69 percent, perinatally in 8 percent, postnatally in 1 percent, and at an unknown age in 22 percent. Dale and Stanley[10] found that decreased neonatal mortality among low birth weight infants in Western Australia coincided with an increase of spastic cerebral palsy in surviving infants, despite an overall decrease in the incidence of cerebral palsy.

Intelligence is a polygenic phenomenon; in other words, at least 10 pairs of genes, and probably more, determine intelligence. With severe and profound levels of retardation, there are almost always diffuse brain abnormalities. One study reported autopsies conducted on 1410 severely and profoundly mentally retarded individuals over a 14-year period and found that 97.5 percent had neurologic damage.[11] The abnormalities of the central nervous system may be congenital or acquired, and causes may be genetic, degenerative, hypoxic, traumatic, or endocrinologic.

Since retardation represents a diffuse neurologic insult, most children who are severely or profoundly retarded also have serious physical handicaps. Conley[7] states that almost 95 percent of individuals with IQ's less than 30 and almost 78 percent of those individuals with IQ's between 30 and 55 suffer from at least one major physically handicapping condition. Among the severely and profoundly retarded, the handicaps are proportionately more common and more severe.[12] Capute and associates[6] examined the major presenting symptoms of mentally retarded children at a nonresidential facility and found them to be (1) overall slowness, (2) motor disability, (3) language disorder, and (4) behavioral disturbances.

Although there are classes of mentally retarded children in which there is no stunting of linear or skeletal development, this condition is rather common among the retarded, particularly among the lower levels of retardates. The degree of stunting is roughly proportional to the degree of IQ deficit.[13]

Weisz and Zigler[14] have summarized the theories about the development of retarded individuals compared to normal (based on Piagetian concepts) and developed the "similar sequence hypothesis." The hypothesis holds that "during development retarded and nonretarded persons traverse the same stages in precisely the same order and differ only in the rate of development and in the ultimate ceiling they attain."[14] Some theorists believe that the hypothesis is valid only for nonretarded and cultural-familial retarded persons, thus, in essence, proposing a different sequence of cognitive development for severely and profoundly retarded individuals who may have brain damage or genetic impairment. Weisz and Zigler,[14] however, drew evidence from 3 longitudinal and 28 cross-sectional studies of developmental phenomena described by Piaget, and found that the evidence supported their hypothesis with respect to every subject group, with the "possible exception of individuals with pronounced electroencephalogram abnormalities."

Severely and profoundly retarded children reach an ultimate mental age of less than 6 years, which means they will always need supervision, and because of associated handicaps, they seldom achieve independence in activities of daily living.

SOCIAL POLICIES AND PROGRAMS

Public awareness, political support, and legal action are important for progress in the management of mental retardation. A historical perspective on these issues is necessary to understand the direction of current programs for the mentally retarded. Two informative publications are the 1977 report of the President's Committee on Mental Retardation, entitled *Mental Retardation: Past and Present*,[15] and Rosen's *The History of Mental Retardation* (Volumes I and II).[16] From 1956 to 1961 federal support for mental retardation services and research increased from $14 million to $94 million.[17] President Kennedy's appointment in 1962 of a panel of experts to make recommendations for national action to combat mental retardation was the beginning of new social and political awareness that resulted in a dramatic surge in activity related to treatment, research, education, and legal action.

The so-called normalization movement of the 1970s was a concerted attempt to end the segregation of mentally retarded individuals in large state institutions and had its roots in political, social, and legal activities. The push was for community-based programs that allowed individualized attention for handicapped persons and access to services that allowed "longitudinal, comprehensive, systematic and chronological age appropriate interactions with persons without identified handicaps."[18] Special education programs were among the recommendations of President Kennedy's panel in 1963. But more dramatic in its impact and the legal direction it provided was "The Education for All Handicapped Children Act of 1975" (Public Law 94-142), signed into law by President Gerald R. Ford.[19]

There are four major purposes of Public Law 94-142[20]:

1. Guarantee the availability of special education programming to handicapped children and youth who require it
2. Assure fairness and appropriateness in decision-making about providing special education to handicapped children and youth
3. Establish clear management and auditing requirements and procedures regarding special education at all levels of government
4. Financially assist the efforts of state and local government through the use of federal funds

The basic civil rights provision with respect to terminating discrimination against America's handicapped citizens was passed in 1973 as part of the Vocational Rehabilitation Act amendments.[21] The rights of the mentally retarded are being tested in the country's legal system by a tremendous number of legal suits. Landmark decisions in the 1970s guaranteed the right to education, the right to treatment, and the right to be free from institutional peonage and involuntary servitude. Mental retardation was the "civil rights movement of the decade."[22] Publications available from the United States Government Printing Office and the Council for Exceptional Children provide interesting documentation of the legal issues in mental retardation.[23,24] Herr[25] optimistically predicts that the 1980s will see an international effort to turn "broad rights into realities" for disabled people, *if* legal advocacy services are strengthened.

There are many groups, both governmental and nongovernmental, that have a significant impact on the population of mentally retarded citizens in the United States. Several deserve mention as they can provide valuable resources for professionals:

Association for Retarded Citizens (National Headquarters, P.O. Box 6109, Arlington, TX 76011): The largest national voluntary health organization, comprised of over 300,000 parents, educators, and professionals (organized in 1950). Influential as a political lobby group for public policy issues.

American Association on Mental Deficiency (5101 Wisconsin Avenue, NW, Suite 405, Washington, DC 20016): A multidisciplinary organization of professional practitioners and researchers. Responsible for the publication of the research journal, *American Journal of Mental Deficiency*; the applied research and public opinion journal, *Mental Retardation*; the *AAMD Monograph Series*; and the *Manual on Terminology and Classification in Mental Retardation*.

Council for Exceptional Children (1920 Association Drive, Reston, VA 22091): Comprised of about 70,000 teachers. Has made significant contributions to the education of the mentally retarded.

President's Committee on Mental Retardation (U.S. Department of Health and Human Services, Washington, DC 20201): Established by executive order in May, 1966 with a mandated function of providing assistance and advice concerning mental retardation to the President and the Secretary of Health and Human Services. Reports are submitted to the

President annually and are available to the public. (Twenty-one citizen members and six ex-officio members appointed by the President.)

Joseph P. Kennedy Foundation (1701 K Street NW, Suite 205, Washington, DC 20006): A private foundation that has provided funding for a wide range of programs, including the Special Olympic Games.

Prevention and the application of research to the development of public policy are two additional issues requiring concerted action. Prevention has been a major goal of the President's Committee on Mental Retardation.[26] Many authorities believe that the incidence of mental retardation could be reduced by half if all of the existing medical and scientific knowledge could be effectively applied. This goal may be overly optimistic, but research has enabled more effective treatment for some of the following causes of mental retardation: (1) Rh-factor incompatibility, (2) inborn errors of metabolism such as phenylketonuria, galactosemia, and hypothyroidism, (3) lead poisoning, (4) rubella, and (5) hydrocephalus and craniosynostosis. All members of the medical team must accept responsibility for the provision of good prenatal care for mothers, genetic screening and counseling, and the management and follow-up of high-risk infants. Although economics is certainly only one aspect of prevention, it is interesting to note that for each case of severe retardation averted in a male, the undiscounted gain to society is almost $900,000 (1970 dollars).[7]

Support for research has been a major thrust of government and privately sponsored programs. Two excellent resources that provide a review of the advances in applied behavioral and biomedical research are an issue of the *American Journal of Mental Deficiency* (Vol. 77, No. 5, 1973) devoted entirely to this subject, and a 1981 article by Schroeder and Schroeder that updates this information.[22] Some of the problems with the research effort are addressed by Baumeister.[27] It is his opinion that despite considerable support over the past two decades, the impact of research on policy has not been marked. He believes that the nature of the process is such that research is secondary to economic, political, and social considerations and that the research enterprise is fragmented and uncoordinated.

MEDICAL MANAGEMENT

Care for the health of severely and profoundly retarded individuals has been less than optimal. It is more a matter of neglect than abuse—a laissez-faire attitude. Indeed, if one uses a functional definition of health, it is often hard to diagnose poor health among the severely handicapped, and difficult to judge whether a specific treatment will improve the quality of life for these individuals. Particularly for the institutionalized mentally retarded, however, medical management has been "marginal."[28]

Orthopedic Surgery

Because of the high incidence of physical handicaps among the severely and profoundly retarded, orthopedic surgery is often a consideration in their management. A recent volume of *Orthopedic Clinics in North America* (Vol.

12, No. 1, January, 1981) was devoted entirely to the subject of orthopedic surgery in the mentally retarded. The question arises, however, whether the potential benefits are worth the risks. Hoffer and Bullock[29] estimate that the length of hospital stay for the severely mentally retarded is two to four times longer than normal, and the rehabilitation period is complicated by the patient's inability to comprehend what has occurred or to cooperate maximally.

Pettitt[30] listed what she believed to be the legitimate reasons for considering surgery for the severely mentally retarded: (1) alleviation of pain, (2) improvement of posture for wheelchair mobilization, and (3) increased ease of nursing care. Lindsey and Drennan[31] would add to that list the achievement or maintenance of ambulation.

Drug Therapy

The use of medication to moderate or alter behavior, to control seizure activity, and to manage a wide variety of concurrent medical problems is often a necessity in this population, but the drugs are powerful and the side effects marked. One of the most alarming discoveries from close scrutiny of the quality of life among the mentally retarded was the widespread use of powerful neuroleptic drugs, primarily to suppress undesirable or aversive behavior. In New Zealand, Pulman and colleagues[32] assessed the prevalence of drug use among institutionalized mentally retarded individuals and found that 60 percent of the total were on some type of drug therapy, and 40 percent were on psychotropic drugs specifically. Lipman[33] estimates that more than 100,000 mentally retarded individuals are on neuroleptic drugs in the United States, and that more than 50 percent have been on them for more than two years. The most commonly prescribed are chlorpromazine and thioridazine. A disturbing side effect of neuroleptic drugs is tardive dyskinesia.[34]

Neuroleptic drugs control behavior by general sedation and tranquilization, but Nyhan and associates[35] took a more definitive approach to controlling aversive behavior. They attempted to alter pharmacologically the balance of biogenic amines in the central nervous system and thereby alter the self-mutilative behavior typically seen in patients with Lesch-Nyhan syndrome. The initial results were dramatically successful, although unfortunately the subjects developed a tolerance for the drug, which negated its long-term effectiveness. Research of this type gives hope for an alternative to sedation as a means of behavior control.

In a study by Richardson and colleagues,[36] almost half of the individuals with an IQ of less than 50 had experienced one or more seizures by the age of 22, most occurring during the first year of life. The drugs used to control seizure activity (anticonvulsants) are powerful central nervous system depressants whose side effects can include paresthesias, drowsiness, anorexia, nausea, dizziness, ataxia, tremor, nystagmus, diplopia, lethargy, irritability, and nervousness.[37] Since so many of these side effects can interfere with psychomotor development, knowledge about their use is an important part of obtaining a medical history.

Nutrition

Altering diet or using nutritional supplements to affect the actual intellectual functioning or behaviors of the mentally retarded is an area of continuing controversy. Critics maintain that the results have been exaggerated and the treatments turned into a profitable market directed at families who are clutching at any offering of hope. Proponents speak to the relatively harmless side effects of a basic approach they believe is proven effective. Harrell and associates[38] maintain that nutritional supplements can improve both the IQ scores and functioning of some severely mentally retarded children. They conducted a partially double-blind experiment with 16 retarded children (initial IQ's ranging from 17 to 70), who were given nutritional supplements or placebos over an 8-month period. Those children receiving supplements had statistically significant increases in their IQ scores when compared with those on placebos. The experimenters had particular success with Down syndrome and believe that their results support the hypothesis that mental retardation is in part a genotrophic disease.

Hutchings[39] reported several case studies where the basic diet was changed to one high in protein and low in carbohydrates and supplemented with megadoses of vitamins and minerals. His clinical impression was that this treatment approach is beneficial for children with autism, schizophrenia, brain damage, and the learning disabilities that may arise as a result of these disorders.

A good basic review of the literature on the advocacy of additive-free diets for hyperkinetic children (popularized by Feingold) is presented by Mailman and Lewis.[40] They are skeptical about the benefits, stating that there was no significant difference noted in well-controlled studies. Good basic nutrition is important for the mentally retarded child, however, and can be a problem area because of associated problems with feeding.

PHYSICAL THERAPY EVALUATION

Physical therapy evaluation of the multiply handicapped severely profoundly retarded child must be comprehensive and as objective as possible. Flexibility in assessment must be maintained in order to recognize and appropriately adapt to behavioral problems, unique or absent communication, and limited capacity to cooperate. Several approaches to evaluation of the neurologically impaired child are covered in other chapters and are applicable to this population. In this section we will review assessment tools that are particularly useful for the severely and profoundly retarded populations, and discuss characteristic problem areas that must be considered when conducting a definitive evaluation. For organizational purposes, various aspects of the assessment are discussed separately, but these various functions cannot and should not be isolated.

Background Information

It is essential to obtain a general knowledge base by reviewing available records and talking with family, teachers, and other connections because of the complexity of multiple handicaps in the client, including poor receptive and expressive communication skills and the decreased capacity to cooperate. These children are an emotional strain on the best of families. What is the structure of the basic family unit and what attitudes are displayed by various members? Multiple problems often make them eligible for a variety of services and programs. What agencies are involved? In what programs is the child participating? For what services and financial support systems is the child eligible?

What medical care has the child received and by whom? Is there a history of seizures, and if so, what type? Are the seizures controlled with medication, or is the child on any other type of medication? Have side effects from these medications been observed? Is there evidence of recurrent problems as one reviews the medical history? For example, recurrent pneumonia is a red flag to carefully assess oral motor function and feeding behaviors. Has there been surgical intervention for physical deformities or other problems? Have hearing and vision been evaluated, and with what result? What equipment is available for the child's use and how is it being used?

Obtaining accurate and complete information in areas such as these provides the basis for planning a comprehensive assessment.

Communication

It would seem, at times, that the specialty skill one needs most in pediatrics is the ability to establish sufficient rapport to gain the cooperation of the child in performing activities and allowing handling or positioning. Carenza[41] compiled a book of strategies successful in gaining the cooperation of children for medical examination and cleverly entitled it *Pediatricks*. Since expressive and receptive communication skills are often absent or delayed, and behavioral problems are common among the severely and profoundly mentally retarded, it is important to obtain information about the child in these areas prior to testing. Are there characteristic behaviors, reinforcement schedules, or communication aids developed for the child that should be employed to facilitate cooperation? The reliability and validity of the assessment may depend on how effectively behaviors are managed and communication established.

Encouraging imitation is one of the "tricks" sometimes used to gain cooperation from children, but it is fairly well-documented that severely mentally retarded individuals lack spontaneous imitative behavior. This may be attributable directly to diminished intelligence, to sensory deficits, or to some experiential concomitant of retardation, such as institutionalization[42]; or it may be the result of perceptual inconsistency and the subsequent difficulty of distinguishing self from the outside world.[43]

Repp and colleagues[44] conducted an interesting study on the effectiveness of various modes of communication with severely mentally retarded persons.

They looked at several types of instruction in various combinations and found that the effectiveness varied depending on the type of secondary problems:

Severely Retarded Population	Most Effective Mode of Instruction
1. No secondary disability	Verbal instruction with physical assistance *or* Nonverbal instruction with physical assistance (depending on setting)
2. Physically handicapped	Nonverbal instruction with physical assistance
3. Hearing impaired	Physical assistance
4. Visually impaired	Nonverbal instruction with or without physical assistance (varied depending on setting)

Language problems in the mentally retarded are four times as common as in the general population, and the frequency and severity is generally inversely proportional to IQ.[6] Difficulties with language may be symptomatic of physical or cognitive problems.

Piaget[45] believes that the cognitive structures necessary for the development of meaningful expressive language are not present until an individual is functioning at Stage 6 of the sensorimotor period. He based this belief on the premise that no mental images are formed during Stages 1 through 5 of sensorimotor imitation. Because many profoundly mentally retarded individuals function at levels below Stage 6,[46] a logical correlate was comparison of language abilities in profoundly retarded persons with their sensorimotor level of function. Kahn[47] used the Uzgiris-Hunt Ordinal Scales of Psychological Development to test two groups (eight subjects each) of severely and profoundly retarded children: one group with expressive language (vocabulary of at least 10 words) and the other group with complete absence of expressive language. His results supported Piaget's hypothesis in that seven subjects in the expressive language group demonstrated Stage 6 functioning on all four subtests, and five subjects with no expressive language were functioning below Stage 6; the remaining three subjects in this group functioned at Stage 6 on only two of the four subtests.

Many nonverbal children have been instructed in alternative modes of communication. Nonspeech communication modes used with the mentally retarded include mime, manual sign language, Blissymbolics, or a variety of communication boards.[48] Basic familiarity with these systems is strongly recommended for anyone working with severely and profoundly retarded children.

Assessment Instruments

One of the most important aspects of the Education for All Handicapped Children Act of 1975 is that it provided legal direction and guidelines for the assessment of handicapped children. The law requires that all initial and reevaluation assessments be multifactored. Section 121a 532 (f) states: "The child is assessed in all areas related to the suspected disability, including, where appropriate, health, vision, hearing, social and emotional status, general intelligence, academic performance, communicative status, and motor ability."[19]

According to Section 121a 532 (a) (2) of Public Law 94-142, tests and other evaluation procedures used in a multifactored evaluation must "have been validated for the specific purpose for which they are used."[19] The intent of this section is to assure more comprehensive and valid assessment of the multiply handicapped, severely or profoundly retarded population, for whom testing previously, if it was done at all, was a hodgepodge of modified instruments, originally designed for a less severely involved group; consequently, marked discrepancies in results from one test to another have been found.[49]

The result of the legal mandate regarding assessment has been a plethora of new tests over the past five years. Most are multidisciplinary in scope and include a section on motor development. These tests seldom include more than a gross assessment of motor abilities, however, and should supplement, not replace, a detailed physical therapy evaluation for the severely or profoundly retarded child with multiple handicaps.

Several resources are available that provide annotated listings of assessment programs for the multihandicapped child.[50,51] Some of the more current tests, designed specifically for the severely or profoundly retarded population, are listed below:

1. Adaptive Behavior Curriculum: Prescriptive Behavior Analyses for Moderately, Severely and Profoundly Handicapped Students (Popovich, Laham, 1982): A curriculum of 3500 behavioral objectives, designed primarily for use by teachers. (Publisher: Paul H. Brooks Publishing Co., P.O. Box 10624, Baltimore, MD 21204)

2. AAMD Adaptive Behavior Scales (Nihara et al., 1975): Provides information on adaptive behavior functioning in 12 essential categories of daily living. (Publisher: American Association on Mental Deficiency)

3. Balthazar Scales of Adaptive Behavior (Balthazar, 1976): Appropriate for assessing ambulatory severely or profoundly retarded individuals ages 5 to 57. Scales on functional independence and social (coping) behaviors. (Publisher: Research Press Company, 2612 North Mattis Avenue, Champaign, IL 61820)

4. Bayley Scales of Infant Development (Bayley, 1969): Useful for young children who are severely or profoundly retarded. Naglieri[52] has extrapolated the developmental indices below 50 for the lower functioning group. (Publisher: The Psychological Corporation, 757 Third Avenue, New York, NY 10017)

5. Behavior Rating Inventory for the Retarded (Sparrow and Cicchetti, 1978): Assesses skills in areas of communication, self-help, and physical and social behavior. (Available from: Child Study Center, Department of Psychology, 333 Cedar Street, New Haven, CT 06511)

6. Camelot Behavioral Checklist (Foster, 1974): Checklist of 339 behavioral objectives arranged in age-expectancy order, all ages. (Publisher: Camelot Behavioral Systems, P.O. Box 3447, Lawrence, KS 66044)

7. Gestural Approach to Thought and Expression, An Index of Nonverbal Communication and Its Critical Prerequisites (Langley, 1968): Data regarding child's communication system, collected in a variety of natural settings,

from birth to 36 months. (Available from: Box 158, Child Study Center, Peabody College for Teachers, Nashville, TN 37203)

8. Prescriptive Behavioral Checklist for the Severely and Profoundly Retarded (Popovich, 1977): Checklist ratings on motor development, eye-hand coordination, and physical eating problems. (Publisher: University Park Press, Baltimore, MD 21202)

9. Programmatic Guide to Assessing Severely/Profoundly Retarded (Crebo and Heifetz, 1981): Provides information in self-help, communication, gross motor, fine motor, sensory discrimination, preacademics and prereading. (Available from: Experimental Educational Unit, WJ-10, Child Development and Mental Retardation Center, University of Washington, Seattle, WA 98195)

10. TMR Performance Profile for the Severely and Moderately Retarded: Scales in the areas of social behavior, self-care, communication, basic knowledge, practical skills, and body usage for severely multihandicapped children. (Publisher: Educational Performance Associates, 563 Westview Avenue, Ridgefield, NJ 07657)

11. Vulpe Assessment Battery (Vulpe, 1969): Performance analysis and developmental assessment in basic senses and functions, gross and fine motor behaviors, language behaviors, cognitive processes, organizational behaviors, activities of daily living, and assessment of the environment. (Publisher: National Institute on Mental Retardation, Ontario, Canada)

Motor Development

Many of the published assessments for the severely and profoundly retarded include a motor performance checklist, which is essentially a yes/no format for accomplishment of the basic motor milestones. What the physical therapist can and *must* contribute to completion of that checklist is a description of motor behaviors and deductive reasoning as to the causes of delays. The physical therapist's role is analysis of the contribution to deficient sensorimotor performance being made by behavior, motivation, cognition, perception, strength, muscle tone, contractures, joint limitation or reflexes.

Reports in the literature vary about the extent of motor deficit in mentally retarded persons. The variability seems to exist, however, because of inconsistencies in what is meant by the term "mental retardation." It is important to determine the level(s) of retardation being discussed (i.e., mild, moderate, severe, or profound) and whether the population being studied was inclusive, or excluded specific subgroups (e.g., those with neurologic dysfunction). In general, research indicates delays in sensorimotor development among the mentally retarded—the extent of the delay roughly paralleling the extent of intellectual impairment.[13,53]

Reflex Development

A comprehensive reflex assessment is essential because the often extensive brain damage may be manifested in the persistence of primitive reflexes that interfere with normal development and predispose to asymmetries in muscle tone, sometimes leading to serious deformity.[54] Recognition of a child's inability to suppress the effect of primitive reflexes on motor behavior can be the key to making appropriate recommendations about positioning, handling, the use of adaptive equipment, and general treatment.

Muscle Tone

The tonus of muscles must be carefully evaluated and some judgments made as to the interference of abnormal tone with functional abilities and how this contributes to musculoskeletal deformity. Since primitive reflexes can greatly influence tone, assessment should be based on observation and handling of the child in a variety of positions and postures. Hypotonia is a commmon characteristic of the severely mentally retarded population when cerebral palsy and other defined neuromusculoskeletal problems are excluded.

Muscle Strength and Function

It is very difficult to test muscle strength with any objectivity in the severely and profoundly retarded. One must extrapolate muscle capabilities from observation of general motor activity and posture.

Joint Range of Motion and Muscle Length

The functional mobility of each joint should be carefully assessed as well as the length of key muscle groups. Awareness of problems in these areas can prevent serious deformity later.

Samilson[54] investigated the incidence of hip subluxation or dislocation among severely involved, neurologically immature, developmentally retarded individuals and found it to be about 28 percent. The mean age when hip problems were discovered was 7 years and 62 percent of those with hip problems were quadriplegic total bed-care patients. Postures that predisposed to dislocation were hip flexion, adduction, and medial rotation, scoliosis, and pelvic obliquity, with rotation and inclination.

Lindsey and Drennan[31] conducted a study of institutionalized mentally retarded persons, which excluded cerebral palsy and other recognizable neuromuscular disorders. Hypotonia, ligamentous laxity, and delayed motor milestones were general characteristics in this population. From a total of 1600 mentally retarded patients, they found 48 (24 with Down syndrome) who had either isolated major foot problems or a combination of significant foot and knee disorders. The use of appropriate foot orthoses to permit proper weight-bearing alignment until skeletal and ligamentous maturity has been achieved is recommended.

Lindsey and Drennan[31] found that knee problems were uniformly associated with antecedent foot problems. The most common problem was genu valgum, associated with varying degrees of joint laxity and sometimes with chronic patellar dislocation, but normally no interference with function. The

Table 9-3. Percentages of Severely Mentally Retarded Persons Having Each Posture as Measured by the New York Posture Rating Chart[a]

Posture	Normal	Mild	Moderate/Severe
Head tilt	88.41	10.14	1.45
Shoulder obliquity	59.42	39.13	1.45
Scoliosis	59.42	36.23	4.35
Hip obliquity	62.32	33.33	4.35
Ankle valgus	28.99	59.42	11.59
Protrusion of abdomen	20.29	46.52	23.19
Lordosis	31.88	56.52	11.60
Kyphosis	57.97	40.58	1.45
Forward head	27.53	62.32	10.15

[a] Adapted with permission from Sherrill C: Posture training as a means of normalization. Mental Retardation 18:136, 1980.

most common functional knee deformity was flexion contracture, which can be attributed to the prolonged part-time use of a wheelchair and the stance adaptation of a crouch gait.

An extensive review of upper extremity problems in spastic cerebral palsy, the indications for surgical intervention, and successful operative procedures, is provided by Mital and Sakellarides.[55]

Posture

Sherrill[56] defines posture as "good body alignment and proper body mechanics" and stresses that posture evaluation should be based on dynamic postures (e.g., walking, sitting, stair climbing, and lifting and carrying objects) rather than a single static stance. Table 9-3 summarizes her findings from a posture assessment done on 69 severely mentally retarded persons, using the New York Posture Rating Chart.

A pictorial description of positions that predispose to posture problems is provided by Kendall and Kendall[57] and is helpful in evaluating the severely and profoundly retarded who may be "locked in" to positions as a result of abnormal tone and primitive reflex posturing.

Samilson[54] provides a comprehensive review of the incidence, etiology, and management of problems in the spine among the mentally retarded. He found that the incidence of scoliosis in ambulatory patients with cerebral palsy was 7 percent and in total bed-care patients, 39 percent. Of a total 232 scoliotics, 193 were spastic quadriplegics: 68 percent had fixed pelvic obliquity, and 81 percent demonstrated deformity of one or both hips that ranged from soft tissue contracture to dislocation.

Under what conditions surgery is indicated for scoliosis is often a difficult decision. Rinsky[58] believes that the most common indications for spinal fusion in neurogenic curves of retarded patients include the following:

1. Pelvic obliquity interfering with sitting tolerance with impending ischial breakdown

2. Collapsing curves requiring use of the upper extremity to maintain sitting balance
3. Pain (usually rib impingement against the iliac crest)
4. Interference with respiration
5. Progressive curves where use of a brace is not feasible
6. Interference with the ability of others to care for the patient

Even with the above problems, Rinsky does not believe that the profoundly retarded, multihandicapped child would realize enough benefit from the surgery to warrant the risks involved.

Kyphotic deformities in the mentally retarded may be secondary to tight hamstrings (with absence of the normal lumbar lordosis) or to an increased lumbar lordosis (with hip flexion contractures).[54] Surgical release of shortened thigh muscles is recommended as a consideration for correction.

Excessive lumbar lordosis, like kyphosis and scoliosis, may be functional or structural. Tight hip flexors, weak hip extensors, and weak abdominals are commonly associated problems.

Sensory Processes and Integration

Sensory integrative dysfunction, a basic problem in the mentally retarded, is the subject of increasing attention in the literature, and it is implicated as a major causative factor in everything from learning disorders and self-abusive behavior to abnormal and delayed motor development.

Ayres[59] has written one of the primary references on the topic of sensory integration (Sensory Integration and Learning Disorders, 1976). An excellent resource for physical and occupational therapists, which condenses the applicable theories of Ayres, is an article by Montgomery[60] on the assessment and treatment of the child with mental retardation. Although general principles are discussed, the emphasis is on sensory integration with specific assessment and treatment strategies for visual, auditory, tactile, olfactory-gustatory, proprioceptive-kinesthetic, and vestibular functions.

Gait

It is difficult to predict the ambulatory potential of mentally retarded children. Illingworth[61] predicts that mentally retarded children without cerebral palsy may walk with an IQ less than 20 and will walk with an IQ above 20. Of those with an IQ less than 40 who do learn to walk, the onset will be delayed in approximately one third.[6]

Because it is generally accepted that the lower the IQ, the less the probability of developing ambulation, the results of two studies investigating the ambulatory capabilities of mentally retarded children with and without cerebral palsy are somewhat confusing. In a study of mentally retarded individuals with IQ's less than 50, Donoghue and associates[62] found that only 10 percent of those with cerebral palsy walked, while 79 percent of those without cerebral palsy walked. One would expect lower percentages in a study by Shapiro and colleagues,[63] which focused on children with IQ's of less than 25. Their results, however, indicated that 11 percent of those children with cerebral palsy walked (at a median age of 63.5 months), and 92 percent of those without cerebral palsy walked (at a median age of 20 months).

Molnar[64] conducted a prospective longitudinal study with 53 infants and young children having mental retardation primarily in the mild to moderate range and delayed motor development without evidence of neuromuscular disability. She found that primitive reflexes did not seem to persist beyond the expected age, but that postural adjustment reactions were significantly delayed. Once specific postural reactions appeared, the attainment of the appropriate motor milestone followed within 1 to 4 weeks.

If one looks at the population of mentally retarded individuals who do not have identified neuromuscular problems, some characteristic gait patterns are evident. Lindsey and Drennan[31] refer to the "Chaplinesque" gait of the mentally retarded. The hips are in moderate functional lateral rotation, the knees are in flexion and valgus, the tibias are in lateral rotation, and the feet are placed with the medial longitudinal arch as the presenting aspect of the foot accompanied by marked valgus of the heel and forefoot pronation.

Many mentally retarded children walk in a crouched posture, which can lead to fixed flexion deformities of the hips and knees. One reason for the development of this type of gait pattern is the delay in motor maturation and balance.[31] Some children will initially stand with a normal posture of full extension at the hips and knees but develop a crouched posture as they approach adolescence. An interesting postulate for this, proposed by Lindsey and Drennan,[31] is that children have a "predetermined functional height." Once they reach that functional height, they compensate for continued skeletal growth by assuming a crouched posture, which enables them to maintain their head position at a constant distance from the floor. It would seem to be an attempt to maintain consistency in specific types of sensory feedback.

It is also common to see mentally retarded children walk with a wide base of support and arms held in a high guard posture. Grady and Gilfoyle[65] theorize that the child is using the basic pivot prone posture in an upright position to facilitate extensor tone.

Toe walking is a typical isolated finding in severely and profoundly retarded populations. Some people believe that this is a behavioral aberrancy, although Capute and colleagues[6] note that it is usually accompanied by "unsustained ankle clonus, equivocal toe signs and mildly limited range of motion at the ankle." Montgomery and Gauger[66] believe that toe walking, as seen in the absence of cerebral palsy or spasticity, is a problem of sensory dysfunction. The children are generally hypotonic and hyperflexible, and demonstrate vestibular dysfunction exacerbated by tactile defensiveness. This type of toe walking must be differentiated from that seen in individuals with spasticity in the gastrocnemius-soleus muscle group. Whereas surgical release and bracing may be indicated in the spastic child, it would be of no benefit to the child with primarily sensory dysfunction.

Several other aspects of gait should receive attention as part of an observational assessment of gait. Are the arms held high, as in the early walker, for increased balance and stability? Is there overflow of muscle tone when upright, evidenced possibly by tight elbow flexion with retraction of the scapulae, and subsequent interference with normal use of the arms for balance? Is there reciprocal, coordinated movement of the arms with the legs?

Where is the focal point of the eyes? Montgomery and Richter[67] believe that children with poor equilibrium often keep their eyes on the floor as they walk, rather than looking straight ahead. Is the head maintained in midline? Tilting of the head to one side or the other may indicate sensory dysfunction, poor integration of primitive reflexes, or asymmetrical muscle tone. Are the hips relatively stable? Is there a good heel-toe pattern? The common foot problems of the mentally retarded child often result in flat feet and concomitant inability to establish a good heel-toe gait. What type of shoes are usually worn? Is there a difference in the gait with and without shoes?

Oral Motor Function

The development of normal oral motor patterns for feeding, respiration, phonation, speech, and language is a complex process influenced by reflexes, muscle tone, positioning, sensory integration, and behavior. It is one of the most important areas in evaluation of the severely handicapped because problems are so common. Aspiration of food was found to be the direct cause of 3.5 percent of deaths of profoundly retarded individuals (the seventh leading cause).[68] Pneumonia, frequently the result of a chemical reaction to the aspiration of food in the profoundly retarded, accounts for 30 to 50 percent of the deaths in this population.[69] Malnutrition is another serious health-related problem. Diet is often deficient in calories, iron, vitamins, and minerals.

Behaviors like drooling or messy eating, over which the child has no control, may be aversive to caretakers, and may affect social interaction, possibly resulting in isolation. Feeding, which should be a pleasurable experience for the child and a time of positive interaction, becomes instead a tension-filled experience. The lack of speech as a result of oral motor dysfunction can prevent meaningful communication and affect the type of interaction in which the child is engaged.

Much has been written on the assessment and treatment of oral motor problems. One of the most comprehensive resources is the proceedings of a 1977 conference, *Oral Motor Function and Dysfunction in Children.*[70] Detailed information on oral motor assessment cannot be included in this chapter, but the following guidelines may be useful as a basis for organizing the approach to this important area of development.

Guidelines for Oral Motor Assessment

    I. General. An assessment should begin by observing the child and caregiver in a typical feeding situation and attending to positioning;

the use of special equipment (e.g., chairs, spoons, cups, plates); the type, texture, and temperature of food; the sequence of presenting food; and the quality of social interaction that occurs. Information should also be obtained about the child's basic diet to ensure that there is adequate intake of calories and nutrients. Dietary supplements may be indicated.

II. Oral reflexes. (Refer to chapter on oral reflexes in *Oral Motor Function and Dysfunction in Children.)*[70]

Reflexes that should be assessed include (1) rooting, (2) sucking, (3) swallowing, (4) gag, (5) bite, (6) Babkin.

III. Muscle tone and sensitivity of the oral structures (cheeks, lips, and tongue).

IV. Feeding behaviors. Knowledge of the normal developmental sequence is essential to determine the difference between normal, delayed, and abnormal patterns. Regardless of other variations in position, the child's head should be in midline, stabilized if necessary, during this part of the assessment.

A. Sucking
   1. Smooth, rapid initiation?
   2. Rhythmical pattern?
   3. Good coordination with breathing and swallowing?
   4. Effect of positioning (e.g., flexion may improve the child's oral motor function)

B. Food from a spoon (try various textures and tastes)
   1. Mouth quiet until food presented?
   2. Graded mouth opening to receive spoon?
   3. Good lip closure around spoon?
   4. Food cleaned from spoon with upper lip?
   5. Stable position of head maintained?
   6. Effective mobility of tongue and jaw?
   7. Swallow and breathing coordinated?

C. Drinking from a cup
   1. Jaw excursion graded?
   2. Jaw sufficiently stabilized to allow normal placement of cup?
   3. Lip closure adequate?
   4. Coordination of drinking, breathing, and swallowing?

D. Biting and chewing
   1. Description of jaw movement (progresses normally from up and down "munching" movement to a more mature rotary movement)
   2. Ability of tongue to move laterally (keep food between teeth)
   3. Adequacy of lip closure

E. Self-feeding

V. Associated behaviors
   A. Frequent gagging or choking
   B. Vomiting (when and how often?)

    C. Drooling
    D. Attitude toward feeding
    E. Expression of food preferences

Respiratory Function

Respiratory problems are common in the multihandicapped retarded child and can interfere with phonation, feeding, and general good health. A single cause of respiratory problems is uncommon; they frequently result from a combination of (1) improper positioning, which can cause deformities of the rib cage, pooling of secretions in dependent areas of the lung, and poor chest excursion; (2) weakness or spasticity in the respiratory muscles, resulting in an ineffective, weak cough and poor chest excursion; (3) incoordination of oral motor and respiratory movements with frequent aspiration; (4) increased saliva production and ineffective means of clearing the saliva so that it tends to collect in the throat; and (5) increased incidence of allergies causing respiratory symptoms (milk products are often implicated).

"Noisy" respirations are a frequent finding. Most often this is the result of secretions or saliva in the upper airways gurgling as the inspired and expired air tries to pass through. The only way to differentiate upper airway congestion from the more serious lobar congestion (pneumonia) is to auscultate the chest. Experience allows one to distinguish true rales, rhonchi, and wheezes from transmitted sounds originating in the upper airways.

Careful observation of the child's respiration in various positions can be diagnostic of many problems and provide the key to effective remediation. The normal infant uses primarily the diaphragm for breathing, so that one sees significant rise and fall of the abdomen. As the child gains the upright position there is a gradual transition to thoracic breathing, the normal adult pattern. Normal rate per minute for a newborn is 35–50, decreasing to about 30 for a 2-year-old, and about 16 for a normal adult. The ability to breathe through the nose is important, as the obligatory mouth breather will have problems coordinating respiration and feeding, and a tendency to aspirate food. As mentioned earlier, aspiration and aspiration pneumonia are significant causes of death among the mentally retarded.

Activities of Daily Living

The severely and profoundly retarded are unable to be independently functioning members of society, but many will be capable of independence in at least some of the activities of daily living and their independence should be encouraged by all possible means. They will be proud of their accomplishments and their family or primary caretakers will be relieved of some of the many time-consuming aspects of basic care. The appropriate use of adaptive equipment and behavior modification can be very helpful in developing skills for daily living.

Adaptive Equipment Needs

Assessment of the child's function with the various pieces of equipment designated for his or her use as well as a projection of potential benefit from other types of adaptive equipment is critical. Especially for the multihandicapped, nonambulatory child, the proper use of adaptive equipment can be one of the most important aspects of a therapeutic program. The process of selecting appropriate equipment requires consideration of the following areas: (1) availability, (2) cost, (3) source of funding, (4) portability, (5) stability, (6) ease of adjustment, (7) ease of modifications, and (8) construction, materials, and aesthetics.[71]

Several published resources are available to stimulate a therapist's creativity and provide some guidelines for construction of homemade equipment: Bergen, *Selected Equipment for Pediatric Rehabilitation*;[72] Slominski, *Please Help US Help Ourselves*;[73] Robinault, *Functional Aides for the Multiply Handicapped*;[74] and Dubose and Deni[75] *Easily Constructed Adaptive and Assistive Equipment*. Skills in correctly identifying equipment needs, locating resources for financial support, and obtaining the right piece of equipment (whether it is purchased or made) are some of the most important within the speciality area of pediatrics.

A child should have a variety of positioning alternatives available that are comfortable, enable him or her to interact maximally with the environment, and provide the support necessary for the activity intended, but still stimulate independent mastery of the necessary postural stabilization. The following areas should be assessed:

1. *Floor positions*. Several alternatives should be available for positioning on the floor or mat.
   a. Prone. The child may benefit from a properly sized bolster or wedge. Size selection and positioning on the equipment will depend on the developmental readiness of the child for head control, forearm support, or extended arm support.
   b. Sidelying. Commercially made sidelyers are available, but the appropriate use of bolsters and pillows may be sufficient.
   c. Seating. A seating arrangement at floor level may help the child to participate in group activities.
2. *Seating*. Several different seating arrangements may be necessary for the multihandicapped child. For instance, a severely involved child with athetosis may need a chair that provides maximum support (head, trunk, and legs) for eating or for fine motor activities. At other times during the day, a chair with less support will allow the child to practice the necessary cocontraction of postural muscles for head and trunk control. Attention should be given to optimal seating for the following activities:
   a. Feeding. A chair that supports the head in midline and helps to normalize muscle tone can be critical in allowing safe, effective feeding behavior.

    b. Fine motor skills. In the hypertonic child, a seat that provides secure flexion at hips and knees may normalize tone and enable significant increase in the functional use of arms and hands.

    c. Interactive play.

3. *Mobility.* If possible, some form of mobility is desirable for independence and exploration. Possibilities include tricycles, Irish mails, scooter boards, walkers, or wheelchairs—adequately adapted and fitted for effective use. Creativity is essential; for example, a specially designed sled enabled a profoundly retarded girl to ice skate and thereby experience the pride, fun, and stimulation of participating in a recreational activity with her peers.[76]

4. *Supported weight bearing.* Options include a prone board, which enables multiple adjustments for standing or kneeling with optimal alignment, or a standing box, which provides more behavioral than physical control.

Finally, the physical therapist or occupational therapist must evaluate procedures for toileting, bathing, and dressing, assess safety and availability of transportation, and identify the presence of architectural barriers preventing access to opportunities for recreation, education, and medical care.

Behavior

The behavior of mentally retarded children and behavioral approaches to management have received considerable attention in the literature. Webster[77] defines behavior as, first, "the manner of conducting oneself," and, second, "anything that an organism does involving action and response to stimulation."

The behavior manifested at any particular time has its origins in an intricate matrix of physiologic and environmental systems. Hutt and Gibby[78] devoted several chapters in their book, *The Mentally Retarded Child*, to discussion of social, emotional, and psychologic development, comparing and contrasting normal and mentally retarded children and factors in their environment that influence personality and may contribute to maladaptive behavior. Behavior is the substrate of a child's response system and must therefore be assessed and taken into consideration when determining potential and establishing a treatment program. Deviant behavior can be more of a deterrent to the success of a treatment program than deficient intelligence.

Stereotypic behaviors among the retarded can interfere with functional behaviors and can be harmful to the individual. Stereotyped mannerisms of mentally retarded children vary with environmental setting and the nature of ongoing activities, and the frequency of stereotyped behavior appears to be inversely related to the potential for alternative activity. This is true for infants as well as older persons. MacLean and Baumeister[79] found that several stereotypes are dependent upon a particular physical positioning of the child, which suggests that stereotypic movements are related to motor development.

PHYSICAL THERAPY

The markedly reduced capacity of the severely or profoundly retarded child to cooperate at a cognitive level with treatment objectives will definitely limit the ultimate level of achievement. Short-term goals may be achieved in minute increments and at a frustratingly slow pace. Studies that have investigated the effectiveness of various treatment regimens have found relatively better results with children functioning at higher cognitive levels. For example, Scherzer and colleagues[80] investigated physical therapy as a determinant of change in the infant with cerebral palsy and found definite changes in motor, social, and management areas, "particularly among children expected to show higher intelligence."

This is not meant to discourage those who work with severely and profoundly retarded children, but it does point to an important premise for treatment. Mentally retarded individuals characteristically have a short attention span and require extensive repetition for learning; therefore, consistency of treatment with frequent opportunity for practice and reinforcement is crucial. Isolated therapy sessions of relatively short duration will be minimally effective without the cooperation of those primarily responsible for the child's care and education. Westervelt and Luiselli[81] found, in trying to establish standing and walking behaviors in a profoundly retarded, institutionalized 11-year-old, that they were unsuccessful until the independent efforts of the clinician were relinquished and the attendant staff were taught how to work on target behaviors. Goals of the treatment program should be based on the development of appropriate adaptive behaviors and should be formulated in cooperation with the child, parents, teachers, aides, and others regularly involved with the individual. Awareness of, and adherence to, any already planned programs for communication or behavior modification is necessary.

Since learning is often at a very basic level and consistency of approach is critical, highly specialized treatment regimens may not be appropriate. The emphasis of treatment programs should be on activities that can be performed by all levels of personnel and easily incorporated into various aspects of the daily routine, so that frequent repetition can be accomplished with relative ease. Professionals will commonly assume a multidisciplinary rather that interdisciplinary team approach, depending, of course, on the training and experience of the team members and the type of setting. Published curricula for the severely and profoundly retarded, which are usually multidisciplinary in design, are available and can be helpful as a focus for a team of professionals in an educational or institutional setting. A good source of information about available curricula is the Technical Assistance Development System (University of North Carolina, 500 NCNB Plaza, Chapel Hill, NC 27514).

Positive reinforcement for appropriate behavior and the integration of treatment objectives with pleasurable experiences are important for children at any level of cognitive development. Kielhofner and Miyake[82] describe "play" itself as a learning and survival behavior and conducted an exploratory study on the therapeutic use of games with a group of moderately and severely retarded adults. The clients who participated showed improvement in motor behavior, cognitive abilities, affect, attention, self-confidence, and social interaction.

Motor Activity

The use of motor activity to enhance the learning process of mentally retarded individuals has been popularized by the many publications of Newell Kephart and Bryant Cratty. According to Kephart,[83] learning is "dependent upon motor activities and the ability to control motor responses." He believes that the "efficiency of the higher thought processes can be no better than the basic motor abilities upon which they are based."[84] He has developed a comprehensive theoretical framework for the evaluation of "slow learners" and a program of remediation based on the use of various types of motor activities.[85]

Although Cratty[86] is a proponent of facilitation of motor activity for a variety of reasons, he questions Kephart's major hypothesis, that movement is the basis of intellect. He stresses that the child must be able to think about the movement he is doing and be involved in a way that encourages the process of decision-making.[87] He suggests the use of perceptual motor activities presented in a specified sequential fashion to enhance the educational process of mentally retarded children.[88]

The basic theories of Kephart and Cratty help us to understand the importance of the interaction between reflex, motor, and sensory systems and the learning that occurs from the direct and immediate feedback resulting from a motor act on the environment. However, the specific programs they suggest require a level of cognitive development beyond that of the severely and profoundly retarded.

Facilitation of Neuromotor Development

The basic neurophysiologic approaches to the neurodevelopmental treatment of the pediatric patient are appropriate for the severely or profoundly mentally retarded child or adult. What is required is an approach that is based on the normal developmental sequence, attempts to normalize postural tone before demanding specific motor responses, requires a minimum of cooperation at a cognitive level, and seeks to integrate sensory and motor functions. As stated by Montgomery, the neurodevelopmental, sensorimotor, and sensory integrative techniques of the Bobaths, Rood and Stockmeyer, and Ayres seem particularly appropriate for the retarded child because all of these approaches emphasize functions that are relatively automatic for the individual (i.e., based on normal reflex and sensorimotor development) and therefore demand learning at a subcortical level.[60] Patterning is another treatment approach that has been widely used for the multiply handicapped child, although it has been surrounded by controversy.

Neurodevelopmental Therapy. Neurodevelopmental therapy was developed by Karl and Berta Bobath[89] as an approach to the management of the sensorimotor disorders seen in patients with cerebral palsy. By definition, cerebral palsy is a nonprogressive lesion affecting the immature brain and "interfering with the normal process of neurodevelopment." The Bobaths' treatment approach is applicable to that relatively large segment of the severely and profoundly retarded population in whom there is involvement of the portion of the brain that integrates and controls sensorimotor activity.

In upper motor neuron lesions producing cerebral palsy, tonic and spinal reflexes are released from the normal integrative and control functions of the brain. Movement is uncoordinated and tends to occur in primitive, synergistic patterns. Sensory and perceptual deficits are common and affect the feedback mechanism, which, when functioning normally, enables refinement of movement activity. Neurodevelopmental therapy is based on the premise that the primary deficit in cerebral palsy is a derangement in the normal postural reflex mechanism.[90]

The aim of treatment is to normalize postural tone and improve the quality and control of movement, following the normal developmental sequence as closely as possible. This is accomplished by using reflex-inhibiting patterns with manual control at key points (e.g., shoulder girdle or pelvis) to normalize postural tone. With tone normalized, then active automatic reactions are facilitated to develop elements of the normal postural reflex mechanism.

The handling techniques used in neurodevelopmental therapy are designed to elicit active, automatic movements from the child, and therefore do not require that the child cooperate at a cognitive level. As the Bobaths[89] state, "It is this aspect of the approach which has made this (Bobath) treatment so eminently adaptable to the needs of the mentally subnormal and uncooperative child."

Sensorimotor Therapy.   Stockmeyer[91,92] has described in the literature an interpretation of Rood's approach to the treatment of neuromuscular dysfunction. Theirs is an approach that "seeks to activate the movement and postural responses of the patient in the same automatic manner as they occur in the normal, without need for conscious attention to the response itself."[91] Reliance on automatic reactions makes Rood's approach, like the Bobaths', applicable to the severely or profoundly retarded child.

Several premises form the basis for Rood's approach to treatment.[91,92] First, motor and sensory functions are inseparable. Stimuli, carefully chosen to activate, facilitate, or inhibit motor responses, are an important part of the treatment program. The effect of various stimuli on not only somatic, but also on autonomic and psychic, function is an ongoing consideration. Second, there are two major sequences in motor development that are distinctly different and yet inextricably interrelated: skeletal functions and vital functions. Third, skeletal function can be separated into four sequential levels of control: (1) mobility (shortening and lengthening of the agonist with its antagonists), (2) stability (cocontraction of agonists and antagonists), (3) mobility superimposed on stability in a weightbearing position (proximal part moving on fixed distal part), and (4) mobility superimposed on stability in a non-weight-bearing position (free distal part moving on a proximal part that is dynamically holding). Fourth,

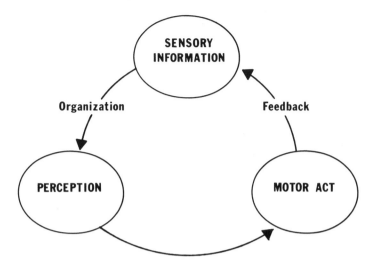

Fig. 9-1. Sensory integration. Diagrammatic representation of the basic process.

children normally traverse a specific skeletal function sequence (also termed ontogenetic motor patterns). This sequence is the guideline Rood proposes for the assessment and subsequent treatment of neuromuscular dysfunction.

Sensory Integrative Therapy. The basis for Ayres's use of sensory integrative therapy is rooted in the Piagetian theory that concrete action precedes and makes possible the use of the intellect and that sensorimotor experiences are the foundations of mental development.[93] Stated another way, intelligence may be viewed as a progressive transformation of motor patterns into thought patterns. The results of an interesting longitudinal study with normal infants and infants with Down syndrome conducted by Bradley-Johnson and associates[94] provide support for Piaget's basic theory. They found that children's performance on the Stanford-Binet at age 3½ years was significantly correlated with the length of time spent on the exploration of novel objects at age 6 months.

Ayres[59] developed a comprehensive theoretical basis for sensory integrative therapy and a rationale for its use with brain-damaged children. She informally defines sensory integration as the ability to organize sensory information for functional use in producing an adaptive response and believes that this ability is the essence of perception. A motor act is a typical response to a perception, and the sensory feedback gained from the motor act enables the child to evaluate the accuracy of the perception and the effectiveness of the response (Fig. 9-1). Ayres believes that a strong relationship exists among cognitive function, motor development, and reflex integration, but that the child first experiences the environment through information conveyed by afferent pathways. Inability to accurately receive or organize sensory input causes dysfunction in the whole process of learning via sensorimotor experience. Sensory integrative therapy is not directed toward the mastery of specific tasks or skills, but toward improving the brain's capacity to perceive, to remember, and to plan motor activity.

Although sensory integrative therapy was not specifically designed for use with the retarded, it can be applied effectively to this population. Montgomery and Richter[67] published a handbook for physical and occupational therapists based on the principles of sensorimotor integration and other neurophysiologically based intervention techniques.

Several studies have investigated the effectiveness of sensory integrative therapy with the severely and profoundly retarded. Clark and colleagues[95] compared the results of operant and sensory integrative methods of promoting development with a population of 27 profoundly retarded institutionalized adults who were minimally vocal. They used three treatment groups: (1) an operant approach, (2) a modified sensory integration approach, and (3) a combination of the two therapies. They found that when they combined the results of the three groups, there were significant gains in the frequency of eye contact, the frequency of vocalizations, and the quality of postural adaptation. They found no differences, however, in the effectiveness of the respective therapies.

Magrun and colleagues[96] used vestibular stimulation prior to a monitored free play situation to increase the spontaneous use of verbal language in trainable mentally retarded children. Effects were generally positive and better results were obtained with younger children who were more severely language disabled. Evans[97] was able to reduce the hyperactive behavior of three profoundly retarded adolescents by increasing the visual and auditory stimulation in their environment.

Two theories have wide currency regarding the basis for the self-injurious behaviors often seen in the severely and profoundly retarded. One theory postulates the behaviors are learned and therefore are most effectively treated with contingency-based management techniques (i.e., behavior modification). The other theory suggests that self-injurious behavior is a type of self-stimulation and should be ameliorated by treatment with various forms of sensory and environmental enrichment. Bright and associates[98] assumed sensory deprivation was at least a partial cause of the self-injurious behavior of a profoundly retarded adult, and they were successful in reducing the frequency of the behavior using sensory integrative techniques.

Trainable mentally retarded children (IQ's less than 50) were the subjects of Montgomery and Richter's[99] study, which compared the effectiveness of three different motor programs on neuromotor development. On a test battery that assessed gross, fine, and perceptual motor skills and reflex integration, the children receiving sensory integrative therapy showed the greatest gains, followed by those who participated in a developmental physical education program, and finally those in an adaptive physical education and arts and crafts program. Montgomery and Richter concluded that neuromotor development may be enhanced more effectively by activities that facilitate improved postural responses than by practice of specific motor skills.

Patterning. Temple Fay was the first to use patterning therapeutically. His approach, termed "neuromuscular reflex therapy," was based on the concept that primitive movements resulting from reflexes, spinal automatisms, and tonic responses to stimuli were possible without a highly developed cerebral cortex.[100] He believed that these lower levels of mobility had to be learned or developed before higher levels of function could be achieved. Doman and Delacato expanded Fay's basic patterning procedures and developed a popular method of treatment they claim can benefit children with neuromuscular disorders, learning disabilities, behavioral disturbances, and mental retardation.

Delacato[101] believes that the ontogenetic development of normal humans recapitulates the phylogenetic process. He has categorized a developmental progression based on that belief. The progression starts with truncal movements of the newborn, which correspond to the swimming movements of the fish and represent a medullary level of function, proceeds through homolateral crawling, cross-pattern creeping and crude walking, and ends with cross-pattern walking, which is considered to be a distinctly human form of locomotion and is identified with mature cerebral function and the establishment of hemispheric dominance. Important to the theory is the premise that each of the levels is stage dependent and that adequate organization at any subsequent level is dependent upon mastery of the coordination requisite for the antecedent stages.

Basic to the treatment method is the application of a variety of sensory and motor experiences directed toward facilitation of "neurologic organization."[101] The patterning aspect of the regimen involves three to five adults passively manipulating the child's arms, legs, and head in a rhythmical pattern, according to a meticulously ordered sequence. Other aspects of the regimen include visual, tactile, and auditory stimulation; a breathing technique designed to increase the amount of carbon dioxide inhaled; expressive activities; gravity, antigravity activities (e.g., rolling, somersaulting and inverted hanging); and a plan of restriction and facilitation of selected experiences to foster the establishment of left hemispheric dominance.[101,102]

The patterning treatment has remained relatively popular for severely and profoundly handicapped children because it does not require any cognitive level of participation by the child, is prescribed for use at home (after a period of training), and has been credited with miraculous cures in the popular press. Criticism has centered around the lack of scientific evidence to support the effects claimed for the treatment regimen and the tremendous emotional, psychologic, and financial burden it places on families. Zigler[103] recently published an article, "A Plea to End the Use of Patterning Treatment for Retarded Children." He regrets the appeal this type of program holds for parents who are seeking a "last hope" and then are faced with the emotional burden of failing to see results from a program whose success was presented to them as strongly dependent on their perseverance. If fully implemented, the program demands many hours of treatment each day, it must be done 7 days a week, and it usually necessitates involving friends as well as family members in a demanding schedule.

Cohen and associates[104] attempted an objective evaluation of the theoretical bases for the patterning system of treatment and the results proclaimed by Doman and Delacato. They concluded that "the data thus far advanced are insufficient to justify affirmative conclusions . . ." and that the theoretical premises of the method were inconsistent with generally accepted views of the nature of neurologic development.

Sparrow and Zigler[105] conducted an intensive longitudinal study on patterning in which they compared the performance of three groups of moderately to profoundly retarded children. One group participated in a modification of the program devised by Doman and Delacato at the Institute for the Achievement of Human Potential; the second was a motivational control group, which participated in activities with foster grandparents designed to improve their self-esteem; and a third group received no treatment. No significant differences were found in posttest performance among the three groups on the majority of measures.

Behavior Modification

Consideration of treatment of the mentally retarded is impossible without discussion of behavior modification. The basic principles of behavior modification as described by Skinner[106] are simple. A target behavior is selected, and the specific responses that are desired are selected and defined. Correctly completed responses are immediately reinforced. By continued specific reinforcement and by successive and more generalized reinforcement procedures, the learning sequence is established, leading to accomplishment of the target behavior. Clinical researchers have used it to shape a variety of gross motor behaviors, including reduction of time in reverse tailor sitting,[107] development of standing and walking,[81,108–113] raising an arm to pull a ring,[114] reduction of drooling,[115] and cessation of crawling.[116] Behavior modification has also been used to reduce or eliminate self-injurious behaviors[117–119] and stereotypic behaviors.[120]

A sophisticated type of behavior modification is biofeedback. Electrodes are placed on the child, which are sensitive to the electrical activity in underlying muscles or to the positioning of the body part in space. Feedback can be given immediately in a variety of modalities. Researchers have used biofeedback devices with cerebral palsied and mentally retarded individuals for reinforcement of head posture,[121,122] range of motion training,[123,124] finger praxis training,[125] prehension skill,[126] and digital exercise.[127]

Other Treatment Priorities

In addition to the facilitation of neuromotor development and behavior modification, consideration must be given to the prevention of deformity, prevention of respiratory complications, and treatment of oral motor problems as priorities in the establishment of a comprehensive treatment program.

Prevention of Deformity.   The more common types of deformity and the forces that tend to cause deformity in the mentally retarded were summarized in the section on assessment. To prevent deformity and the subsequent loss of function, an effective treatment program must be developed that includes sug-

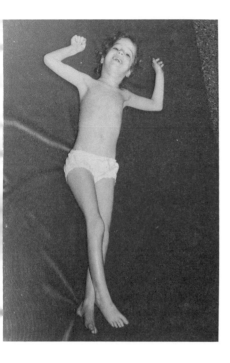

Fig. 9-2. Case study: Sarah. Increased muscle tone in supine.

gestions for handling and positioning, exercise, and the appropriate use of adaptive equipment.

Two case examples might help to illustrate these points.

Sarah is an 8-year-old spastic quadriplegic with profound retardation. Extensor tone predominates in the lower extremities with a posturing of adduction, medial rotation and extension of the hips, extension of the knees, and plantar flexion of the feet (Fig. 9-2). Other prominent patterns are strong retraction of the neck and shoulder girdle; flexion of the elbows, wrists, and fingers, and pronation of the forearms. Primitive reflexes are not integrated, with particular influence on postural tone from persistence of the crossed extension, tonic labyrinthine, positive support, and asymmetrical tonic neck reflexes. Oral motor function is markedly abnormal. Mouth opening is associated with neck extension, and there is profuse drooling. Chest excursion is minimal and she almost always has upper airway congestion.

Priority for Sarah would be a well-fitted chair to be used for feeding and other activities. To reduce the extensor tone in her legs, the chair should have foot rests that promote full contact of the soles of her feet (to avoid stimulating a positive support reaction), an abduction wedge with sufficient depth to generalize the contact with the adductors and help to keep her hips back in the chair, a seat that is tilted back at a slight angle to promote hip flexion of slightly more than 90 degrees, and a pelvic strap to keep her hips securely back in the chair and flexed. To inhibit the retraction of the arms, a padded support to bring the shoulders forward and a lap board for arm support would be helpful. Any control needed to keep the head in midline and slightly flexed should also be used.

The supine position should be avoided because of the influence of the tonic labyrinthine reflex. Sidelying with hips and knees well flexed would be a good position to use to work on hand function, or for general positioning, because it provides stabilization in midline and inhibits the tonic labyrinthine reflex. The prone position, supported under the chest with a bolster or wedge with shoulders forward for elbow propping, would help to stimulate head and upper trunk control and inhibit retraction of the shoulder girdle.

Other equipment that might provide positioning alternatives are a hammock, a bean bag chair, a prone board, or a scooter board (with a good abductor wedge).

Carrying suggestions might include straddling the adult's hip or fully flexed at hips and knees and facing away from the adult. Support should be used as minimally as possible to stimulate independent head and trunk control.

> Tony is a 17-year-old student with a nonspecified genetic disorder characterized by hypothyroidism, absence of sweat glands (causing hypersensitivity to heat and susceptibility to skin breakdown), partial blindness, musculoskeletal abnormalities, and profound mental retardation. General hypotonicity and ligamentous laxity are present. Tony has no means of communication and is upset by movement and handling. He demonstrates distress with a throaty scream and self-inflicted blows to his head. He is ambulatory with assistance (required primarily because of his blindness). Figure 9-3 illustrates his severe kyphoscoliosis and the deformities of his feet.

Ideally, Tony should have received orthopedic care (surgery and/or bracing) at an early age to help prevent his present deformities, but he was discharged from orthopedic follow-up at the age of 3 because of his "lack of potential." His parents, intelligent and caring people, were faced with a difficult decision among the following alternatives concerning his kyphoscoliosis: surgical correction with postoperative immobilization for 6 to 9 months in either a full body cast or skeletal traction, bracing (e.g., Milwaukee), or palliative exercise and positioning. The fear of skin breakdown with full body casting or bracing eliminated all but the surgery followed by skeletal traction. The closest medical center that could perform the surgery was 6 hours from home, and Tony's parents were apprehensive about his emotional response to separation from them, as well as the discomfort and strangeness of the immobilization. They decided that the benefits of surgery did not outweigh the risk of severe emotional trauma. Because the arches of the feet were thought to have collapsed maximally, and since these deformities were unlikely to progress, surgery and/or bracing were presented as alternatives for the future should his

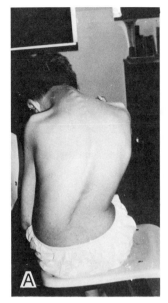
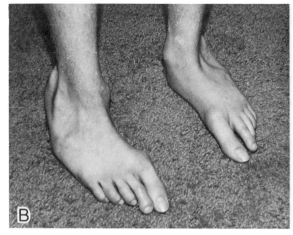

Fig. 9-3. Case study: Tony. (A) Severe kyphoscoliosis in unsupported sitting. (B) Bony collapse of the feet.

continued ability to ambulate become jeopardized or the feet cause pain or discomfort.

The "rightness or wrongness" of the orthopedic physician's decision not to follow Tony at an early age and the parent's decision not to allow spinal surgery at this point are not at issue. Therapists are frequently presented with "regrettable" situations.

In a case like this, a realistic explanation of the purpose of exercise and positioning should be given to the classroom teacher and the parents. They should be made aware that exercise and positioning are not likely to affect the progression of the scoliosis, but should be encouraged to follow a basic program to prevent soft tissue contractures, maintain flexibility in the trunk, and minimize impingement of the rotated thorax and twisted spine on the lungs and other vital organs.

Several different suggestions for positioning could be made. In general, Tony should avoid sitting on the floor and should always have a chair with a firm back and a table or lap board of an appropriate height to allow arm support, thereby decreasing the kyphosis. A small firm cushion placed under one hip may counter the lumbar curve and result in some improvement of the scoliosis. Positioning in prone over a large wedge with arms forward will minimize the kyphosis, stimulate use of the extensor muscles of the neck and upper trunk, and reduce the scoliosis by the mild traction effect of gravity pulling against fixed shoulders. Sidelying with the convexity of the major curve down is often recommended for children with scoliosis, but positioning on either side may be effective in reducing the curve.

Instruction to caregivers should be given in basic exercise to stretch the soft tissue in the feet, legs, and trunk, which are at risk for shortening because of the persistent deforming forces. Handling should include activities to stimulate Tony's ability to support himself in the prone and four-point positions.

A program of appropriately graded stimulation to decrease Tony's sensitivity to touch and a program of sensory stimulation or behavior modification to eliminate his self-abusive behavior should also be included.

Prevention of Respiratory Problems.   Frequent change of position in the severely handicapped child is probably the single most important measure for preventing respiratory problems. Proper positioning will help to prevent rib cage deformity and pooling of secretions and facilitate improved chest excursion. For feeding, the child should be positioned with the trunk at a minimum of a 45-degree angle (seated at 90 degrees is preferable), with the head balanced in a neutral position between flexion and extension. If the neck is allowed to extend in what has been termed the ''bird feeding'' position, the glottis is not able to close effectively over the trachea, and there is essentially an open channel for the aspiration of food into the lungs.

Inverted positioning is of value in promoting the drainage of secretions from the airways. Traditional postural drainage, however, with specific positioning to drain various lung segments, accompanied by percussion and vibration to those areas, is not indicated for upper airway congestion. Theoretically, the effect of postural drainage is to remove secretions, such as are produced in a lobar pneumonia, from the alveoli of specific lung segments. Its use for less serious upper airway congestion is not harmful, but neither is it likely to be particularly beneficial.

Treatment of Oral Motor Problems.   Following a careful assessment of oral motor problems, remediation of the problem areas can be accomplished following the guidelines provided by Morris (in Wilson,[70] Mueller[128]) or others. Consistency is particularly important in an oral motor program. Rarely can a therapist be available for all, or even most, of a child's feeding sessions, so that provisions for carryover to other mealtime situations is essential. It may be that the therapist will choose not to instruct others in highly specialized techniques like jaw control, but, if at all possible, consistency in the position the child is in, the utensils used and the type, texture, and temperature of foods offered should be provided.

It is important for therapists to support families or other primary caregivers in what can be initially a frustrating experience. Somehow, eating seems to be such a basic function that we just expect children to eat well. In the face of a sloppy, slow eater who may have poor nutrition and choke frequently, this unmet expectation may lead to serious feelings of personal inadequacy or nonacceptance of the child on the part of a parent. Patience is essential. Feeding is such a habitual process that any change will at first seem to worsen rather than improve the situation and it takes time—sometimes as much as an hour and a half–to complete a meal when a new program is initiated.

Mealtime should be a relaxed time, a sometimes rare opportunity for one-to-one interaction. In a book entitled *Mealtimes for Severely and Profoundly Handicapped Persons: New Concepts and Attitudes*, more than 50 professionals, as well as parents, volunteers, and handicapped persons themselves, describe and interpret the value of mealtimes.[129] Creative situations and meal-time atmospheres are described that can be the strata for positive interaction, development, and education.

PARENT AND STAFF EDUCATION

Parents of severely and profoundly mentally retarded children are faced with tremendous emotional strains, the need to make critical decisions (sometimes from birth), and the responsibility for a person who will all of his or her life require supervision and have special needs. Prior to the normalization movement of the 1970s, parents had basically two alternatives: to send their children away to large state or private institutions (often a choice encouraged by professionals because of a generally hopeless outlook), or to keep them at home with virtually no support and no services. Fortunately, alternatives are being created that bridge the large gap between home care and institutionalization. These alternatives include group homes, foster home care, home care with day school, home care with respite care (either community-based or in an institution), and short-term institutionalization for the purpose of intensive training or respite for the family.

Enactment of Public Law 94-142 guaranteed privileges that other parents take for granted—assistance with the education and social development of their offspring and a break from the 24-hour-a-day responsibility for their supervision and care. The law also mandated that parents be included in the formulation of appropriate goals and effective programs for their children.

Substantial government and public support have also been provided for multidisciplinary intervention programs starting at birth for high-risk infants and continuing until school age. Denhoff[130] states that one of the major benefits of infant stimulation or enrichment programs is that they enable severely handicapped infants to stay at home. "A good (infant enrichment) program not only instructs and supports parents in carrying out a therapeutic regimen at home, but also helps them to cope with irregularities of feeding, sleeping, crying, and other problems which lessen the chances of survival of the family."

Educational materials specifically addressed to parents have been published by a wide variety of public organizations and private citizens. Bibliographies listing publications of interest to parents are available from The Association for the Severely Handicapped and the Association for Retarded Citizens. Both of these associations provide excellent support to parents and effective advocacy for their handicapped chaildren. More is needed.

The passage of laws does not guarantee that the rights of mentally retarded individuals will be supported in philosophy and practice. Parents need to know what the rights of their children are and how to become effective advocates in their behalf. They need opportunities to meet parents of other handicapped children and assistance in developing support groups. The concept of community-based programs is an important one for parents, but ideas can be a long way from reality. Too many families do not have access to group homes, respite care, or other support services in their community. Although, in general, public awareness and concern for mentally retarded individuals has improved, parents still often feel isolated and guilty. The persistence of architectural barriers in public facilities is a too-frequent reminder that society is not yet concerned enough. Many of the programs and much of the research effort that benefits mentally retarded individuals is funded through government sources. With severe cuts in state and federal budgets, it is more important than ever that citizens in every community become advocates for the mentally retarded and help support the children and their families.

Professionals must resist the tendency to make prejudgments about what is appropriate for the severely handicapped and to give parents "stock" answers.[131] The ability to listen and to consider compassionately not only the financial but the emotional economy of each family is vital. Parents must be encouraged to voice their own needs and concerns, guided to an understanding of their child's many problems, assisted in finding constructive ways to interact with and "teach" their handicapped child, and supported in their efforts to work in the child's behalf.

With the development of new types of programs—new facilities as well as traditional institutional settings—paraprofessionals with a variety of job descriptions are providing care for the profoundly and severely retarded. These workers need to receive instruction in how to develop effective patient management skills, so that the mentally retarded can benefit from their consistency and the workers themselves can receive the positive feedback of seeing development and growth in the children under their care.

Another group that needs guidance in how to love and support the mentally retarded are the normal children, who, as a result of mainstreaming, are interacting with their mentally retarded peers in school on a regular basis. Successful attempts at shaping positive attitudes have been achieved with group discussion, role playing, and the use of audiovisuals.[132–134]

CONCLUSION

The severely and profoundly retarded are people with needs and rights like all of us. Caring for and about them adequately simply demands a little extra insight, creativity, resourcefulness, and patience.

"Cortical function can be curtailed in a great variety of patterns, but barring the totally comatose state, there are always residual perceptions and expressions. These latter elements can be reached, usually in stimulation and training programs, and the expression of such established function is the core of 'fulfillment' at any level. Gratification of this need for fulfillment will add grace to what can otherwise be a dismal atmosphere."[131]

REFERENCES

1. Humphrey H: Quoted in, The Problem of Mental Retardation. President's Committee on Mental Retardation, U.S. Department of Health and Human Services (79-21021), Washington, 1977.

2. Grossman H (ed): Manual on Terminology and Classification in Mental Retardation. Garamound/Pridemark Press, Baltimore, 1973.

3. Hobbs N (ed): Issues in the Classification of Children. Vols 1, 2. Jossey-Bass, San Francisco, 1975.

4. Roszlowski M, Spreat S: A comparison of the psychometric and clinical methods of determining level of retardation. Appl Res Ment Retard 2:359, 1981.

5. Dingman HF, Tarjan G: Mental retardation and the normal distribution curve. Am J Ment Defic 64:991, 1960.

6. Capute AJ, Shapiro BK, Palmer FB: Spectrum of developmental disabilities: Continuum of motor dysfunction. Orthop Clin North Am 12:3, 1981.

7. Conley RW: The Economics of Mental Retardation. John Hopkins University Press, Baltimore, 1973.

8. "The Truth About Mental Retardation," a brochure published by the Association for Retarded Citizens (National Headquarters, PO Box 6109. Arlington, TX 76011).

9. Gustavson KH, Holmgren RJ, Son Blomquist HK: Severe mental retardation in children in a northern Swedish county. J Ment Defic Res 21:161, 1977.

10. Dale A, Stanley FJ: An epidemiological study of cerebral palsy in Western Australia, 1956–1975, II: Spastic cerebral palsy and perinatal factors. Dev Med Child Neurol 22:13, 1980.

11. Malamud N: Neuropathology. In Stevens HA, Heber R (eds): Mental Retardation, A Review of Research. University of Chicago Press, Chicago, 1964.

12. Conway JW, Durr KE: Survey and analysis of the habilitation and rehabilitation status of the mentally retarded with associated handicaps. Department of Health and Human Services, Washington, DC, 1971.

13. Hardman ML, Drew CJ: The physically handicapped retarded individual: A review. Ment Retard 15:43, 1977.

14. Weisz JR, Zigler E: Cognitive development in retarded and nonretarded persons: Piagetian tests of the similar sequence hypothesis. Psychol Bull 86:831, 1979.

15. President's Committee on Mental Retardation: Mental Retardation—Past and Present. U.S. Department of Health and Human Services, Washington, DC, 1977.

16. Rosen M (ed): The History of Mental Retardation. Vols I, II. University Park Press, Baltimore, 1976.

17. Association for Retarded Citizens: Mileposts. Arlington, TX.

18. The Association for the Severely Handicapped: "Deinstitutionalization Policy." Seattle, WA.

19. "The Federal Education for All Handicapped Children Act" (P.L. 94-142): Signed, November 29, 1975. Council for Exceptional Children, Reston, VA, 1976.

20. Ballard J: Public Law 94-142 and Section 504—Understanding What They Are and Are Not. Governmental Relations Unit, Council for Exceptional Children, Reston, VA, 1977.

21. Vocational Rehabilitation Act Amendments (Sect 504, P.L. 93-112), Fed Regist May 4, 1977.

22. Schroeder CS, Schroeder SR: Mental retardation in the United States: assessment, program development and applied research. Appl Res Ment Retard 2:181, 1981.

23. Levine JM (ed): Mental Retardation and the Law—A Report on the Status of Current Court Cases. President's Committee on Mental Retardation, Washington, DC, 1980.

24. Council for Exceptional Children: A continuing summary of pending and completed litigation regarding the education of handicapped children. State-Federal Information Clearinghouse for Exceptional Children, Reston, Virginia.

25. Herr SS: From Rights to Realities—Advocacy By and For Retarded People in the 1980's. President's Committee on Mental Retardation, Washington, DC, 1980.
26. President's Committee on Mental Retardation: Report to the President. Mental Retardation: Prevention Strategies that Work. U.S. Department of Health and Human Services, Washington, DC, 1980.
27. Baumeister AA: Mental retardation policy and research: The unfulfilled promise. Am J Ment Defic 85:449, 1981.
28. Gaines RF, Tobis JS: Rehabilitation recommendations for institutionalized motor-disabled patients. Arch Phys Med Rehabil 62:180, 1981.
29. Hoffer MM, Bullock M: The functional and social significance of orthopedic rehabilitation of mentally retarded patients with cerebral palsy. Orthop Clin North Am 12:185, 1981.
30. Pettitt B: Surgery of the lower extremity in cerebral palsy: Considerations and approaches. Arch Phys Med Rehabil 57:443, 1976.
31. Lindsey RW, Drennan JC: Management of foot and knee deformities in the mentally retarded. Orthop Clin North Am 12:107, 1981.
32. Pulman RM, Pook RB, Singh NN: Prevalence of drug therapy for institutionalized mentally retarded children. Aust J Ment Retard 5:212, 1979.
33. Lipman RS: The use of psychopharmacological agents in residential facilities for the retarded. In Menolascino FJ (ed): Psychiatric Approaches to Mental Retardation. Basic Books, New York, 1970.
34. Gaultieri CT, Hawk B: Tardive dyskinesia and other drug-induced movement disorders among handicapped children and youth. Appl Res Ment Retard 1:55, 1980.
35. Nyhan WL, Johnson HG, Kaufman IA, et al: Seratonergic approaches to the modification of behavior in the Lesch-Nyhan Syndrome. Appl Res Ment Retard 1:25, 1980.
36. Richardson, SA, Koller H, Matz M: Seizures and epilepsy in a mentally retarded population. Appl Res Ment Retard 1:123, 1980.
37. Gever LN (Clinical Pharmacy Ed.): Nursing 81 Drug Handbook. Intermed Communications, Horsham, PA, 1981.
38. Harrel RF, Capp RH, Davis DR, et al: Can nutritional supplements help mentally retarded children? An exploratory study. Proc Natl Acad Sci USA 78:574, 1981.
39. Hutchings WD: Megavitamins and diet. In Feingold B, Bank C (eds): Developmental Disabilities of Early Childhood. Charles C Thomas, Springfield, IL, 1978.
40. Mailman RB, Lewis MH: Food additives and developmental disorders: The case of Erythosin (FD and C Red # 3) or guilty until proven innocent? Appl Res Ment Retard 2:297, 1981.
41. Carenza EC: Pediatricks. Van Nostrand Reinhold, New York, 1974.
42. Altman R, Talkington LW, Cleland CC: Relative effectiveness of modelling and verbal instruction on severe retardates' gross motor performance. Psychol Rep 31:695, 1972.
43. Ritvo ER, Ornitz EM, La Franchi S: Frequency of repetitive behaviors in early infantile autism and its variants. Arch Gen Psychiatry 19:341, 1968.
44. Repp AC, Barton LE, Brulle AR: Correspondence between effectiveness and staff use of instructions for severely retarded persons. Appl Res Ment Retard 2:237, 1981.
45. Piaget J: The origins of intelligence in children. Norton, New York, 1963.
46. Woodward M: The behavior of idiots interpreted by Piaget's theory of sensori-motor development. Br J Educ Psychol 29:60, 1959.
47. Kahn JV: Relationship of Piaget's sensorimotor period to language acquisition of profoundly retarded children. Am J Ment Defic 79:640, 1975.

48. Silverman FH: Communication for the Speechless. Prentice-Hall, Englewood Cliffs, NJ, 1980.
49. Gould J: The use of the Vineland Social Maturity Scale, the Merrill-Palmer Scale of Mental Tests (non-verbal items) and the Reynell Developmental Language Scales with children in contact with the services for severe mental retardation. J Ment Defic Res 21:213, 1977.
50. Langley MB: Assessment of the Multihandicapped, Visually Impaired Child. Stoelting, Chicago, 1980.
51. Murray JN (ed): Developing Assessment Programs for the Multi-handicapped Child. Charles C Thomas, Springfield, IL, 1980.
52. Naglieri JA: Extrapolated developmental indices for the Bayley Scales of Infant Development. Am J Ment Defic 85:548, 1981.
53. Francis RJ, Rarick GL: Motor characteristics of the mentally retarded. Am J Ment Defic 63:792, 1959.
54. Samilson RL: Orthopedic surgery of the hips and spine in retarded cerebral palsy patients. Orthop Clin North Am 12:83, 1981.
55. Mital MA, Sakellarides HT: Surgery of the upper extremity in the retarded individual with spastic cerebral palsy. Orthop Clin North Am 12:127, 1981.
56. Sherrill C: Posture training as a means of normalization. Ment Retard 18:135, 1980.
57. Kendall HO, Kendall FP: Developing and maintaining good posture. Phys Ther 48:319, 1968.
58. Rinsky LA: Perspectives on surgery for scoliosis in mentally retarded patients. Orthop Clin North Am 12:113, 1981.
59. Ayres AJ: Sensory Integration and Learning Disorders. Western Psychological Services, Los Angeles, 1976.
60. Montgomery PC: Assessment and treatment of the child with mental retardation: guidelines for the public school therapist. Phys Ther 61:1265, 1981.
61. Illingworth RS: The Development of the Infant and Young Child. 5th Ed. Churchill Livingstone, London, 1974.
62. Donoghue E, Kirman B, Bullmore GH: Some factors affecting age of walking in a mentally retarded population. Dev Med Child Neurol 18:71, 1976.
63. Shapiro BK, Accardo PJ, Capute AJ: Factors affecting walking in a profoundly retarded population. Dev Med Child Neurol 21:369, 1979.
64. Molnar GE: Motor deficit of retarded infants and young children. Arch Phys Med Rehabil 55:393, 1974.
65. Grady A, Gilfoyle E: A developmental theory of somatosensory perception. In Henderson A, Coryell J (eds): The Body Senses and Perceptual Deficit. Boston University, Boston, 1973.
66. Montgomery P, Gauger J: Sensory dysfunction in children who toe walk. Phys Ther 58:1195, 1978.
67. Montgomery PC, Richter E: Sensorimotor Integration for the Developmentally Disabled Child: A Handbook. Western Psychological Services, Los Angeles, 1980.
68. Cleland CC, Powell HC, Talkington LW: Death of the profoundly retarded. Ment Retard 9:36, 1971.
69. Chaney RH: Respiratory complications in the profoundly retarded compared to those in less retarded. In Schwartz JD, Eyman PC, Cleland CC, O'Grady R (eds): The Profoundly Mentally Retarded. Vol. IX. Western Research Conference, Austin, TX, 1978.
70. Wilson JM (ed): Oral Motor Function and Dysfunction in Children (Proceedings of a Conference). University of North Carolina, Chapel Hill, 1977.

71. Wilson JM: Selection and use of adaptive equipment for children. Totline 6:4, 1980.
72. Bergen A: Selected Equipment for Pediatric Rehabilitation. Blythdale Children's Hospital, Bradhurst Avenue, Valhalla, New York, 10595, 1974.
73. Slominski A: Please Help Us Help Ourselves: Inexpensive Adapted Equipment for the Handicapped. Cerebral Palsy Clinic, Indiana University Medical Center, Indianapolis, 1970.
74. Robinault I: Functional aides for the multiply handicapped. Harper and Row, New York, 1973.
75. Dubose RF, Deni K: Easily Constructed Adaptive and Assistive Equipment. The Council for Exceptional Children, Reston, VA, 1980.
76. Capecchi J: Skater sled for retarded persons. Phys Ther 58:181, 1978.
77. Webster M: Webster's New Collegiate Dictionary. Merriam, Springfield, MA, 1979.
78. Hutt ML, Gibby RG: The Mentally Retarded Child: Development, Training and Education. 4th Ed. Allyn and Bacon, Boston, 1979.
79. MacLean W, Baumeister A: Observational analysis of the stereotyped mannerisms of a developmentally delayed infant. Appl Res Ment Retard 2:257, 1981.
80. Scherzer AL, Mike V, Ilson J: Physical therapy as a determinant of change in the cerebral palsied infant. Pediatrics 58:47, 1976.
81. Westervelt VD, Luiselli JK: Establishing standing and walking behavior in a physically handicapped, retarded child. Phys Ther 55:761, 1975.
82. Kielhofner G, Miyake S: The therapeutic use of play with mentally retarded adults. Am J Occup Ther 35:375, 1981.
83. Godfrey B, Kephart N: Movement Patterns and Motor Education. Appleton-Century-Crofts, New York, 1969.
84. Chaney C, Kephart N: Motoric Aids to Perceptual Training. Merrill, Columbus, OH, 1968.
85. Kephart N: The Slow Learner in the Classroom. 2nd Ed. Merrill, Columbus, OH, 1971.
86. Cratty BJ, Martin MM: Perceptual Motor Efficiency in Children. Lea and Febiger, Philadelphia, 1969.
87. Cratty BJ: Motor Activity and the Education of Retardates. Lea and Febiger, Philadelphia, 1974.
88. Cratty BJ: The use of movement activities in the education of retarded children. In: Physical Therapy Services in the Developmental Disabilities, eds. Pearson PH, Williams CE. Charles C Thomas, Springfield, ILL, 1972.
89. Bobath K, Bobath B: Diagnosis and assessment of cerebral palsy. In Pearson PH, Williams CE (eds): Physical Therapy Services in the Developmental Disabilities. Charles C Thomas, Springfield, ILL, 1972.
90. Semans S: The Bobath concept in treatment of neurological disorders: A neurodevelopmental treatment. Am J Phys Med 46:732, 1967.
91. Stockmeyer SA: An interpretation of the approach of Rood to the treatment of neuromuscular dysfunction. Am J Phys Med 46:900, 1967.
92. Stockmeyer SA: A sensorimotor approach to treatment. In Pearson PH, Williams CE (eds): Physical Therapy Services in the Developmental Disabilities. Charles C Thomas, Springfield, IL, 1972.
93. Ginsburg H, Opper S: Piaget's Theory of Intellectual Development. Prentice-Hall Englewood Cliffs, NJ, 1969.
94. Bradley-Johnson S, Friedrich DD, Wyrembelski AR: Exploratory behavior in Down's syndrome and normal infants. Appl Res Ment Retard 2:213, 1981.

95. Clark FA, Miller LR, Thomas JA, et al: A comparison of operant and sensory integrative methods on developmental parameters in profoundly retarded adults. Am J Occup Ther 32:86, 1978.

96. Magrun WM, Ottenbacher K, McCue S, et al: Effects of vestibular stimulation on the spontaneous use of verbal language in developmentally delayed children. Am J Occup Ther 35:101, 1981.

97. Evans RG: The reduction of hyperactive behavior in three profoundly retarded adolescents through increased stimulation. AAESPH Rev 4:259, 1979.

98. Bright T, Bittick K, Fleeman B: Reduction of self-injurious behavior using sensory integrative techniques. Am J Occup Ther 35:167, 1981.

99. Montgomery P, Richter E: Effect of sensory integrative therapy on the neuromotor development of retarded children. Phys Ther 57:799, 1977.

100. Page D: Neuromuscular reflex therapy as an approach to patient care. Am J Phys Med 46:816, 1967.

101. Delacato CH: The Diagnosis and Treatment of Speech and Reading Problems. Charles C Thomas, Springfield, IL, 1963.

102. Doman RJ, Spitz EB, Zucman E, et al: Children with severe brain injuries. Neurologic organization in terms of mobility. JAMA 174:157, 1960.

103. Zigler E: A plea to end the use of the patterning treatment for retarded children. Am J Orthopsychiatry 51:388, 1981.

104. Cohen HJ, Birch HG, Taft LT: Some considerations for evaluating the Doman-Delacato "Patterning" method. Pediatrics 45:302, 1970.

105. Sparrow S, Zigler E: Evaluation of a patterning treatment for retarded children. Pediatrics 62:137, 1978.

106. Skinner BF: Science and Human Behavior. Macmillan, New York, 1953.

107. Bragg JH, Houser C, Schumaker J: Behavior modification: Effects on reverse tailor sitting in children with cerebral palsy. Phys Ther 55:860, 1975.

108. Banks SP: Behavior therapy with a boy who had never learned to walk. Psychother Theory Res Pract 5:150, 1968.

109. Chandler LS, Adams MA: Multiply handicapped child motivated for ambulation through behavior modification (case report). Phys Ther 52:399, 1972.

110. Hester SB: Effects of behavior modification on the standing and walking deficiencies of a profoundly retarded child: Case report. Phys Ther 61:807, 1980.

111. Kolderie ML: Behavior modification in the treatment of children with cerebral palsy. Phys Ther 51:1083, 1971.

112. Loynd J, Barclay A: A case study in developing ambulation in a profoundly retarded child. Behav Res Ther 8:207, 1970.

113. Miller H, Patton M, Henton K: Behavior modification in a profoundly retarded child: A case report. Behav Ther 2:375, 1971.

114. Rice HK, McDaniel MW, Denney SL: Operant conditioning techniques for use in the physical rehabilitation of the multiply handicapped retarded patients. Phys Ther 48:342, 1968.

115. Garber NB: Operant procedures to eliminate drooling behavior in a cerebral palsied adolescent. Dev Med Child Neurol 13:641, 1971.

116. O'Brien F, Azrin T, Bugle C: Training profoundly retarded children to stop crawling. J Appl Behav Anal 5:131, 1972.

117. Vukelich R, Hake DF: Reduction of dangerously aggressive behavior in a severely retarded resident through a combination of positive reinforcement procedures. J Appl Behav Anal 4:215, 1971.

118. Corte HE, Wolf MM, Locke BJ: A comparison of procedures for eliminating self-injurious behavior of retarded adolescents. J Appl Behav Anal 4:201, 1971.

119. Luiselli JK: Controlling self-inflicted biting of a retarded child by the differential reinforcement of other behavior. Psychol Rep 42:435, 1978.
120. Barret R, Matson J, Shapiro E, et al: A comparison of punishment and DRO procedures for treating the stereotypic behavior of mentally retarded children. Appl Res Ment Retard 2:247, 1981.
121. Ball TS, McCrady RE, Hart AD: Automated reinforcement of head posture in two cerebral palsied retarded children. Percept Mot Skills 40:619, 1975.
122. Silverstein L: Biofeedback with young cerebral palsied children. In Feingold B, Bank C (eds): Developmental Disabilities of Early Childhood. Charles C Thomas, Springfield, IL, 1978.
123. Ball TS, Combs T, Rugh J, et al: Automated range of motion training with two cerebral palsied retarded young men. Ment Retard 15:47, 1977.
124. Skrotzky K, Gallenstein JS, Osternig LR: Effects of electromyographic feedback training on motor control in spastic cerebral palsy. Phys Ther 58:547, 1978.
125. Ball TS, McCrady RE: Automated finger praxis training with a cerebral palsied retarded adolescent. Ment Retard 13:41, 1975.
126. Frielander BZ, Kamin P, Hesse GW: Operant therapy for prehension disabilities in moderately and severely retarded young children. Train Sch Bull (Vinel) 71:101, 1974.
127. Sachs DA, Martin JE, Fitch JL: The effect of visual feedback on a digital exercise in a functionally deaf cerebral palsied child. J Behav Ther Exp Psychol 3:217, 1972.
128. Mueller HA: Facilitating feeding and pre-speech. In Pearson PH, Williams CE (eds): Physical Therapy in the Developmental Disabilities. Charles C Thomas, Springfield, IL, 1972.
129. Perske R, Clifton A, McLean B, et al (ed): Mealtimes for Severely and Profoundly Handicapped Persons: New Concepts and Attitudes. University Park Press, Baltimore, 1977.
130. Denhoff E: Current status of infant stimulation or enrichment programs for children with developmental disabilities. Pediatrics 67:32, 1981.
131. Crocker AC, Cushna B: Pediatric decisions in children with serious mental retardation. Ped Clin North Am 19:413, 1972.
132. Gottlief J: Improving attitudes toward children by using group discussion. Except Child 47:106, 1979.
133. Kitano M, Chan KS: Taking the role of retarded children: Effects of familiarity and similarity. Am J Ment Defic 83:37, 1978.
134. Westervelt VD, Turnbull AP: Children's attitudes toward physically handicapped peers and intervention approaches for attitude change. Phys Ther 60:896, 1980.

10 | Learning Disabilities

Barbara H. Connolly

As few as 1 percent and as many as 28 percent of elementary school children have been described as learning disabled.[1-7] The percentage of children labeled as having learning disabilities is contingent on the definition. After 25 years of diligent work by many professionals and lay persons, the accepted definition of children with learning disabilities is as follows:[8]

> [those who] exhibit a disorder in one or more of the basic psychological processes involved in understanding or in using spoken or written language. These may be manifested in disorders of listening, thinking, talking, reading, writing, spelling or arithmetic. They include conditions which have been referred to as perceptual handicaps, brain injury, minimal brain dysfunction, dyslexia, developmental aphasia, etc. They do not include learning problems which are due primarily to visual, hearing or motor handicaps, to mental retardation, emotional disturbances or to environmental disadvantage.

Three major events have profoundly influenced the study and treatment of learning disabilities: (1) the passage of Public Law 94-142, (2) regulations in the 1977 Federal Register, and (3) proposed regulations in the 1982 Federal Register. The passage of Public Law 94-142 mandated a precise definition of specific learning disabilities for dispersion of federal monies for children with learning disabilities. The United States Office of Education relied on the definition previously stated in the Learning Disabilities Act of 1969 but believed that further refinement in the criteria was needed for accurate identification of the disorder.

The 1977 Federal Register outlined a procedure to be used in identifying learning disabilities in children which no longer relied on identification of psychologic process disorders but instead focused on the discrepancy component. Criteria used for identification included the following[9]:

317

A team may determine that a child has a specific learning disability if: (1) The child does not achieve commensurate with his or her age and ability levels in one or more of the areas listed in the paragraph below . . . when provided with learning experiences appropriate for the child's age and ability levels and (2) The team finds that a child has a severe discrepancy between achievement and intellectual ability in one or more of the following areas: oral expressions, listening comprehension, written expression, basic reading skills, reading comprehension, mathematics calculation or mathematics reasoning.

The proposed regulations in the 1982 Federal Register currently under debate may have profound effects upon the service that are to be provided to children with learning disabilities and on the involvement of parents in the planning for delivery of those services. In particular, the inclusion of related services, such as physical therapy and occupational therapy, may be deleted or related services may be restricted to only certain types of children.

CHARACTERISTICS OF LEARNING DISABILITIES

Hyperactivity and distractability are characteristic of children with mental retardation, emotional disturbances, and learning disabilities. To be identified as learning disabled, a child must have low- to above-average IQ scores, a characteristic that distinguishes him or her from the mentally retarded child. Other characteristics of learning disabled children include impairments of perception and concept formation, soft neurologic signs, disorders of speech and comprehension, disorders of motor functions, problems in academic achievement, disorders of the thinking processes, poor emotional control, poor peer relationships, and variations from normal in physical development.[10] Examples of perceptual problems include visual perceptual disorders, manifested primarily through problems with form perception, position in space, and visual closure. Tactual, kinesthetic, and vestibular dysfunctions may create problems in academics and may interfere with the development of bilateral integration, lateralization, form and space conceptualization, eye-hand coordination, praxis, and speech and language. Common speech and language dysfunctions include problems with the reception or decoding and expression or encoding of written or spoken language. Children may have oral dyspraxia resulting in articulation difficulties. Auditory processing problems may create difficulties in the child's ability to attend to his environment. Auditory memory problems may produce difficulties with memory for spoken word sequences or with retrieval of words. Teachers and parents often complain that this type of child cannot follow commands. Motor disorders are usually described as gross or fine motor incoordination. Gubbay and his associates[11] identified the severely incoordinated child as having the clumsy child syndrome. These children, predominantly males, were identified as having difficulties in motor coordination as well as in cognition.

Attentional deficits, often attributed to children with learning disabilities, may create difficulties in the child's ability to orient to tasks and to screen out extraneous stimuli, which leads to behaviors such as hyperactivity, distractibility, and short attention span. Academic problems in basic reading skills, reading comprehension, mathematical calculations and mathematical reasoning are seen singularly or in combination in children with learning disabilities. The academic problems may occur as end products of dysfunctions in other areas such as somatosensory perceptions.

Wallace and McLoughlin[12] identified the most prevalent social/emotional problems in learning disabled children as excessive dependence upon parents, teachers, and other adults, distractibility, poor self-concept, physically disruptive behaviors, difficulty in changing tasks, withdrawal, and hyperactivity. Bryan and Bryan[13,14] attempted to explain some of the children's social problems by suggesting that the child has difficulty in interpreting social situations. The child may be unable to discriminate subtle affective cues and may react inappropriately to peers and to adults. Aggression, as a form of interaction, may be used to attract the attention the child desires. Poor self-concept, ego, and self-esteem in the learning disabled child may be a reflection of a lack of positive self-regard generated by the child's repeated failures.

THEORETICAL CAUSES OF LEARNING DISABILITIES

The exact cause(s) of learning disabilities is unknown. Theories of causation offered in the past have met with varying degrees of acceptance. In the following sections we will discuss those theories that have been most important in the advancement of our knowledge of learning disabilities, although some are obsolete at this time.

Maturational Lag

In the 1930s, Bender[15] proposed that the brain may develop at different rates and that if the rate is altered in certain ways, the child may develop learning disabilities. Reitan and Ball,[16] in 1973, supported Bender's early theory through their clinical research indicating that, in the absence of actual brain damage, academic or perceptual deficits may be related to a lag in the normal developmental organization of the brain. Birch[17] stated that the sensory systems develop in a sequential pattern as the child learns to associate or integrate stimuli from one system with those of another. He believed that children with learning disabilities might have a delay in their ability to integrate information from the various sensory systems. Myklebust and Johnson[18] further speculated that children had two semiautonomous systems for learning; the intraneurosensory and the interneurosensory systems. The two systems were thought to be able to function either independently or in concert. Learning disabilities were thought to be caused by a dysfunction within the brain which specifically altered processing in the area of interneurosensory learning; however, the child's general capacity to learn was not affected by the dysfunction because the intraneurosensory system remained intact.

Neurologic Patterning

The "patterning" theory of enhancing neurologic organization, the Doman-Delacato method, has been the cause of much debate among professionals. Delacato[19] hypothesizes that development of the human neurologic system is a recapitulation of phylogenetic development. Delacato[19-21] proposes that training in specific locomotor tasks (patterns of movement) will positively influence brain centers such as the midbrain and the cerebral cortex. This influence in turn will enhance the child's learning abilities. Language and reading are thought to be the end products in the continuum of neurologic organization. Therefore, dysfunctions in these areas are thought to represent dysfunctions at lower levels in the neurologic system. However, Robbins and Glass,[22] after reviewing research on the Doman Delacato approach, stated that (1) the tenets of the theory are refuted by internal inconsistencies, lack of supporting evidence, and direct contraindications by existing knowledge; (2) the studies cited by the Institute for the Achievement of Human Potential lack proper control and statistical analysis; and (3) no empirical evidence has been produced to substantiate the values of theory or practice of neurologic organization.

Cerebral Hemispheric Specialization

Recent brain research suggests that understanding of cerebral hemispheric organization or hemispheric specialization may provide a new key to comprehending alterations in brain physiology. Invasive and noninvasive studies have shown that the right hemisphere is responsible for visual spatial functions, tactile spatial relations, and auditory functions such as music and melodies. The left hemisphere is thought to be responsible for the processing of language and for motor planning.[23,24] In general, the right hemisphere is thought to perform a "Gestalt" function, while the left hemisphere is more responsible for analytical functioning. Interestingly, in an autopsy study of dyslexic patients, Galaburda and associates[25] found that Wernicke's language area was not larger on the left side of the brain as in normals but was the same size on both sides.

Information Integration

Senf's[26] information integration theory is based on the individual's ability to organize and integrate information to generate behavior. The integration of the information is based upon the individual's internal environment which consists of the store of memories, mental reactions to salient features of events such as the magnitude of incoming stimuli, and feedback from bodily sensation and motoric behavior. Senf's model assumes that learning disabilities involve a dysfunction in information processing and in information integrating, which occurs if the child is not able (1) to receive incoming stimuli correctly, (2) to interpret incoming stimuli correctly, (3) to produce an appropriate neural response to the stimuli, or (4) to screen out task-irrelevant stimuli. The model stipulates that a feedback loop be present within the system thus supplying continuity between thinking and sensory processing.

Sensory Integrative Dysfunction

Ayres[27] proposes a sensory integration theory similar to Senf's information integration theory. Ayres states, as does Piaget, that early sensory motor learning provides a basis for later cognitive functioning. She stresses the importance of both sensory integration and adaptive motor responses as the basis for facilitation of learning. Ayres[28] views praxis, eye-hand coordination, form and space perceptions, and lateralization as outcomes of sensory integration with the eventual end products being academic achievement and psychosocial skills (Table 10-1). The sensory integrative theory does not advocate the teaching of specific skills but instead has the more general goal of enhancing the brain's ability to learn. Sensory integration is defined as the organization and interpretation of sensory stimuli for the production of an adaptive response. Organization here means the translation of stimuli into meaningful percepts. Interpretation is defined as the link between perception and the adaptation or motor behaviors of the organism which make possible successful interaction with the environment and promote survival.

Based upon selected concepts and principles of central nervous system functioning, the three primary assumptions of the sensory integrative theory are as follows:[29]

1. The integration of performance of the parts is necessary for the functioning of the whole brain. The simultaneous provision of various types of sensory input via the tactile, somatic, proprioceptive, and vestibular systems is assumed to enhance sensory integration.

2. The maturation of the human brain is thought to be comprised of a series of hierarchical stages. The functioning of the cerebral cortex is influenced by the integrative processing of sensory information by the lower levels of the central nervous system such as the brainstem or spinal cord.

3. Plasticity in the central nervous system is present throughout the organism's life span. Based upon this premise, sensory integration techniques may have the capacity to alter the function of the central nervous system of the child. The approach does not propose to cure the basic neurologic problem interfering with learning, but attempts to modify the neurologic dysfunction identified through the use of sensory integrative tests and other clinical observations.

Ayres[28] states that sensorimotor dysfunction may be caused by either brain damage or by sensory deprivation, either real or internal. She speculates that some children experience sensory deprivation not because the experiences are

Table 10-1. The Senses, Integration of Their Inputs, and Their End Products

The Senses	Integration of Their Inputs		End Products
Auditory (hearing)		Speech	
		Language	Ability to concentrate
Vestibular (gravity and movement)	Eye movements Posture Balance Muscle tone Gravitational security	Body percept Coordination of two sides of the body Motor planning	Ability to organize Self-esteem Self-control Self-confidence Academic learning ability
Proprioceptive (muscles and joints)		Activity level Attention span Emotional stability	Capacity for abstract thought and reasoning Specialization of each side of the body and the brain
Tactile (touch)	Sucking Eating Mother-infant bond Tactile comfort	Eye-hand coordination Visual perception Purposeful activity	
Visual (seeing)			

Reprinted by permission of Western Psychological Services. Ayres AJ: Sensory Integration and the Child. p 60. Western Psychological Services, Los Angeles, 1979.

not available to them but because they are unable to process the stimuli appropriately. Disorders that are identified by Ayres as exemplary of sensory integrative problems include the vestibular system dysfunctions, bilateral integrative disorders, tactile defensiveness, somatosensory dysfunctions, developmental dyspraxia, and visual perceptual disorders.

Validation of the effectiveness of any treatment approach is necessary for acceptance by professionals. The effectiveness of the sensory integrative approach has been examined by both the medical and educational communities. Ayres'[29] early study with learning disabled children with auditory language deficits produced statistically significant increases in reading scores after the implementation of sensorimotor training as compared with the control group. In 1976, a study by Ayres[30] with 92 learning disabled children revealed that those children who received six months of sensory integrative therapy made greater gains in reading and spelling than did children in the control group.

In a recent study on hyporeactive nystagmus following vestibular stimulation in learning disabled children, Ottenbacher and colleagues[31] found that children with hyporeactive postrotary nystagmus also had reduced oculomotor control. After a program of sensory integrative therapy that emphasized vestibular and somatic proprioceptive activities, improvements were noted in the duration of postrotary nystagmus and in ocular fixation skills. Ottenbacher and associates[31] speculated that sensory integrative therapy would be beneficial to those children whose eye movement control deficits might be associated with reading problems. Other studies have not shown statistically significant results but provide information that should stimulate further research.[32]

CONCEPTS FOR TREATMENT OF LEARNING DISABILITIES

Kephart: Perceptual Motor Match

The perceptual motor match concept as proposed by Kephart[33-35] states that perception and movement must be matched if learning is to take place effectively. The matching supposedly occurs when a wide variety of sensory experiences and movement opportunities are provided. Kephart further asserts that motor development precedes visual development and that kinesthetic input from motor activities serves as a feedback device for the monitoring of visual activities.

Kephart believes that poor development in eight motor bases or generalizations are related to learning problems. These motor generalizations include posture, balance, locomotion, directionality, body image, laterality, contacting and receiving objects, and propelling objects. Kephart considers posture to be a primary pattern of movement through which the child maintains a relationship to gravity. Locomotion enables the child to learn about the dynamics of movement and the relationship of his or her body to surrounding objects. Kephart defines contact skills as reaching, grasping and releasing objects. He believes that knowledge gained from the manipulation of objects enables the child to develop skills in form perception and in figure-ground discrimination. Additionally, practice of receipt and propulsion skills is thought to teach the child how objects move and about velocities, sizes and distances in space. Laterality, according to Kephart, is related to directionality and is defined as the child's recognition of the right and left sides of the body. Directionality is viewed as an expression of laterality and is the ability to locate objects outside the body. If laterality or directionality skills are deficient, Kephart asserts that letter reversals and incorrect placement of letters in words may occur. Body image as a motor generalization is thought to be necessary if the child is to understand the relationship of his or her body to the surrounding space. Kephart's therapeutic program can be divided into four ageas of activities: chalkboard, sensorimotor, ocular motor, and form-perception training. Ocular training or the establishment of adequate visual perceptual skills are thought to assist in the establishment of all of the motor generalizations proposed by Kephart.[35]

Controversy has arisen over the effectiveness of the perceptual motor program that was proposed by Kephart, particularly in relationship to the effect upon reading. A study by Haring and Stables[36] compared the perceptual and motor skills in two groups of children, one group having been involved in a perceptual motor program and the other not having been involved. They found that various perceptual and motor skills were improved, but they did not assess reading abilities at any time in these children. Roach[37] and Brown,[38] in an assessment of reading skills before and after the use of a perceptual motor program found no difference in the reading skills of either group. More recently, Vellutino and colleagues[39] reported that a link between poor reading and linguistic deficits was found in their study, rather than a relationship between perceptual deficits and poor reading.

Even though perceptual motor programs have been criticized, portions of the programs seem to have demonstrated value for certain children. Hallahan and Cruickshank[40] critically reviewed 42 studies on the efficacy of perceptual motor programs and found only 17 percent to be free from errors of faulty reporting, unsound methodological procedures, or both. Of the seven sound studies, there was no consensus on the positive or negative effects of the training. Hallahan and Cruickshank[40] concluded that

> although no persuasive empirical evidence has been brought to face in support of perceptual motor training, neither has there been solid negative evidence. Owing to the lack of satisfactory research studies with proper methodological controls, it is injudicious to decide whole heartedly that perceptual motor training deserves or does not deserve approval. The ultimate acceptance or rejection of these theorists and their procedures ought to depend upon systematic, empirical investigations yet to be done.

Barsch: Movigenic Curriculum

Barsch[41,42] developed the "movigenic curriculum" based upon his belief that the development of spatial orientation improves the child's learning abilities. Barsch's[41] techniques in the movigenic curriculum are based upon ten basic constructs:

1. Humans are designed for movement.
2. The objectives for movement is survival, thus survival chances are improved with efficient mobility.
3. Movement takes place in a gravitational field, and thus information is received through movement.
4. The mechanism for receiving the information is the perceptocognitive system.
5. Since movement takes place in space, humans must learn to move efficiently in space.
6. Developmental momentum pushes the learner toward maturity.
7. Movement causes some degree of stress but a degree of stress is necessary for learning.
8. Feedback is necessary for efficiency of movement.
9. Development occurs in sequential progression from simple to complex.
10. Language, a visual and spatial phenomenon, is the communicator of movement efficiency.

Based upon these constructs, Barsch described the three components of normal motor development as postural-transport orientation (muscular strength, dynamic balance, body awareness, spatial awareness, and temporal awareness); perceptocognitive modes (gustatory, olfactory, tactile, kinesthetic, auditory, and visual), and degrees of freedom (bilaterality, rhythm, flexibility, and motor planning). Barsch speculated that the three components of movement blend together to give the child an adequate body image, which is important to the learning process.

Activities suggested by Barsch[43] include rolling, crawling, walking, jumping, and moving to the pace of a metronome, progressing the child through unilateral to bilateral and finally to cross-diagonal movements. Other training activities suggested by Barsch include chalkboard work stressing bilaterality, muscular strengthening; equilibrium practice using the balance beam and balance board; spatial and body activities such as "angel in the snow" activities; and activities stressing flexibility and motor planning.

Cratty: Perceptual Motor Program

Cratty's[44-46] perceptual motor program was developed for the enhancement of motor skills and for increasing a child's cognitive abilities. Cratty, unlike Kephart and Barsch, does not agree that reading or learning improvements are accomplished through the use of perceptual systems. He does agree that an inability to effectively participate in gross motor activities can produce unpleasant socialization experiences for the child which may lower his self-esteem and peer acceptance, which in turn may adversely affect motor and cognitive functioning. Cratty does maintain that, by associating a child's movements with higher level thinking, gross motor activities can benefit intellectual development.

Cratty's model of maturation in the infant attempts to map how specific abilities diffuse, collect together and interact in the maturing individual. Attributes as defined by Cratty[46] are "clusters of scores in similar tasks denoting a relatively specific ability trait." According to Cratty, bonds connect the various facets of the child's attributes or skills. The formation of a new bond between the skills may signal the emergence of a new skill.

The conceptual schema of development advocated by Cratty is presented in the form of assumptions and of propositions derived from the assumptions. Basically, Cratty[46] divides skill development into four areas, cognitive, verbal, motor, and perceptual (Fig. 10-1). In each of these areas, individual skills mature at different times and may be influenced by the child's external environment and by self-perceptions. Cratty[46] states that as the child matures, connections occur between skill areas and within skill areas. For example, the ability to balance has a strong bond or connection with the child's ability to walk, to run, and to jump (Fig. 10-2). Cratty also states that the speed at which the connections are made between skills and the speed of development of skills may be affected by the child's cognitive abilities. A third assumption or axiom proposed by Cratty is that a slowing of the acquisition of skills may occur if the child is not offered appropriate experiences during the critical periods of learning.

Cratty believes that some skills in the child that originally involve observation or imitation are eventually overtaken by cognitive functioning as the child matures. As the child matures, bonds or connections may develop between previously independent skills and sometimes even between two or three skills at the same time. However, with multiple bonding, each bond may not be equally well established at the same time. In addition, some bonds must disappear as the child no longer needs the bonds or if the bonds interfere with effective functioning. Cratty states that the clinician or educator may assist the child in the formation or deletion of bonds by offering experiences to the child. The effectiveness of the clinician, educator or parent depends upon their recognition of the connections which are weak or ineffective in the child.

Based on his theoretical model, Cratty[45] designed games and exercises enhance the development of skill areas in the child. His activities, although primarily motor, are aimed at the development of all skill areas: motor, verbal, perceptual, and cognitive. Cratty divides his activities into those for (1) perceptions of body and position in space, (2) balance, (3) locomotion, (4) agility, (5) strength, endurance, and flexibility, (6) catching and throwing balls, (7) manual abilities, and (8) moving and thinking.

Frostig–Horne: The Move–Grow–Learn Program

Remedial programs providing activities designed to strengthen the child's abilities in the areas of ocular motor coordination, visual figure-ground discrimination, form constancy, position in space, and spatial relations were developed in the 1960s and 1970s based upon the Frostig Developmental Test of Visual Perception[47,48] (Table 10-2). Frostig[47] states that both classroom ob-

(*Text continues on page 330.*)

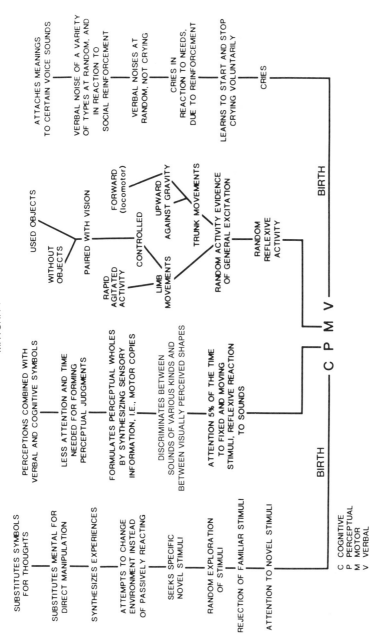

Fig. 10-1. Attribute channels according to Cratty, illustrating examples of behaviors contained by each. (Redrawn from Cratty B: Perceptual and Motor Development in Infants and Children. 2nd ed. p 14. Prentice-Hall, Englewood Cliffs, NJ, 1979.)

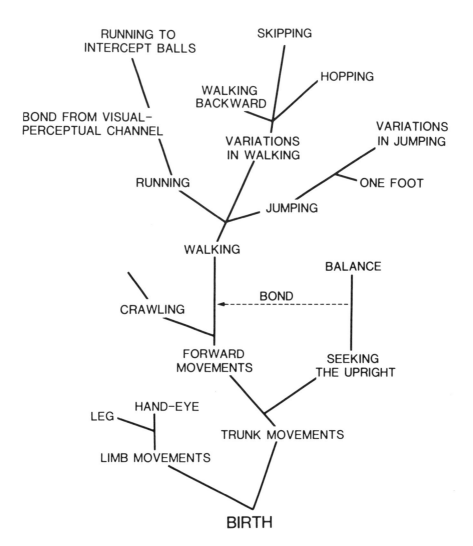

Fig. 10-2. The differentiation, diffusion, and bonding that occur within the attribute branch containing locomotor and trunk behaviors. (Redrawn from Cratty BJ: Perceptual and Motor Development in Infants and Children. 2nd ed. p 18. Prentice-Hall, Englewood Cliffs, NJ, 1979.)

Table 10-2. Frostig Developmental Test of Visual Perception (Brief Summary)

Subtest Name	Example	Some Functions Covered	Some Suggested Training Procedures
Eye-motor coordination	Draw straight lines horizontally. Stop and start on target.	Eye-hand coordination. Necessary for handwriting, drawing, arts and crafts, manipulatory and self-help activities.	Eye-movement training. Arts and crafts. Manipulatory exercises. Handwriting exercises. Physical education program.
Figure-ground	Find a hidden figure. Find one of two or several intersecting figures.	Ability to focus visually on relevant aspects of visual field and disregard irrelevant background.	"Finding" games; e.g., hidden figures included in many children's activity books. Sorting exercises. Unscrambling intersecting words such as *(symbols)*
Form constancy	Find all the squares on a page regardless of color, background, tilt, size.	Ability to see sameness of essential form despite changes of image on retina. Has implication for learning to identify letters presented in various printing styles.	Identifying objects or drawings at different distances or angles. Drawing diagrams of three-dimensional patterns. Finding all objects of a certain shape in the room.
Position in space	Find the form that is reversed or rotated.	Ability to discriminate position; to differentiate letters such as "*d*" and "*b*," "*w*" and "*m*."	Exercises promoting awareness of body position in relation to objects—go under the table, over chair, around the desk, and so on. Physical education program. Learning directions in space: right, left.
Spatial relations	Duplicate a dot pattern by linking dots with a line.	Ability to see spatial relationships of objects to one another; related to ability to perceive the sequence of letters in a word.	Copying patterns with pegs, beads, marbles; puzzles.

Frostig M, Maslow P: Learning Problems in the Classroom. pp 126–127. Grune & Stratton, New York, 1973.

servation and experimental studies indicate that these five abilities are relevant to the child's progress in school and in the development of perceptual skills. The use of movement in combination with visual perception is considered an important aspect of the remedial program, particularly in sustaining the child's attention and in channeling his or her energies.

Frostig and Horne[48] state that the effectiveness of the visual perceptual training programs is dependent upon the age of the child when the program is initiated and in the transference of skills learned in the perceptual training to use in other environments. The training should assist the child in paying attention for longer periods of time, increasing his or her awareness of the environment and gathering more information from the surroundings.

Numerous studies have been reported on the effectiveness of the Frostig-Horne program. In an evaluation of 62 studies on the effectiveness of perceptual motor programs, 31 assessed the effectiveness of the Frostig-Horne program.[49] Only 32 percent of these studies had significantly positive results. Of the remaining 31 studies, which addressed the effectiveness of the Kephart, Getman, Cratty and Barsch approaches, only 20 percent of these studies had positive results. However, even of those studies with positive results, methodology problems were present. Myers and Hamill concluded that perceptual motor programs such as the Frostig-Horne program continue to be experimental and not data-based. They stressed that more research needs to be done considering (1) characteristics of the children who can be helped by such programs, (2) the amount of time needed for achieving effectiveness, and (3) whether perceptual motor abilities can be improved via training.[49]

The Feingold Diet

Feingold[50] proposes that the use of food additives, colors, and preservatives contribute to hyperkinesis and learning disabilities in some children. Feingold claims that with proper dietary controls, improvements in hyperactivity, aggression, impulsivity and attention span are seen within one week after the diet is initiated. The age of the child tends to influence the speed and degree of response to the dietary management; however, children between 5 and 12 years of age should respond within 10 to 14 days. Feingold's initial research produced much criticism and stimulated research in many laboratories.[51-53] Spring and Sandoval,[51] in a detailed examination of the research on the Feingold diet, concluded that (1) no reliable data were available to prove that the use of synthetic colors and flavors cause hyperactivity, (2) the diet may cause placebo effects with only perceived reduced hyperactivity in children, and (3) further public advocacy should be curtailed until the efficacy of the diet is established through clinical research.

Orthomolecular (Megavitamin) Therapy

Controversy continues to exist in the professional community about the use of the "orthomolecular" or megavitamin approach to treatment. Cott[54] observed that massive doses of vitamins given to children with hyperactivity, academic problems, and perceptual disturbances were beneficial; however, other studies using Cott's regimen of vitamins have failed to produce the same results.[55,56] Opposition to the use of megavitamins has been voiced by physicians who stress the dangers of the side effects of megavitamin therapy. Jelliffe[57] cautions that megavitamins may be "poisoning" the system. He speculates that not enough is known about the harmful effects of vitamin megadoses (A and D excluded) and that megadoses could lead to cumulative and harmful effects.

In 1977 The American Academy of Pediatrics Committee on Nutrition[58] issued a statement on megavitamin therapy for childhood psychoses and learning disabilities. The committee concluded that "megavitamin therapy as a treatment for learning disabilities and psychoses in children, including autism, is not justified on the basis of documented clinical results."

Visual Motor Training

Visual motor training programs are based primarily on the beliefs of Getman,[59] which state that academic performance depends heavily on form and symbol recognition and intepretation; form and symbol recognition can be developed and trained; the development of these perceptual skills is related to the levels of coordination of the body systems; and when perceptual skills are developed, the child is able to profit from instruction and to learn independently.

Activities described by Getman are aimed at improving visual perception and in particular ocular motor activities. Six general divisions of activities are proposed: general coordination, balance, eye-hand coordination, eye movement, form perception, and visual memory.

The validity of the visual motor programs advocated by Getman and others has been questioned. In 1972, a Joint Organizational Statement on the value of eye exercises was issued by the American Academy of Pediatrics, the American Academy of Opthalmology and Otolaryngology, and the American Association of Opthalmology. Basically, the statement stressed that (1) learning disabilities require a multidisciplinary approach and eye exercises should not be done in isolation; (2) no peripheral eye defect causes reading problems or learning disabilities; (3) treatments that depend on visual training (muscle exercises, ocular pursuits, glasses) have no scientific support for claims of improving academic skills; (4) children with learning disabilities have the same incidence of ocular abnormalities as normal children; and (5) learning disorders are basically educational problems.[60]

INTERDISCIPLINARY COOPERATION IN THE TREATMENT OF LEARNING DISABILITIES

The physical therapist has the opportunity and responsibility to interact with other professionals in the treatment of learning disabled children. The interdisciplinary approach, strongly recommended in the treatment of learning disabled children, allows the therapist to interact with a number of other professionals on an ongoing basis with the goal being to provide the child with the most beneficial comprehensive program.[61-63]

The passage of Public Law 94-142[64] has had implications for greater involvement of professionals and parents in the educational programs of handicapped children including those children with learning disabilities. Public Law 94-142 mandates that each child be evaluated by a multidisciplinary team prior to the placement of the child in a special education program. Public Law 94-142 further states that parents must also be allowed to be involved in the diagnostic and the prescriptive decisions made for their children.

The role of each of the disciplines with chidren with learning disabilities may vary from school system to school system. Additionally, roles of the various disciplines are often more flexible in dealing with handicapped children than with handicapped adults with some disciplines performing tasks traditionally attributed to other disciplines; however, an overview of the basic role of each of the major disciplines is provided in the following paragraphs.

Medicine

The medical evaluation performed by the physician contributes much information to the interdisciplinary evaluation of and to the program developed for the child. The physician assists by obtaining a detailed medical history consisting of prenatal, perinatal, and postnatal information; developmental history; and familial social information such as the family constellation, interpersonal family relationships and psychological stresses within the family. The physician may also supply information on the child's visual and auditory acuity status. The presence of "soft" neurologic signs such as clumsiness, dysdiadochokinesis, minor involuntary movements, sensorimotor incoordination, dysarthria, and impaired left-right awareness, should alert the physician to underlying neurologic dysfunctions which might interfere with the child's educational or therapeutic program. Other tests commonly performed by the physician include tests for eye movement, facial apraxia, eye-hand coordination, involuntary movements, synkinesis, double tactile stimulation, finger to nose and heel to knee tests, rapid alternating movements, finger agnosis, and right-left orientation.[65]

The following responsibilities of the physician with the learning disabled child are advocated: (1) knowledge of special education services available in the community, (2) maintain a cooperative relationship with other service agencies, (3) diagnose and treat physical and psychological handicaps that may interfere with learning, (4) interpret pertinent medical findings to others, (5) specify appropriate medical treatment for any identified problems, and (6) use all services available for prevention such as screening programs.[66-67] Many physical therapists also continue to need a physician's referral prior to the initiation of physical therapy services in order to comply with their state's laws.

Education

Referrals from classroom teachers are extremely important in the early identification of children with learning disabilities. Although screening programs for learning disabled children are in the process of being developed, the teacher will probably continue to be the first to identify many children with potential or actual problems.[68] The responsibility of the classroom teacher is to be aware of the early signs of dysfunction such as coordination problems irregular eye pursuits, choreoathetosis, and decreased muscle tone.[68]

Communication with the teacher while a child is enrolled in a physical therapy is a necessity. The therapist can provide information about the child's sensorimotor and perceptual motor systems and explanations of why the child has difficulties in certain activities in the classroom. The teacher can offer suggestions about the emotional and behavioral status of the child and provide information on the motivation and management of individual children. Jointly, the teacher and the therapist can adjust the child's overall program to utilize the child's strengths and not penalize him or her for weaknesses.

Parents. The involvement of parents in the educational and therapeutic programs of their children has been stressed more than ever since the passage of Public Law 94-142. In the modern school setting parents are encouraged now to become active participants beginning with the evaluative sessions and ending with active participation in the treatment programs. Parents can provide historical information about their child's development and can assist the therapist and other professionals in the development of the child's program by sharing their concerns and expectations. In addition, the goals and objectives of the child's overall program must be mutually agreed upon by the school staff and the parents if the guidelines of Public Law 94-142 are followed. Even if the child is seen in a clinical setting, the parents should be encouraged to participate in the child's evaluation and overall programming if optimal effectiveness of the therapeutic program is to be realized.

Psychology

Two tests commonly administered by psychologists provide the physical therapist with information that is beneficial in the planning of appropriate therapeutic programs for learning disabled children. The Illinois Test of Psycholinguistic Abilities (ITPA) provides information in the areas of auditory reception, visual reception, auditory association, visual association, verbal expression, manual expression, visual closure, grammatical closure, auditory closure, sound blending, auditory sequential memory, and visual sequential memory.[69] Although much controversy has been raised about the use of the ITPA as a diagnostic tool for identifying specific psycholinguistic strengths and weaknesses, the subtest on visual perception provides useful information to the therapist particularly in the interpretation of the Southern California Sensory Integration Test.[70-72]

The Bender Gestalt Visual Motor Test with the Koppitz adaptation, appropriate for children between five and eleven years of age, is administered by showing the child eight figures and having him reproduce them.[73,74] Results from the test can be utilized by the therapist in understanding the child's visual perceptual and visual motor skills.

Interactions between the physical therapist and the school psychologist would be of particular importance if behavioral or emotional problems are present in the child with learning disabilities. Information on behavior modification on management programs that are being used would be helpful to the therapist in maintaining an adequate learning environment during physical therapy.

Speech Pathology and Audiology

Three tests of auditory discrimination commonly used by the speech pathologist, the Wepman Auditory Discrimination Test, the Goldman-Fristoe-Woodcock Test of Auditory Discrimination and the Flowers-Costello Tests of Central Auditory Abilities provide the physical therapist with useful information about the child's auditory skills.[75-77] Dichotic listening tests may also be utilized by the speech pathologist to assess the difference in the capacity of the right and left ears to report accurately an auditory stimulus under perceptual rivalry conditions. Ayres suggests that the results of auditory tests such as those identified above can assist the therapist in the interpretation of the results of the sensorimotor evaluation of the child.

OCCUPATIONAL THERAPY AND PHYSICAL THERAPY

Public Law 94-142 introduced, for the first time in many states, the provision of related services in the individual educational plans for children with handicaps. Each service that is necessary for maintaining the child in school and for enabling him or her to participate maximally in the classroom is to be provided.

Physical therapists and occupational therapists, utilizing their knowledge of the nervous system, human development, and human behavior, are becoming more involved with the learning disabled child since the implementation of the public law. These two disciplines may participate in the screening process, which may include a review of the child's developmental/medical/academic history; an observation of the child; a discussion of the child's problems with the child, the parents and/or the teachers; and an evaluation of the child's abilities using nonstandardized and standardized screening tools. Once screening is performed and the need for further testing is determined, either the occupational therapist or the physical therapist may administer formal testing to the child. These tools may include the Southern California Sensory Integration Tests, the Southern California Postrotary Nystagmus Test, Harris Test of Lateral Dominance, and the Bruininks-Oseretsky Test of Motor Proficiency. The

raining and skill of the individual therapist should be the determining factor
of who should administer the test to the child. Evaluative tools that might be
utilized will be further discussed under the section on physical therapy evaluation. One tool, however, that is more frequently used by occupational therapists than by physical therapists is the Frostig Developmental Test of Visual
Perception.[78] This test, in process for several years and copyrighted in 1963,
was developed as a tool to assess visual perception, hand-eye coordination and
motor skills as they relate to visual configuration. The test was normed on 2116
children between the ages of three years and nine years who were primarily
from Caucasian and middle-class families. Validity tests have been done but
poorly controlled; however, the initial reliability study (test-retest) produced
a Pearson product moment correlation coefficient of 0.98.[78]

The Developmental Test of Visual Perception is appropriate for screening
children in preschool, kindergarten and first grade, and for other children for
diagnostic testing. The developers of the test state that the results of the test
allows the examiner to determine if problems are present in ocular motor coordination, figure-ground perception, constancy of shape, position in space,
and spatial relationships. Table 10-2 illustrates some of the items from the
subtests and suggested activities for programming.[78]

After evaluation, using the standardized tools as well as nonstandardized
procedures such as clinical observations, treatment may be initiated by either
the occupational therapist or the physical therapist, depending upon the therapist's skill and training. Treatment should consist of self-directed, purposeful
activities which provide selected sensory input through a variety of somatosensory or vestibular channels. More discussion on treatment is included in
the section on physical therapy.

Physical therapists have historically been members of the team dealing
with handicapped children but have often been overlooked as members of the
team dealing with learning disabled children. With more physical therapists
becoming certified in the sensory integrative approach and with the passage
of the Education for All Handicapped Children Act (PL 94-142), physical therapists have the opportunity to become more involved in the management of
children with learning disabilities.

CLINICAL OBSERVATIONS OF LEARNING DISABILITIES

Careful evaluation of a number of areas is required prior to the initiation
of a treatment program for learning disabled children. Many of the traditional
tests performed by physical therapists, such as assessment of muscle tone and
muscle strength, and general sensory testing may be appropriate for learning
disabled children. Coordination and balance activities such as finger movements, foot patting, and heel-toe walking might additionally be appropriate.
Using the coordination tasks listed above, DeHaven and associates[79] found

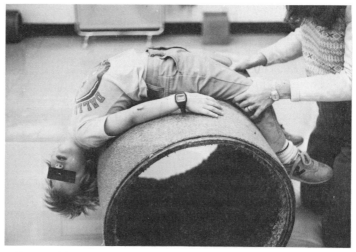

Fig. 10-3.   Test position for assessment of postural security according to Ayres. (Cour
tesy of Barbara Brooks.)

that children between the ages of 7 and 18 years who were diagnosed as learning
disabled differed from normal children in their performance on the tasks. A
similar study by Kendrick and Hanten[80] revealed that the rates of performance
of opposition and foot patting were significant variables and could be used to
differentiate between learning disabled and normal children.

Ayres suggests numerous clinical observations that should be made with
children suspected of having sensorimotor dysfunctions.[81] These clinical observations include assessment of activity level; muscle tone: cocontraction in
the upper extremities and the neck; and postural background movements. The
child's eye and hand preferences should be assessed as a means of determining
establishment of laterality. Assessment of the child's ability to pursue objects
visually across midline, to converge on a moving object and to quickly localize
a moving object provides the therapist with information on the child's visual
and vestibular systems as well as on motor planning and laterality. Coordination
activities such as slow movements of the arms, rapid forearm rotation, and
thumb-finger touching should be assessed quantitatively and qualitatively.
These coordination activities, when performed by the two upper extremities
separately and then together, allow the therapist to assess right-left differences.
Tongue to lip movements may be used to assess the presence of adequate oral
motor planning.

Ayres advocates the assessment of postural security with the child in supine and in sitting on an unstable surface such as a large ball[28] (Fig. 10-3).
When the surface is moved, the degree of fearfulness is noted as an indicator
of vestibular functioning, equilibrium reactions, and postural mechanisms.
Equilibrium and protective reactions should be tested in different positions,
such as prone, quadruped, sitting, kneeling, and standing, and on different

surfaces such as a large ball or a vestibular board. Testing of the reactions yields information on the vestibular, somatic, proprioceptive and visual systems; optical righting; motor planning; and postural mechanisms. Asymmetries can also be easily assessed when examining equilibrium and protective reactions.

Assessment of the asymmetric tonic neck and symmetric tonic neck reflexes are included by Ayres in her clinical observations.[81] The symmetric tonic neck reflex is assessed with the child in the quadruped position. A positive symmetric tonic neck reflex is indicated by definite changes in joint extension or flexion as the head is extended or flexed. The asymmetric tonic neck reflex may be assessed in three different positions. In the Schilder's arm extension position, the child is asked to stand with the feet together, the arms out in front of the body at shoulder level, the fingers spread apart and the eyes closed.[81] The child is asked to maintain this position while the examiner counts to 20. Choreoathetoid movements, hyperextension of the elbows and raising or lowering of the arms are noted. Difficulties with the position may indicate problems with processing the vestibular and somatic proprioceptive information or with postural mechanisms. This position additionally allows the therapist to observe whether the child is able to dissociate head and trunk movements and to maintain cocontraction in the shoulders. In the same position as described above, but with the examiner turning the head, observations of the arms lowering, flexing and/or extending may provide information about the presence of the asymmetric tonic neck reflex. A second position for assessment of the asymmetric tonic neck reflex is the quadruped position. The child is asked to assume a four-point position with the elbows slightly flexed. The examiner turns the child's head to the right and then to the left. Observations of the amount of flexion and extension in the arms are made. Studies have shown that up to 30 degrees of elbow flexion on the occipital side of the asymmetric tonic neck reflex is normal for children up to nine years of age.[82,83] A third position is the quadruped reflex inhibiting posture with the child on hands and knees. One hand is then placed on the hip on the same side and the opposite leg is raised. The child is asked to turn the head from side to side while the therapist observes the effect of the asymmetric tonic neck reflex on equilibrium. Ayres states that the body's weight on one hand stimulates conscious maintenance of extension in an arm that would have normally had flexion facilitated by the asymmetric tonic neck reflex.[81] Once the leg is lifted, the child begins to activate his equilibrium reactions. Ayres believes that the equilibrium reactions may be affected if the asymmetric tonic neck reflex is present, and that the extra stress of this position may elicit the asymmetric tonic neck reflex when it has not been seen in any other position.

The antigravity positions of prone extension and supine flexion are important postures to be evaluated.[81] (Fig. 10-4). Ayres states that the inability of the child to hold the prone extension posture may be due to insufficient vestibular processing. She further states that the difficulty some children have in holding the supine flexed posture may be caused by motor planning and motor execution problems.[84]

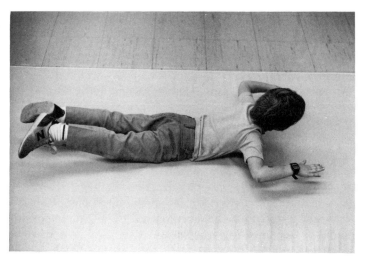

Fig. 10-4. The pivot prone position. (Courtesy of Barbara Brooks).

The process of tactile defensiveness should be assessed by the therapist during all clinical observations and during the administration of any formal tests. Agitation and increasing irritability during the administration of tactile tests may be particularly indicative of tactile defensiveness.

GROSS MOTOR ASSESSMENT

Although the child's motor assessment will primarily yield a developmental age and not explain the underlying cause of dysfunction, the current level of functioning is necessary for baseline information. For some children, a screening of their motor abilities may be sufficient to determine if motor dysfunction is present. Three tests available for screening such children are the Stott Test of Motor Impairment, the Hughes Basic Gross Motor Assessment, and the Bruininks-Oseretsky Test of Motor Proficiency.[85-97]

The Stott Test of Motor Impairment was developed from the Gollnitz revision of the Oseretsky. Five tasks for each age group between 5 and 13 years were selected from the Gollnitz revision and normed for 6 to 15 years of age for the Stott. Validity of the test was demonstrated by Moyes[88] who tested 35 children between 6 and 8 years of age who had been identified by their teachers as having motor impairments. A tetrachoric correlation of 0.85 was obtained between the test results and the teachers' ratings.[85]

The Hughes Basic Gross Motor Assessment (BGMA), was normed on 1260 children between the ages of 5 years and 6 months and 12 years 5 months in the Denver, Colorado area.[86] Gross motor tasks on the test included standing balance on one foot with the eyes open, tandem walking, hopping on one foot, skipping, target throwing with bean bags, and ball handling. According to

Hughes and Riley,[86] use of the BGMA can assist therapists in differentiating children with minor motor problems from normal children; however, no motor age can be assigned from the results of the test.

The Bruininks-Oseretsky Test of Motor Proficiency was designated for use with children functioning between 4½ years and 14½ years in their motor abilities.[87] The test is comprised of subtests in running speed and agility; balance; bilateral coordination; strength; upper limb coordination; response speed; visual motor control; and upper limb speed and dexterity. Although the complete test consists of 46 test items, 14 items from the test have been identified for use in screening of children.

More comprehensive evaluations of perceptual motor and sensorimotor skills can be performed through the use of one or more of the instruments commercially available, including the full version of the previously mentioned Bruininks-Oseretsky Test of Motor Proficiency. A brief description of two of the other tests most commonly used by physical therapists, the Purdue Perceptual Motor Survey, and the Southern California Sensory Integration Tests follows.

The Purdue Perceptual Motor Survey was designed for use with children between 6 and 9 years of age and included the following activities[89] (Fig. 10-5):

1. Walking forward, backward, and sideward on a balance beam
2. Hopping on both feet and on each foot alone
3. Identifying parts of the body
4. Imitating arm movements
5. Moving through an obstacle course
6. Moving arms and legs into various positions while supine
7. Drawing on a chalkboard
8. Performing visual achievement tasks such as copying shapes

Although the Purdue Perceptual Motor Survey is a relatively simple test to administer, a major problem with the tool is interpretation of the scores. The validity of a particular score or series of scores in terms of defining perceptual motor dysfunctions and predicting classroom abilities is not well documented; therefore, interpretations of what the test results actually means should be done with caution.

The Southern California Sensory Integration Tests (SCSIT) consist of 17 tests which provide information in the areas of somatosensory processing, motor performance, form and space perception, and lateralization. The tests include the following[90]:

1. Space visualization (Fig. 10-6)
2. Figure-ground perception (Fig. 10-7)
3. Position in space
4. Design copy
5. Motor accuracy

BALANCE AND POSTURAL FLEXIBILITY

1. Walking Board

Forward		
		Comments
Steps off board	——	
Pauses frequently	——	
Uses one side of body more consistently than other	——	
Avoids Balance: Runs Long steps Feet crosswise of board	—— —— ——	
Maintains inflexible posture	——	Score ☐

Backward		
		Comments
Steps off board	——	
Pauses frequently	——	
Uses one side of body more consistently than other	——	
Avoids balance: Runs Long steps Feet crosswise of board	—— —— ——	
Twists body to see where he is going	——	
Must look at feet	——	
Maintains inflexible posture	——	Score ☐

Sidewise		
		Comments
Unable to shift weight from one foot to the other	——	
Confusing or hesitation in shifting weight	——	
Crosses one foot over the other	——	
Steps off board	——	
Performs more easily in one direction than the other: Right lead Left lead	—— ——	Score ☐

Fig. 10-5. Example of skills to be tested by Purdue Perceptual Motor Survey. (Roach EG, Kephart NC: The Purdue Perceptual Motor Survey. p 2. Charles E. Merrill, Columbus, OH, 1966.)

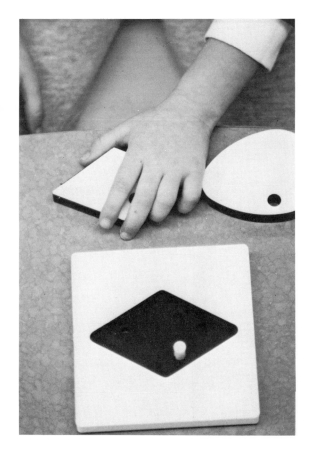

Fig. 10-6. Example from the space visualization test of the Southern California Sensory Integration Tests. (Courtesy of Barbara Brooks).

  6. Kinesthesia (Fig. 10-8)
  7. Manual form perception
  8. Finger identification (Fig. 10-9)
  9. Graphesthesia
10. Localization of tactile stimuli
11. Double tactile stimuli perception
12. Imitation of postures
13. Crossing midline of body
14. Bilateral motor coordination
15. Right-left discrimination
16. Standing balance, eyes open, and
17. Standing balance, eyes closed

The Southern California Postrotary Nystagmus Test (SCPNT) (Fig. 10-10) was normed on 226 children between 5 and 9 years of age in the Los Angeles area.[91] All of the normative sample had nystagmus following rotation. A random sample of learning disabled children in the Los Angeles area showed decreased

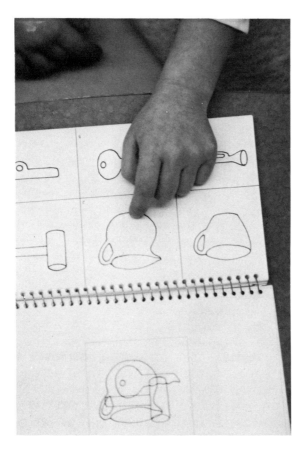

Fig. 10-7. Example from the figure-ground test of the Southern California Sensory Integration Tests. (Courtesy of Barbara Brooks).

postrotary nystagmus when compared with the normative sample. Additionally, 86 percent of the learning disabled children had 10 seconds or less of nystagmus following rotation as compared to only 50 percent of the normal sample. Reliability of repeated measurements of duration of nystagmus in 42 children was 0.84; however, the test-retest coefficient of correlation of estimated eye excursion was only 0.485. Studies by DeQuiros and associates[92,93] supported Ayres' assumption that reduced postrotary nystagmus may be seen in children with learning disabilities. Recent studies by Ottenbacher[94] revealed that some children with learning disabilities have excessive scores on the SCPNT which may be due to subtle central nervous system dysfunction of cerebral cortical, rather than vestibular, origin.

The SCSIT and the SCPNT may assist the therapist in differentiating types of sensory integrative disorders in the nervous system including the following: form and space perception, praxis, vestibular and bilateral integration, eye-hand coordination and tactile defensiveness.[95] Based upon the results of these two tests as well as the therapist's clinical observations, appropriate therapeutic intervention can be planned. Although the tests may appear easy to administer,

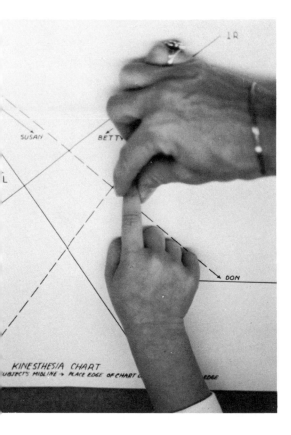

Fig. 10-8. Example from the kinesthesia test of the Southern California Sensory Integration Tests. (Courtesy of Barbara Brooks).

the therapist utilizing the tests should be trained in the administration and interpretation of the tests. The tests must be given in the standardized manner in order to be valid. Accurate interpretation is especially critical to the development of an intervention program and should be done only by those therapists who have been certified in the use of the tests.

PHYSICAL THERAPY

In the treatment of the learning disabled child, the occupational therapist and physical therapist must work closely together in order to provide the child with comprehensive services. Once the child has been thoroughly and accurately assessed by the occupational therapist and the physical therapist through the use of clinical observations and standardized testing, an appropriate treatment program can be implemented. The therapists should seek information from other members of the interdisciplinary team in the planning of the program and should utilize the team as a support system during the actual treatment program.

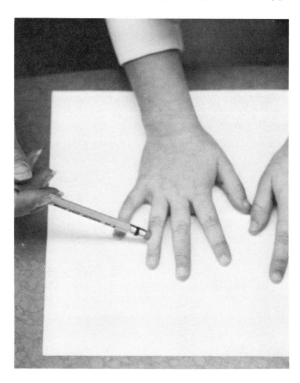

Fig. 10-9.   Example from the finger identification test of the Southern California Sensory Integration Tests. (Courtesy of Barbara Brooks).

A sensorimotor or a perceptual motor approach or a combination of the two may be taken in the treatment of the learning disabled child. In the sensorimotor approach, the goal is to provide and control sensory input to the child in a manner that elicits an adaptive response. The adaptive response is the action or reaction of the child to the environment acting on him or her. In addition, the adaptive response should be a purposeful and goal directed action. Ayres believes that for an adaptive response to occur, intersensory integration must be occurring. Ayres further states "that the most therapeutic situation is that in which the child's inner urge for action and growth drives him toward a response that furthers maturation and integration."[81] The role of the therapist therefore should be to provide an environment that allows for a balance of freedom within a structure that encourages exploration by the child; however, manipulations of the environment by the therapist may be necessary to allow freedom on the part of the child yet lead to higher levels of functioning. Sensorimotor treatment has been shown to be effective in decreasing hypersensitivity or sensory-seeking behaviors in some children. In other children, the treatment can be used to increase alertness or interactions with the environment.

Inputs from the vestibular system, the muscles, joints, and skin are stressed in the sensorimotor approach. Tactile stimuli may be applied through the use of different textured materials with the child. Deep pressure is advocated rather than light touch because of the sympathetic nervous system mediated responses

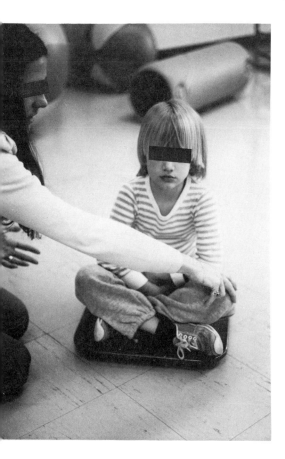

Fig. 10-10. The test position for the Southern California Post Rotary Nystagmus Test. (Courtesy of Barbara Brooks).

o light touch noted in some children. Rubbing, before the application of tactile stimuli, can lessen the interpretation of the stimuli as noxious to some children. Vibration may be used as a tactile and vestibular input with some children. The use of this stimulus seems to guide the child in making an appropriate adaptive response. Proprioceptive stimulation through the joints, ligaments and tendons provides important sensory information to the child about his or her body in relationship to the environment. In addition, enhanced kinesthesia, whereby a combination of input from proprioceptors and information from cutaneous and visual receptors is processed, provides information to the child about the movement of the body in space.

Use of the vestibular system in therapy programs is emphasized by Ayres. The role of activation of the vestibular system in maintaining muscle tone is important for many learning disabled children who demonstrate decreased muscle tone and who have problems in execution of motor activities. In addition, the vestibular system can be utilized for alerting or arousing children who demonstrate attentional problems. Whether the vestibular system has an inhibitory or facilitatory response on the system depends on the type of vestibular input. Slow rhythmical movements tend to be inhibitory, while rapid movements tend to be facilitatory.

Sensory stimulation using the vestibular system can be extremely beneficial to the child; however, caution should be exercised in the administration of the stimuli due to the adverse reactions to such stimulation seen in some children.[96,97] Seizure activity has been cited as a response to vestibular stimulation; however, conflicting information about the incidence of seizures has been reported. Certain rules of using vestibular stimulation should be followed during treatment programs including active involvement of the child in the activities, particularly in allowing the child to determine how long and to what extent he or she will participate. A child should not be forced to participate in the movement activity but should be allowed to participate gradually.

The auditory and visual systems are not specifically stimulated in the sensorimotor approach. Although the importance of these two systems is not negated, the earlier developing systems or phylogenetically old systems are used as a basis for activation of the phylogenetically newer systems of audition and vision.

Activities that are used in the sensory integrative approach depend upon the individual needs of the child. Once the child has been evaluated using tests such as the SCSIT, SCPNT, and clinical observations, the program should be planned according to areas of strengths and weaknesses. Different positions such as prone, supine, sitting, all fours, kneeling and standing may be used with the child in the treatment program. In addition, rolling, crawling, creeping, and locomotion may be used in conjunction with the controlled sensory input. Activities should be based upon the child's needs, for example, the program for the child with tactile based form and space problems would be different from the program planned for the child with vestibular-based bilateral integrative problems.[28] In the approach, use of controlled sensory input is considered primarily for the development of motor skills; however, the presence of poorly integrated primitive reflexes and poorly established equilibrium and balance reactions are addressed in the types of activities that are utilized. Numerous texts have been published with suggestions for activities to be used with children with sensorimotor problems and should be studied by therapists wishing to utilize the sensorimotor approach.[28,98]

PERCEPTUAL MOTOR THERAPY

The perceptual motor programs, although geared more toward the motor skills of the child, also employ sensory stimulation in their approach, especially the use of various textures and movements, e.g. children are urged to perform activities on different surfaces and in different positions. Kephart, Cratty, and Barsch utilize activities in prone, supine, sitting, and standing and all follow a developmental sequence; however, each differs in the types of activities utilized. Examples of activities that might be advocated for the therapist that wishes to use a perceptual motor approach are: walking lines marked on the

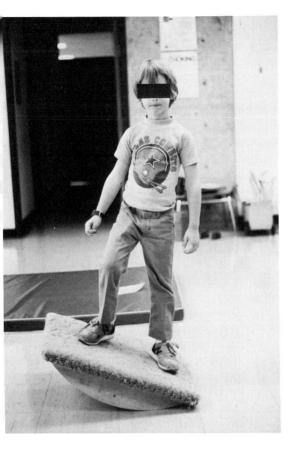

Fig. 10-11. Example of the use of the balance board in a perceptual motor program. (Courtesy of Barbara Brooks).

floor; walking balance beams of various widths; running in all directions; running and stopping quickly; running and changing direction; throwing balls at targets; batting balls with the hands; hitting a ball off a tee; kicking balls; jumping over lines, over ropes, in and out of hoops; tumbling forward, backward, and sideward, down hills or inclines; balancing particularly when on a tilting platform; strengthening activities using push-ups and sit-ups; and trampoline activities[45] (Fig. 10-11). A metronome or music might be used in conjunction with the motor activities if rhythm is needed for the individual child. Numerous texts are available to therapists on perceptual motor programs for children and should be consulted prior to the initiation of a perceptual motor program.[33,45,99]

The type of therapeutic program that is utilized with the child may depend upon the setting in which the child is seen. The therapist may opt to see the child for direct or indirect services through a school program or on an individual basis at a private clinic. Regardless of the type of setting in which the child is seen, the parents should be encouraged to be involved in the treatment of their child. The parents should be urged to observe periodically during the treatment sessions or to meet with the therapists to discuss their child's progress or lack of progress. In many instances, suggestions can be given by the therapist that may improve the parents' handling of the child at home. Suggestions can be made about the types of activities that should be stressed and those activities that should be avoided. Parents as therapists for their children can be very effective if the physical therapist takes the opportunity to guide them; however, not every parent is capable of or willing to work with their child. If the therapist feels that parents are capable and motivated, a written program listing specific activities and general suggestions should be given to the parents. Periodic sessions should be scheduled with the parents to reassess the effectiveness or appropriateness of the activities that are done at home. The importance of making the activity sessions positive experiences should be emphasized with the parents as well as with teachers.

NEED FOR FURTHER RESEARCH

The importance of a perceptual motor or a sensorimotor program to the learning disabled child has been questioned by many educators and administrators. Behavioral and motor results from motor programs for learning disabled children are often hard for educators to accept as being beneficial to the learning process. Even more difficult is the financial justification by school administrators. Current research seems to link the behavioral and motor results to academic improvements, but more research is needed to supply additional support for the efficacy of such programs. The physical therapist who works with the learning disabled population must be willing to interact with other professionals who deal with the same group of children and must be willing to be accountable for the results or lack of results that occur with the therapeutic program. In the area of learning disabilities, perhaps more than any other area, the physical therapist must keep current on research and be able to discuss openly and professionally the rationale for physical therapeutic programs with the learning disabled.

REFERENCES

1. National Advisory Committee on Handicapped Children: Special Education for Handicapped Children: First Annual Report. US Department of Health, Education and Welfare, Washington, D.C., 1968.
2. United States Office of Education: Estimated Number of Handicapped Children in the United States. US Office of Education, Washington, DC, 1971–1972.
3. Myklebust HR, Boshes B: Minimal brain damage in children. Final Report. Contract 108-65-142. Neurological and Sensory Disease Control Program. Department of Health, Education and Welfare, Washington, DC, 1969.
4. Meier JH: Prevalence and characteristics of learning disabilities found in second grade children. J Learn Disabil 4:1, 1971.
5. United States Department of Health, Education and Welfare: Reading Disorders in the United States: A Report of the National Advisory Committee on Dyslexia

and Related Reading Disorders. U.S. Government Printing Office, Washington, DC, 1969.

6. Bruininks RH, Glaman G, Clark C: Prevalence of Learning Disabilities: Findings, Issues and Recommendations. Research Report #20. Department of Health, Education and Welfare, Washington, DC, 1971.

7. Special Study Institute for Special Learning Disabilities: Proceedings. State of Florida Department of Education, Tallahassee, 1975.

8. Children with Specific Learning Disabilities Act of 1969, PL 91-230. The Elementary and Secondary Amendments of 1969.

9. U.S. Office of Education: Education of handicapped children. Fed Regist 42:65083, 1977.

10. Clements SD: Minimal brain dysfunction in children. Monograph No. 3. Public Health Service Bulletin #1415, NINDS. Department of Health Education and Welfare, Washington DC, 1966.

11. Gubbay SS, Ellis E, Walton JN, et al: Clumsy children: A study of apraxia and agnostic defects in 21 children. Brain 88:295, 1965.

12. Wallace G, McLoughlin JA: Learning Disabilities: Concepts and Characteristics. Merrill, Columbus, OH 1975.

13. Bryan T, Bryan J: Understanding Learning Disabilities. 2nd Ed. Alfred, Port Washington, NY, 1978.

14. Bryan T: Learning disabled children's comprehension of nonverbal communication. J Learn Disabil 10:501, 1977.

15. Bender LA: A visual motor gestalt test and its clinical use. Orthopsychiatry Assoc Res Monogr 3, 1938.

16. Reitan RM, Ball TJ: Neuropsychological correlates of minimal brain dysfunction. Ann NY Acad Sci 205:65, 1973.

17. Birch H: Brain Damage in Children. The Biological and Social Aspects. Williams and Wilkins, Baltimore, 1964.

18. Myklebust HR, Johnson DJ: Learning Disabilities: Educational Principles and Practices. Grune and Stratton, New York, 1967.

19. Delacato CH: Treatment and Prevention of Reading Problems. Charles C Thomas, Springfield, IL, 1959.

20. Delacato CH: The Diagnosis and Treatment of Speech and Reading Problems. Charles C. Thomas, Springfield IL, 1963.

21. Delacato CH: Neurological Organization and Reading. Charles C Thomas, Springfield IL, 1966.

22. Robbins MP, Glass GV: The Doman-Delacato rationale: A critical analysis. In Hellmuth J (ed): Educational Jeopardy. Vol 2. Special Child Publications, Seattle, 1959.

23. Geschwind N: The apraxias: Neural mechanisms of disorders of learned movement. Am Sci 63:188, 1975.

24. Wada J, Rasmussen TR: Intracarotid injection of sodium amytal for the lateralization of cerebral speech dominance: Experimental and clinical observations. J Neurosurg 17:266, 1960.

25. Galaburda AM, LeMay M, Kemper TL, et al: Right-left asymmetries in the brain. Science 199:852, 1978.

26. Senf GM: An information integration theory and its application to normal reading acquisition and reading disability. In Bryant ND, Kass CE (eds): Leadership Training Institute in Learning Disabilities: Final Report, Vol 2. University of Arizona, Tucson, 1972.

27. Ayres AJ: The development of sensory integration theory and practice. Kendall-Hunt, Dubuque, IA, 1974.

28. Ayres AJ: Sensory Integration and the Child. Western Psychological Services, Los Angeles, 1979.
29. Ayres AJ: Improving academic scores through sensory integration. J Learn Disabil 5:338, 1972.
30. Ayres AJ: The effect of sensory integrative therapy in learning disabled children. Monograph. The Center for the Study of Sensory Integrative Dysfunction, Pasadena, CA, 1976.
31. Ottenbacher K, Watson PJ, Short MA, et al: Nystagmus and ocular fixation difficulties in learning disabled children. Am J Occup Ther 33:717, 1979.
32. Ayres AJ: Effect of sensory integrative therapy on the coordination of children with choreoathetoid movements. Am J Occup Ther 31:291, 1977.
33. Kephart NC: The Slow Learner in the Classroom. Merrill, Columbus, OH, 1960.
34. Kephart NC: The perceptual motor match. In Cruickshank WM, Hallahan DP (eds): Perceptual Learning Disabilities in Children. Vol 1: Psychoeducational Practices. Syracuse University Press, Syracuse, NY, 1975.
35. Kephart NC: The Slow Learner in the Classroom. 2nd Ed. Merrill, Columbus, OH, 1971.
36. Haring NG, Stables JM: The effect of gross motor development on visual perception and eye-hand coordination. Phys Ther 46:129, 1966.
37. Roach EG: Evaluation of an experimental program on perceptual motor training with slow readers. In Figurel JA (ed): Vistas in Reading. International Reading Association Conference Proceedings, IX, 1966.
38. Brown RC: The effects of a perceptual motor education program on perceptual motor skills and reading readiness. Presented at Research Section, AAHPER, St. Louis, MO, 1968.
39. Vellutino FR, Steger BM, Mayer SC, et al: Has the perceptual deficit hypothesis led us astray? J Learn Disabil 10:375, 1977.
40. Hallahan DP, Cruickshank WM: Psychoeducational Foundations of Learning Disabilities. Prentice Hall, Engelwood Cliffs, NJ, 1973.
41. Barsch RH: Achieving Perceptual-Motor Efficiency. Special-Child Publications, Seattle, 1967.
42. Barsch RH: Ray H. Barsch. In Kauffman JM, Hallahan DP (eds): Teaching Children with Learning Disabilities: Personal Perspectives. Charles E. Merrill, Columbus, 1976.
43. Barsch R: Achieving Perceptual-Motor Efficiency. Vol. 2. Special Child Publications, Seattle, 1968.
44. Cratty BJ: Movement Behavior and Motor Learning. 2nd Ed. Lea and Febiger, Philadelphia, 1967.
45. Cratty BJ: Active Learning. Games to Enhance Academic Abilities. Prentice-Hall, Englewood Cliffs, NJ, 1971.
46. Cratty BJ: Perceptual and Motor Development in Infants and Children. 2nd Ed. Prentice Hall, Englewood Cliffs, NJ, 1979.
47. Frostig M, Maslow P: Learning problems in the classroom. Grune and Stratton, New York, 1973.
48. Frostig N, Horne D: The Frostig Program for the Development of Visual Perception: Teacher's Guide. Follett, Chicago, 1964.
49. Myers PI, Hammill DD: Methods for Learning Disorders. Wiley, New York, 1976.
50. Feingold BF: Hyperkinesis and learning disabilities linked to the ingestion of artificial food colors and flavors. J Learn Disabil 9:551, 1976.
51. Spring C, Sandoval J: Food additives and hyperkinesis: A critical evaluation of the evidence. J Learn Disabil 9:560, 1976.

52. Harley JP, Ray RS, Tomasi L, et al: Hyperkinesis and food additives: Testing the Feingold hypothesis. Pediatrics 61:818, 1978.
53. Williams JI, Cram DM, Tausig FT, et al: Relative effects of drugs on hyperactive behaviors: An experimental study. Pediatrics 61:811, 1978.
54. Cott A: Megavitamins: The orthomolecular approach to behavioral disorders and learning disabilities. Acad Ther 7:245, 1972.
55. Arnold LE, Christopher J, Huestis RD, et al: Megativamins for minimal brain dysfunction. JAMA 240:2642, 1978.
56. Kershner J, Hawke W: Megavitamins and learning disorders: Controlled double blind experiment. J Nutr 109:819, 1979.
57. Jelliffe DB: The megavitamin scene. Lancet 4:1217, 1974.
58. American Academy of Pediatrics, Committee on Nutrition: Megavitamin therapy for childhood psychoses and learning disabilities. Postgrad Med 61:230, 1977.
59. Getman GN: Gerald N. Getman. In Kauffman JM, Hallahan DP (eds): Teaching Children with Learning Disabilities: Personal perspectives. Merrill, Columbus, OH, 1976.
60. Joint Organizational statement: The eye and learning disabilities. Pediatrics 49:454, 1972.
61. Gottlieb MI: The learning disabled child: Controversial issues revisited. In Gottlieb MI, Zinkus PW, Bradford LJ (eds): Current Issues in Developmental Pediatrics: The Learning Disabled Child. Grune and Stratton, New York, 1979.
62. Gonzalez ER: Learning disabilities. Lagging field in medicine. JAMA 234:1891, 1980.
63. Lerner JW: Children with learning disabilities. Theories, Diagnosis and Teaching Strategies. 2nd Ed. Houghton Mifflin, Boston, 1976.
64. Public Law 94-142, Education for all handicapped children. 20 USC 1401 et seq, 1977.
65. Grossman HJ: Neurologic assessment and management of learning disorders. Pediatr Ann 7:326, 1978.
66. Bateman B, Frankel H: Special education and the pediatrician. J Learn Disabil 5:176, 1972.
67. Richmond J, Walzer S: The central task of childhood—Learning. The pediatrician's role. Ann NY Acad Sci 205:390, 1973.
68. Goldstein PK, O'Brien JD, Katz GM: A learning disability screening program in a public school. Am J Occup Ther 35:451, 1981.
69. Kirk SA, McCarthy JJ, Kirk WD: Illinois Test of Psycholinguistic Abilities. Rev. Ed. University of Illinois Press, Urbana, 1968.
70. Lund KA, Foster GE, McCall-Perez FC: The effectiveness of psycholinguistic training: A re-evaluation. Except Child 44:310, 1978.
71. Hammill DD, Larsen SC: The effectiveness of psycholinguistic training: A reaffirmation of position. Except Child 44:402, 1978.
72. Smead VS: Ability training and task analysis in diagnostic/prescriptive teaching. J Special Educ 11:113, 1977.
73. Bender L: A Visual Motor Gestalt Test and Its Clinical Uses. Research Monograph No. 3. American Orthopsychiatric Association, New York, 1938.
74. Koppitz EM: The Bender-Gestalt Test for Young Children. Grune and Stratton, New York, 1964.
75. Wepman JM: Auditory Discrimination Test. Language Research Associates, Chicago, 1958.
76. Goldman R, Fristoe M, Woodcock RW: Goodman-Fristoe-Woodcock Test of Auditory Discrimination. American Guidance Service, Circle Pines, MN, 1970.

77. Flowers A, Costello MR, Small V: Flowers-Costello Tests of Central Auditory Abilities. Perceptual Learning Systems, Dearborn, MI, 1970.
78. Frostig M, Lefever DW, Whittlesey JRB: The Marianne Frostig Developmental Test of Visual Perception. Consulting Psychology Press, Palo Alto, CA, 1964.
79. DeHaven GE, Mardock JB, Loykovich KM: Evaluation of coordination deficits in children with minimal brain dysfunction. Phys Ther 49:153, 1969.
80. Kendrick KA, Hanten WP: Differentiation of learning disabled children using four coordination tasks. Phys Ther 60:784, 1980.
81. Ayres AJ: Sensory Integration and Learning Disorders. Western Psychological Services, Los Angeles, 1972.
82. Parr C, Routh DK, Byrd MT, et al: A developmental study of the asymmetrical tonic neck reflex. Dev Med Child Neurol 16:329, 1974.
83. Parmenter CL: The asymmetrical tonic neck reflex in normal first and third grade children. Am J Occup Ther 29:463, 1975.
84. Montgomery P, Richter E: Sensory Integrative Theory. Workshop given at the University of Tennessee Center for the Health Sciences, Memphis, 1977.
85. Stott OH, Moyes FA, Henderson SE: Test of motor impairment. Brook Educational Publishers, Ontario, 1972.
86. Hughes JE, Riley A: Basic gross motor assessment: Tool for use with children having minor motor dysfunction. Phys Ther 61:503, 1981.
87. Bruininks R: Bruininks-Oseretsky Test of Motor Proficiency. American Guidance Services, Circle Pines, MN, 1978.
88. Moyes FA: A validational study of a test of motor impairment. Master's thesis. University of Leicester, England, 1969.
89. Roach EG, Kephart NC: The Purdue Perceptual Motor Survey. Merrill, Columbus, OH, 1966.
90. Ayres AJ: Southern California Sensory Integration Tests. Western Psychological Service, Los Angeles, 1972.
91. Ayres AJ: Southern California Postrotary Nystagmus Test. Western Psychological Service, Los Angeles, 1975.
92. DeQuiros JB: Diagnosis of vestibular disorders in the learning disabled. J Learn Disabil 9:50, 1976.
93. DeQuiros JB, Schrager OL: Neuropsychological Fundamentals in Learning Disabilities. Academic Therapy Press, San Rafael, CA, 1978.
94. Ottenbacher K: Excessive postrotary nystagmus duration in learning-disabled children. Am J Occup Ther 34:40, 1980.
95. Ayres AJ: Southern California Sensory Integration Tests Manual Revised. Western Psychological Services, Los Angeles, 1980.
96. Henderson A, Coryell J (eds): The Body Senses and Perceptual Deficits. Boston University, Boston, 1973.
97. Kantner RM, Clark DL, Atkinson J, et al: Effects of vestibular stimulation in seizure-prone children: An EEG study. Phys Ther 62:16, 1982.
98. Montgomery P, Richter E: Sensorimotor Integration for Developmentally Disabled Children: A Handbook. Western Psychological Services, Los Angeles, 1977.
99. Arnheim DD, Sinclair WA: The Clumsy Child: A Program of Motor Therapy. Mosby, St. Louis, 1975.

11 | Cerebral Palsy

Janet M. Wilson

Cerebral palsy may be the most common pediatric neurologic problem referred to physical therapists and at the same time may represent the least well-defined and least-understood pediatric neurologic problem. It is important, first, to understand that the term cerebral palsy is a description, not a specific diagnosis, of the clinical sequelae resulting from a nonprogressive encephalopathy whose etiology may be prenatal, perinatal, or postnatal.[1] Cerebral palsy is characterized by sensorimotor dysfunction, which has as its expression abnormal muscle tone and abnormal posture and movement. While cerebral palsy is caused by a static encephalopathy, the symptoms often appear to be progressive because it affects a changing organism in which a developing, albeit abnormal, central nervous system (CNS) attempts to direct and control other maturing systems, including the musculoskeletal structures. The expression of the disorder can appear worse as the child grows, develops, and attempts to compensate for abnormality while confronting the force of gravity in every effort to move. Cerebral palsy is a developmental disorder affecting the total development of the child either directly, relating to sensorimotor function, or indirectly through associated problems. As a developmental disorder, cerebral palsy has varying effects on children at different stages of development as well as at different chronologic ages. Although the hallmark of cerebral palsy is motor dysfunction, various other problems frequently coexist, including sensory impairments, retrolental fibroplasia, nystagmus, strabismus, seizure disorders, mental retardation, behavior disorders, learning disabilities, sensory integrative dysfunction, speech and language disorders, or oral-dental disorders.[2]

PREVALENCE AND ETIOLOGY

Because cerebral palsy is neither a reportable disease nor a diagnostic entity, figures on prevalence in the literature vary.[3–8] Much of the variation arises from the lack of uniform criteria for diagnosis, sample selection and size,

353

and age at time of outcome assessment. A figure of 2.0 per 1000 live births represents an average of data from prevalence studies reported in a review by Hagberg.[9] The notion of a steady reduction in cerebral palsy prevalence rates corresponding to improved neonatal care is not sustained by the available evidence. Reported changes in rates vary from one country to another as well as within cities and counties within a single country.[4,6] In recent years, neonatal mortality rates for low birth weight infants have declined in neonatal intensive care units; however, considerable variation exists in the reported rates of handicaps in these surviving children.[5]

Etiologic factors underlying cerebral palsy are usually grouped into prenatal, natal, and postnatal categories.[10] Prenatal factors are hereditary or genetic conditions; prenatal infections including viral (rubella, herpes), bacterial, and parasitic (toxoplasmosis); fetal anoxia caused by hemorrhage from premature separation of the placenta, or maldevelopment of the placenta; Rh incompatibility including erythroblastosis fetalis, hemolytic anemia, and hyperbilirubinemia; metabolic disorders such as maternal diabetes and toxemia of pregnancy; and developmental deficits, which include maldevelopment of the brain, vascular, and skeletal structures.

Natal factors include rupture of brain blood vessels, or compression of the brain during prolonged or difficult labor, and asphyxia caused by drug sedation, distress of labor, premature separation of the placenta, placenta previa, or related to prematurity.

Postnatal factors leading to cerebral palsy include vascular accidents and intracranial hemorrhage; head trauma; brain infections, including bacterial or viral encephalopathies; toxic conditions, such as lead poisoning; anoxia from drowning or cardiac arrest; seizures; and tumors. Most children with cerebral palsy are noted to have multiple etiologies with intraventricular and periventricular bleeds or difficulty maintaining adequate oxygenation because of prematurity being the most common associated factors.[10] Certain etiologic factors predispose to specific clinical types of cerebral palsy. For example, O'Reilly and Walentynowicz showed in their study of 2004 children that prematurity or multiple births accounted for 55 percent of children with spastic diplegia while anoxia, respiratory distress and erythroblastosis fetalis accounted for 63 percent of the athetoid children.[10]

The clinical picture resulting from hemorrhagic or ischemic brain damage differs depending on the postconceptional age of the infant at the time of the insult.[11,12] The clinical picture of spastic diplegia in the very young premature infant results from ischemic damage to descending motor pathways in the internal capsule which control the motoneurons to muscles of the legs and trunk. Intraventricular bleeds in the immature infant may cause destruction of the germinal matrix surrounding the cerebral ventricles and result in hydrocephalus. Birth asphyxia in the term infant results in a variety of patterns of damage depending on the extent to which systemic blood pressure and cerebral blood flow are maintained. The clinical picture ranges from spastic quadriplegia or hemiplegia to choreoathetosis.[12,13]

Changes in obstetric management and neonatal intensive care have altered the percentages in the various etiologic categories. For example, O'Reilly and Walentynowicz[10] and Churchill and colleagues[14] report increasing incidence of spastic diplegia related to the problems of prematurity, a decrease in athetosis related to erythroblastosis fetalis, and decrease in hemiplegia associated with cesarian section. Pape and Wigglesworth,[12] however, believe that the incidence of uncomplicated periventricular leukomalacia resulting in clinical spastic diplegia is decreasing with improved management of hypothermia, nutrition, and apnea. In the surviving very low birth weight infants, an increased frequency of severe mutliple defects, including spastic quadriplegia, hemiplegia, and severe mental retardation, is related to massive periventricular lesions.

CLASSIFICATION

Classification of cerebral palsy by clinical types was adopted by the American Academy for Cerebral Palsy (now the American Academy for Cerebral Palsy and Developmental Medicine) and remains the most widely used system of classification.[15] This system, based on a description of topographical distribution of the tone and movement disorder is useful to physical therapists because it provides a picture of the child's motor problem. Appendix A of this chapter summarizes this classification of cerebral palsy. Although this system is well-recognized, it is limited in two aspects. First, it does not take into account changes that occur during development of the child with cerebral palsy. For this reason it is possible for an infant to be described as having hypotonic cerebral palsy, and at 1 year, as he or she begins to crawl and sit, to be described as a spastic diplegic, while at 4 years as he or she pulls to stand, attempts to walk, manipulate toys, and struggles with self-care, the child may be described as a spastic quadriplegic. None of these descriptions are wrong. This child actually presented quite differently at various developmental stages and chronologic ages. Yet the changing "diagnosis" leads to confusion and mistrust between the parents and the professionals and lack of credibility among professionals.

Another system of classification described in Quinton and Wilson[16] classifies children with cerebral palsy according to tonus and changing motor patterns. Quinton classifies cerebral palsy by the development of the child's tone and movement as he or she changes over time with position and movement against gravity. This classification serves three functions. It allows the examiner to (1) recognize normal and abnormal changes in tone and movement as the child grows and develops, (2) observe the progression of symptoms of motor dysfunction and determine which child is recovering from an initial brain insult and which one is developing increasing symptoms of motor dysfunction, and (3) determine if treatment is effectively changing the child's movements to more normal patterns.

A second problem of classifying cerebral palsy according to clinical types is the inability to provide clues for reliable prognosis. This problem is addressed in a classification system proposed by Milani-Comparetti and Gidoni.[17,18] This classification is divided into three syndromes: Regression, Defect, and Disharmony Syndromes.

The Regression Syndromes are abnormalities of movement identical with patterns seen in the early stages of normal fetal development, hence the term. The primary characteristic of these syndromes is limited variety of movement resulting from the overpowering influence of the early fetal movement patterns. The Defect Syndrome is characterized by lack of postural control. This syndrome is often associated with severe mental retardation. The Disharmony Syndrome is characterized by disorganized movement but without any limitation in the variety of movement patterns available.

To some extent, choice of a system of classification of cerebral palsy depends on the reasons for describing the child. Classifications of cerebral palsy that focus on progression of symptoms as the child moves against the force of gravity may provide more information to the physical therapist who is interested in how movement changes (normally and abnormally) and how movement patterns can be affected by treatment. The traditional classification by topographical distribution of tone and abnormal movement does not have this inherent component.

DIAGNOSIS AND PROGNOSIS

In addition to the problems of classifying and describing children with cerebral palsy, the problems of accurate identification and prediction of the extent of motor dysfunction are well known to the reader. Retrospective studies have emphasized a history of pre- and perinatal complications, including prematurity,[19,20] the presence of a number of abnormal neurologic findings in the neonatal period,[21-23] abnormal tone and maintained primitive reflexes,[24-26] failure of development of the postural reflex mechanism and delayed developmental milestones,[2,25,26] as precursors or indications of the diagnosis of central nervous system dysfunction in children. Paine and colleagues[27] followed the natural history of a large number of abnormal infants and described the appearance of abnormal tone, persistent primitive reflexes, and delay in the postural reactions in this population. Data from the Collaborative Perinatal Project in which 53,600 singleton infants born between 1959 and 1969 were periodically examined and followed for 7 years are now being published.[3,28] This study has provided much additional information regarding specific signs as predictors of cerebral palsy. Ellenberg and Nelson[3] report the combination of low birth weight and hypertonus at 4 months as highly predictive of cerebral palsy at 7 years. They also report that the additional presence of delayed motor milestones at four months strengthens the accuracy of this prediction. Campbell and Wilhelm[29,30] have reported their initial data from a longitudinal prospective study of infants at high risk for central nervous system dysfunction during the first year of life and found primitive reflexes and increased tone to be evident for long periods of time in the high-risk infants, but they were not related to motor outcome at 2 years unless very strong or very delayed in resolving. Again, delayed motor milestones in the first 6 months were highly predictive of poor outcome, although not necessarily of cerebral palsy, at 2 years of age. While clinical data are accumulating, the task of early identification as it affects the prognosis of any specific child remains difficult, especially in the case of children with mild central nervous system dysfunction who may not be identified in infancy.

To compound the problem of accurate early identification, modern neonatal care and intensive care nurseries are rapidly changing the distribution of types of infants who survive severe birth trauma with major motor deficits. The actual incidence of infants surviving with handicaps ranges from 10 percent in inborn units to 30–40 percent in outborn units.[31–33] Follow-up studies confirm that the most immature infants and those requiring ventilatory support have the highest risk of neurodevelopmental sequelae.[31,32,34] Initial reports on the neurodevelopmental outcome of infants surviving neonatal intraventricular hemorrhage documented by computed tomographic (CT) brain scan or sequential ultrasound show similar incidences of neurologic defects.[35–37] Although this information is important for medical management, it actually contributes to the frustration of parents and therapists who have been told by well-informed pediatricians that a specific child will be likely to recover from early insult. In approximately 75 percent of the cases, the physician is correct and fortunately most children do develop normally; but because of the inability to predict which children will fall into the approximately 25 percent who do not recover, the family may experience continued uncertainty and frustration in managing the child, loss of confidence in their own parenting skills, delay in involvement in intervention programs, and loss of confidence in the medical community if an unfavorable diagnosis is finally established.

Accurate diagnosis of cerebral palsy at a young age is important for economic, social, and emotional, as well as medical reasons. Because the value of early intervention has not been clearly established, accurate identification is essential for evaluation of the independent effects of treatment and maturation.

MEDICAL MANAGEMENT

Various drugs, including meprobamate, mephenesia, and benzodiazpines, have been used over the years to reduce spasticity or control involuntary movement in the child with cerebral palsy. Most recently baclofen, a gamma aminobutyric acid (GABA) derivative has been shown to be an effective inhibitor of mono- and polysynaptic reflexes and gamma motoneuron activity in decerebrate animals and a facilitator of Renshaw cell activity.[38]

Baclofen has been shown to be useful in the control of spinal and cerebral spasticity in adults.[39] More recently, studies have been done to determine the effectiveness of baclofen in reducing spasticity in children with spastic cerebral palsy. Milla and Jackson[38] and McKinlay and associates[40] examined the effects of baclofen in double-blind crossover trials. Both groups examined 20 children between 2 and 16 years of age with spastic cerebral palsy. Milla and Jackson[38] found that baclofen was significantly more effective than placebo in reducing spasticity in children with cerebral palsy. Active movement showed significant improvement and resistance to passive movement decreased. McKinlay and colleagues,[40] however, did not find any significant benefits from baclofen on posttrial examination. Both groups reported side effects of hypotonia, sedation, enuresis, and attention problems.

Young[41] reported on an open trial of baclofen in 27 children between 4 months and 12 years of age with spastic cerebral palsy. He found that baclofen was beneficial in spastic diplegia in improving mobility and ability to wear orthoses. He cautioned that, although independent mobility improved, the gait pattern did not because tonal distribution contributing to scissoring was unchanged by baclofen. The drug was ineffective in mixed types of cerebral palsy or in children with fixed deformities.

Minford and colleagues[42] assessed gait by polarized light goniometry in 15 hemiplegic children between 4 and 15 years of age prior to and following a 4- to 6-week treatment with baclofen. Each child was matched for age and sex with a normal child. A statistically significant decrease in hip and knee flexion at the toe-off phase of the gait cycle was found in both legs of experimental group children. Of the nine children who showed the greatest change upon goniometric assessment, five showed obvious clinical improvement as well. Again, side effects of transient sedation, enuresis, and deterioration in behavior and concentration were reported, and the authors suggest that baclofen should be used with caution and careful supervision.

Dantrolene sodium has also been used to control spasticity in children with cerebral palsy. Joynt and Leonard[43] reported on a double-blind study of 20 children comparing the effects of dantrolene sodium suspension and a placebo. The drug was found to be physiologically active in reducing the force of muscle contraction in response to peripheral nerve stimulation, but objective functional improvement as measured by multiple performance tests, including tests of mobility and manual dexterity, was not significant.

In addition to drugs that affect spasticity, the use of intramuscular alcohol has been used for temporary reduction in spasticity. Carpenter and Sietz[44] reported on the use of intramuscular alcohol injection in 211 patients between the ages of 18 months and 16 years. They found the procedure to be of no effect in athetosis, rigidity or ataxia, or when contracture was involved. The gastrocnemius-soleus muscle group had the highest predictable degree of success with reduction of tone from the alcohol injection.

At this time, pharmaceutical management of spasticity in children with cerebral palsy is not very promising as the complexity of the motor problems prevent predictable outcomes. In selected cases, with careful monitoring, drugs may be beneficial for assessment periods or for management of a specific problem related to overcoming spasticity.

Surgical Management

Orthopedic surgery is an important aspect of the management of the child with cerebral palsy. The current literature describes procedures for the upper extremities, spine, and lower extremities.[45,46] The orthopedic literature is extensive; however, most of the reports are descriptive rather than evaluative. The ages, types, and severity of involvement as well as detailed descriptions of the surgical procedures are mentioned. Postoperative results are usually described in general terms of increased function, improved posture, or improved cosmesis and hygiene, without providing the reader with details regarding how the results are obtained or how they correlate with preoperative status.

In articles on surgery of the upper extremity and hand, only House and colleagues[47] describe the evaluation of various upper extremity surgical procedures. In 56 children with cerebral palsy, they compared each patient's preoperative and postoperative functional status measured on a functional classification scale devised by the authors. They found that patients with a markedly impaired hand showed greatest functional improvement on their scale of functional skills. IQ did not seem to play a very important role in predicting results. Normal sensibility was important but not as useful as voluntary control in predicting outcome. Although the functional scale was an attempt to provide quantitative data, no evidence exists to suggest that this scale actually represents the levels of acquisition of hand skills in the cerebral palsied population.

All authors in the articles reviewed indicated that outcome of surgical treatment of spastic patients was more predictable than in children with athetosis. Patients with hemiplegic cerebral palsy made up the great majority of children for whom upper extremity surgery was indicated. Age and IQ were reportedly not as important as they once were thought to be, so long as the child was old enough and capable of cooperating with the program. Goals for hand surgery generally include improved function and activities of daily living (ADL), and improved cosmesis and hygiene.[47–49]

Hoffer and colleagues[50] indicate that the most difficult factors to document for surgical decision-making are the control and phasic activity of various muscles. These authors suggest that dynamic electromyography (EMG) using needle electrodes can be used to document muscle control and phasic activity. The electromyographic results in 21 patients showed that, in cerebral palsy, muscles are phase-dependent and will not change phase; thus, it is important to transfer a muscle that will operate in the appropriate phase for its intended function. If the electromyogram demonstrated that target muscles were continuously active throughout the grasp-release cycle, lengthening of these muscles, rather than transfer, was indicated.

Surgical management of scoliosis in children with cerebral palsy may be the most difficult problem facing the orthopedic surgeon. Because of the many other problems of cerebral palsy, scoliosis treatment by conventional means is difficult and presents many postsurgical management problems.[51] Harrington rod instrumentation requires prolonged postoperative management in a body cast, a treatment difficult for the child with cerebral palsy to tolerate. Bonnett and associates[52] and, in a separate report, MacEwen,[53] reported poor correction overall as well as various postoperative problems of pseudoarthroses, instrument failures, pressure sores, and poor tolerance to casts. Bonnett and colleagues[52] also described treatment with Dwyer instrumentation and anterior fusion, and again reported pseudoarthrosis and broken cables as problems. Allen and Ferguson[54] reported problems, including pressure sores, of managing patients in a body jacket. Allen and Ferguson[54] also reported on 10 patients with cerebral palsy who had L-rod instrumentation in which L-shaped steel rods were secured by a sublaminar wire at each vertebra. The advantage of this procedure is that the wire fixation was sufficiently secure so that there generally was no need for a patient to wear a postoperative plaster cast or orthosis.

Surgical management of the lower extremities ranges from tenotomies, muscle lengthenings and muscle transplants, to osteotomies, neurectomies, and fusions. The results reported are equally variable. Truscelli and colleagues[55] suggest that the variation in long-term results of elongation of the tendoachilles depends on differences in underlying pathophysiology rather than differences in surgical techniques. The authors suggest that there may be a reduction of the number of sarcomeres or reduction in the length of the sarcomes resulting in varying outcome of muscle lengthening and immobilization.

Castle and associates[56] suggest that abnormalities in the muscle may contribute to variation in surgical outcome. On biopsies of various muscles in the extremities of 85 patients undergoing surgery, they demonstrated various degrees and combinations of Type I and Type II muscle fiber atrophy and hypertrophy. Castle and associates[56] believe that a muscle showing Type II fiber atrophy or Type I hypertrophy will not be appropriately functional if transplanted, but may only serve as a dynamic tenodesis. The normal Type II fiber component of a muscle seems to be required for reeducation of the transplant and the health of Type II fibers appears to serve as an indicator of the quality of neuronal activation of the muscle.

Many authors compare the results of one surgical method to another. Root and Spero[57] compared adductor tenotomy with hip adductor transfer in a 10-year study of 102 patients. With an average of 3.8 years at follow-up, these authors reported that, although the adductor transfer operation takes longer and is associated with a higher incidence of postoperative problems, the transferred muscle provided better pelvic stability, decreased hip flexion contractures, and reduced hip instability in comparison to tenotomized muscle.

Orthopedic surgery is considered essential treatment in many children with cerebral palsy; however, a lack of uniform criteria exists for selection, surgical intervention procedures, and outcome assessment. Studies that incorporate the essential elements of research design are notably absent from the literature and a need exists for systematic longitudinal data on the effectiveness of orthopedic surgical intervention for children with cerebral palsy.

Neurosurgery

Cooper and associates[58] introduced chronic electrical stimulation of the cerebellum to reduce spasticity and improve motor function in patients with cerebral palsy. Numerous articles on this technique have been written, but controversy remains over its effectiveness.[59-62] Double-blind studies have produced little support for the stated effects of cerebellar stimulation.

Penn and Etzel[61] reported on the effects of chronic electrical stimulation of the cerebellum in 14 patients with cerebral palsy, who were studied prospectively for 1 to 44 months; 11 showed improvement in motor function. However, a double-blind test of 10 patients off and on stimulation for an average of 8 weeks produced no significant changes; thus the functional changes may not have been the result of cerebellar stimulation.[63]

Gahm and associates[64] used a double-blind crossover technique to assess the value of chronic cerebellar stimulation in eight children or adolescents with cerebral palsy. Improvements in speech, reduced spasticity, and increased mental alertness occurred during placebo periods as often as with stimulation. Whittaker[65] also used a double-blind crossover experiment with 3-week periods of on-off intervention and was unable to document any changes in function.

Chronic cerebellar stimulation for cerebral palsy remains a controversial procedure, difficult to evaluate objectively because of the complexity of the symptoms in cerebral palsy. The clinical syndrome varies over time, and the patients undergoing the procedure and their families are highly motivated to change. Tests of neurophysiologic function, spasticity, and motor skills have suggested that changes occur but double-blind evaluations have not provided supportive data.[66]

PHYSICAL THERAPY ASSESSMENT

The interdisciplinary, multidisciplinary, or transdisciplinary team approach is the current standard of practice for assessment of cerebral palsy.[67,68] Depending on the child's age, developmental level, and degree of involvement, the system of service delivery, and physical setting, the components of the team may vary, including some or all of the following medical and educational specialists: pediatrician, neurologist, orthopedist; physical, occupational, and speech therapist; special educator, social worker, psychologist, nutritionist, and dentist. The role and degree of involvement for each of these specialists will vary not only with the current needs of the child and family but also with the interest, training, and experience of the individual specialist.

Because the hallmark of cerebral palsy is sensorimotor dysfunction, the physical therapist is always part of the assessment team. If the clinic is designed for evaluation and diagnostics, the physical therapist usually assesses motor patterns and response to sensory input, developmental reflexes, and postural reactions, as well as range of motion and motor milestones. Depending on the role of the physical therapist, the skills of other members of the assessment team, and reasons for assessment, the physical therapist may use a variety of screening tests or tests of general development such as the Denver Development Screening Test, the Wolanski Gross Motor Developmental Examination, Milani-Comparetti Developmental Examination, the Alpern-Boll Development Profile, Movement Assessment of Infants, Gesell or Bayley tests which are described by Stengel and colleagues in Chapter 2 of this book.

Most of these tests will allow a therapist to evaluate the level of motor performance of the child with cerebral palsy in comparison with the total population of children, but because eventually developmental delay is clearly seen in cerebral palsy, motor assessment for specific diagnosis and treatment planning requires additional detailed analysis of posture, movement, and coordination. While much of the information collected during such a motor assessment is descriptive, efforts to summarize these findings in an objective manner will aid in evaluating the direction of change over time as a result of both intervention and development.

The sensorimotor assessment should always provide information important for treating or managing the motor problems of the child. The description of assessment in this chapter will focus on the importance of collecting this information for program planning. Only the sensorimotor components of the assessment will be presented in depth in this chapter. The actual method of assessment of cerebral palsy depends to some extent on the theoretical framework, training, and experience of the individual therapist; however, most authors describe the following components as essential in the motor assessment of children with cerebral palsy.[69-72]

Muscle Tone

Abnormalities of muscle tone have been found to be consistent as predictive findings in young children who are at risk for cerebral palsy, as well as one of the hallmarks of children who are described as having cerebral palsy.[3,73,74] Unfortunately, criteria for objectively evaluating muscle tone in infants beyond the neonatal period and in young children have not been established. In addition, the difficulty of assessing muscle tone is compounded by the fact that muscle tone normally changes drastically in the premature infant as development progresses through the first year of life. Saint-Anne Dargassies[75] has described the changes in muscle tone in the normally maturing premature infant and uses this method of evaluating the distribution of tone in premature infants. Amiel-Tison[76] has used much the same method of evaluating tone in small-for-dates infants. Most examiners evaluate both active and passive muscle tone. Active tone is defined as the power and adaptability of the muscles during spontaneous movement, and passive tone refers to resistance of the muscle when movements are imposed by the examiner.[2,77-79]

The following definitions can be applied when evaluating passive or active tone in children with cerebral palsy:

1. Severe hypotonia
    Active: Inability to resist gravity, lack of cocontraction at proximal joints for stability, weakness, limited voluntary movements
    Passive: Joint hyperextensibility, no resistance to movement imposed by examiner, full or excessive passive range of motion
2. Moderate hypotonia
    Active: Decreased tone primarily in axial muscles and proximal muscles of the extremities; interferes with rate of development and length of time a posture can be sustained
    Passive: Mild resistance to movement when imposed by examiner in distal parts of extremities only; joint hyperextensibility at elbows and knees
3. Mild hypotonia
    Active: Decreased tone interferes with axial muscle cocontraction, delays in initiation of movement against gravity and speed of adjustment to postural change
    Passive: Mild resistance in proximal as well as distal segments; full passive range of motion
4. Normal tone
    Active: Quick and immediate postural adjustment during movement; ability to use muscles in synergic and reciprocal patterns for stability and mobility depends on task of the moment
    Passive: Body parts resist displacement, momentarily maintain new posture when placed in space, and can rapidly follow changing movements imposed by examiner
5. Mild hypertonus
    Active: Increased tone causes delay in postural adjustment; poor coordination, slowness of movement
    Passive: Resistance to change of posture in part of or throughout the range; poor ability to accommodate to passive movements
6. Moderate hypertonus
    Active: Increased tone limits speed, coordination, variety of movement patterns, and active range of motion
    Passive: Resistance to change of posture throughout the range; limited passive range of motion at some joints
7. Severe hypertonus
    Active: Severe stiffness of muscles in stereotypes patterns limits active range of motion; little or no ability to move against gravity; very limited patterns of movement
    Passive: Passive range of motion limited; unable to overcome resistance of muscle to complete full range
8. Intermittent tone
    Active: Occasional and unpredictable resistance to postural changes alternating with normal adjustment; may have difficulty initiating active movement or sustaining posture
    Passive: Unpredictable resistance to imposed movements alternating with complete absence of resistance

Distribution of Tone.   Muscle tone in one part of the body is described relative to other body parts. Generally the head, neck, and trunk tone is compared with that in the extremities, the right side compared with the left, the upper extremities compared with the lower extremities, and the distal parts of the extremities compared with the proximal parts. Any asymmetries, including facial asymmetries, are also described.

Tone Under Stimulation.   Changes in tone with speaking, laughing, crying, excitement, change in environment, and play are noticed. This information is particularly important to a therapist when planning treatment. For example, a child who gets very stiff when asked to talk should not be engaged in complicated language games during difficult movement activities.

Interactions of Tone and Movement Patterns.   The interdependent relationship between muscle tone and movement patterns has been described by several authors.[80,81] During the assessment, the therapist notes what influence tone has on movement in various positions in which the force of gravity must be resisted. Some children get much stiffer when they attempt to move and the degree of tone at rest does not correlate well with the interference experienced during movement. Other children become less stiff with movement. Although movement will not be the only factor affecting the child's tone, treatment planning requires that the therapist know what to expect when the child begins moving. If a child is stiff (or floppy) prior to beginning treatment, and gets stiffer with movement, the therapist will need to find positions and movements that do not increase tone, and alter speed and stimulation to accommodate tone changes. In addition, some children will be much more able to manage movement without abnormal tone change in some positions against gravity than in others. By observing the interaction of tone and movement in various positions, the therapist will be able to decide which positions give the child the greatest opportunity for producing the most normal quality of movement.

Effect of Sensory Input on Tone.   The therapist needs to note the effect of pressure and touch on tonus of the child. Some children may have a low threshold to tactile input so they are unable to inhibit motor response to exteroceptive stimulus. Children who have not been treated are often fearful of movement and become quite stiff when handled. In addition, the therapist will note the influence of speed, direction, and force of vestibular input on the changing patterns on the child's tone. In an initial assessment, it is important to attempt to find the amount and type of sensory input and movement a child can tolerate while maintaining a relatively normal muscle tone.

Patterns of Posture and Movement

Children with cerebral palsy move in patterns that are more or less predictable based on the clinical description, age, extent of involvement, and their own movement experience.[82] Understanding how the patterns of movement develop and how they can be expected to change is based on a thorough understanding of normal development as well as an understanding of abnormal development. (See Chapter 2 by Stengel and colleagues.) This information makes it possible to anticipate how a child's existing posture and movement will influence, either positively or negatively, his or her continued development.

Information on posture and movement is gathered as a child moves spontaneously during an examination and includes the following data.

Posture in Supine, Prone, Sidelying, Sit, Kneel, and Stand. The child should be encouraged through play to assume as many postures requiring resistance to the force of gravity as possible. Given a comfortable situation and adequate time, a child will do what he or she can do. It is possible to gain a representative sample of a child's motor behavior only if he or she is cooperative and unthreatened. The examiner should question the parent as to whether observations represent typical behavior. In each position, the therapist looks for common components that are normal or abnormal. One can either describe each position and then later analyze common problematic patterns (see Wilson, "Analysis of Posture and Mobility," in *Vulpe Assessment Battery*,[83]) or note repeating abnormal patterns as the child moves. For example, rounded upper back in four-point, sit, and kneeling positions; weight on right side in sitting and standing positions; weight on fisted hands in prone on elbows or prone on hands, and in the four-point position. The focus is on the repetition of abnormal components of movement, not the position itself, as repeating patterns will be more predictive of future development and potential movement and orthopedic problems.

This section of the assessment also includes description of the patterns of weight bearing, noting how the child shifts and bears weight in anticipation of movement in each position. The inability to initially shift weight in the direction opposite the anticipated movement is frequently seen in children with cerebral palsy. Symmetry or asymmetry in weight bearing is noted because persistent asymmetrical weight bearing to one side limits movement of that side and can contribute to development of structural scoliosis and other orthopedic problems.

Normal and Abnormal Movement. It is important to note how the child moves, emphasizing both normal and abnormal movement patterns. A mildly involved diplegic child may move quite normally in lower level developmental positions and only show abnormal movement patterns with standing and walking. Knowing the position in which the child has basically normal movement aides selection of positions to be used in treatment. In addition to describing how the child moves, one should note the frequency with which a movement pattern is performed. For example: Does the child *always* support on the left side and reach out with the right? Does the child *always* get to sitting by moving over the left side or pull to stand with the right leg placed forward? This information is valuable both for planning treatment as well as for predicting future outcome.

This section of the assessment also includes information on initiation of movement. Hemiplegic children often initiate movement with the sound side. The diplegic child often initiates movement with the upper trunk and arms while the legs follow through quite passively. Some children attempt to initiate movement with the same side (or extremity) they are using for weight bearing or support. The inability to initiate movement with the body part appropriate for the tasks causes further distortions in movement patterns. In addition, speed of initiation and effort of movements is noted. Many children show long latency of response, which can be confused with lack of understanding directions rather than related to the motor problem. Excessive effort in movement may contribute to poor general exercise endurance.

Finally, this section of the assessment includes identification of primitive movement patterns. Many infants and young children with cerebral palsy who have had little experience of movement retain motor patterns typical of younger children. It is important to differentiate between truly abnormal patterns and patterns that are only immature, because primitive patterns can be easily modified in therapy if treatment begins before they become established habits.

Asymmetries of Movement. Assessment of asymmetry includes observations of differences in amount of movement and stability of one side from the other, the extremities versus the trunk, one extremity from another, or parts of the extremities relative to each other (proximal versus distal). Asymmetries between the two sides of the body are easy to detect in hemiplegic children, but are also commonly found in spastic diplegic and athetoid children.[82] Asymmetries may change with position and stress as well as with development. Facial asymmetries during talking or eating should be recorded.

Effects of Sensory Input on Posture and Movement. Just as it is important to know the effect sensory input has on tone, the therapist also needs to know the effect of exteroceptive or proprioceptive input on posture and movement. Some children are extremely sensitive to auditory or visual stimulus to the point that loud or sudden auditory input or bright visual input may affect their ability to maintain balance in a position. Some children are almost immobilized by multisensory stimulation because they are unable to attend and respond to appropriate cues for movement.

Associated Reactions. Increased tone in certain parts of the body is caused by movement in other body parts. These reactions are clear in hemiplegia[82] but are also seen in the lower extremities in diplegia. The presence of associated reactions indicates lack of disassociation of muscular activity of one body part from that in another and is one sign of increased tone occurring with movement.

Associative Movement. Mirror movements, either partial or complete, in the paired contralateral extremity, are frequently observed in normally developing preschool and early school-age children. The persistence or overpowering nature of these associative movements in children with cerebral palsy prevents them from performing different functions with their two hands, as exemplified by the child who always drops an object held in one hand when trying to release an object in the other hand, or by the child who cannot release an object with one hand while holding something with the other. The predominance of these reactions prevent coordinated, reciprocal hand use.

Influence of Developmental Reflexes and Postural Reactions in Movement

Molnar[84] has described the differences in motor behavior of children with cerebral palsy and those with mental retardation and postulates that the motor deficit of retarded infants is related to disturbance in the postural reflex mechanism, while the motor deficit found in cerebral palsy children is related to both the persistence of developmental reflexes and a disturbance in the postural reflex mechanism. Developmental reflex testing provides information on how a child response to specific sensory input applied in a systematic way. Reflex testing, positions, and procedures have been described by Fiorentino,[85] Wilson,[86] Capute and associates,[87] and Barnes and associates.[88] While each of these tests provide for test-retest comparison of a child, none of them have normative data available. For the severely involved child who has little voluntary or spontaneous movement, a reflex test is essential to see if movement can be elicited through proprioceptive and exteroceptive stimulation. For less involved children, the examiner's ability to recognize the more subtle influence on movement of persistent developmental reflexes or lack of development of the postural reactions is critical.

Developmental Reflexes. The persistence of primitive reflexes as an influence on movement in cerebral palsy has been described by many authors.[27,82,87] If these early reflex patterns dominate the child's movement, the child will have little variety of movement, decreased isolated movement of a body part and inability to inhibit the effect of exteroceptive and proprioceptive input in motor responses. For example, one may see that the only way a child can extend one arm is by initiating it with a head turn toward that arm. The influence of the asymmetric tonic neck reflex prevents other variations of arm extension and prevents disassociation of movements of the head from those at the shoulders. Recognizing the influence of primitive reflex patterns during spontaneous movement requires close observation and a great deal of experience. If the tester records the way a child moves in the second part of the assessment (Patterns of Posture and Movement), examination of the recurring patterns may reveal consistent influence of the primitive reflexes. The importance of recognizing whether arm extension with head turning is in fact the persistence of the asymmetric tonic neck reflex, or a visual problem or habit pattern, is clearly important in treatment and educational planning. Habit patterns often can be modified through a behavioral modification approach, a visual problem can be corrected with lenses or surgery, while a persistent asymmetric tonic neck reflex can be modified only with maturation and specific handling techniques.

Postural Reactions. This part of the assessment includes evaluation of the postural reactions of equilibrium, righting and protective extension which are primarily responsible for a child's ability to gain and maintain mobile posture against the force of gravity and freedom of movement necessary to develop highly skilled activities. Most children with cerebral palsy have at least some components of the postural reflexes, but poorly developed reactions interfere with posture and balance in upright positions and limit the child's movement repertoire. A child who has poor equilibrium reactions in sitting will frequently place one hand on the floor in a protective response, thereby limiting two-hand use for dressing or play. A child who is posturally insecure against gravity will often develop *one* way to perform a task, and his or her movements will be stereotyped and limited in variety. Statements regarding the quality of righting, equilibrium, and protective responses relating to speed, direction, force, frequency, and duration of the stimulus, as well as the quality of response in different positions, are noted.

A rating scale was published in 1977 by this author, as a method for obtaining objective ratings regarding influence of reflexes or reactions on a child's motor performance.[86] This rating scale does not imply that the presence (or absence) of a particular response is good or bad. It can be used to show reliable changes in components of movement with treatment or maturation.

Oral Motor Functions

Many children with cerebral palsy have a history of oral dysfunction including feeding problems, persistent primitive oral reflexes, respiratory problems, drooling, and delayed or abnormal vocalization. As part of the motor assessment, this section includes information regarding the child's oral history, present oral function and influence of tone, posture, and movement on overall oral functions. If oral motor dysfunction is severe, a separate oral motor evaluation should be done. Comprehensive assessment has been described by Morris.[89,90]

Stages of Development

Children with cerebral palsy experience delays in motor development. It is particularly difficult to apply motor age equivalents to a child with cerebral palsy because their development is so uneven. Often, however, this information is requested by educational programs for placement and is sometimes used to document the success of therapeutic programs. General level of development is also important in planning treatment programs because the developmental milestones represent the functional goals of a therapeutic program. Assessment of developmental level includes gross and fine motor skills the child performs independently, regardless of the pattern of movement. This section also includes notation of the influence of tone, reflexes and abnormal movement on the level of skills. Some children show delays which are even greater than would be expected based on evaluation of tone, reflexes or abnormal movements because of a significant degree of mental retardation. It is important to identify the strongest influences on limitations of functional skills because the therapist must adjust his or her methods and expectations for goal achievement according to the findings.

The influence of handling on the level of skills should also be recorded. Often providing minimal support for balance allows a child to pull to stand ven though he or she cannot perform the task independently. This information s important for determining later progress and potential for independence. Vulpe describes a Performance Analysis Scale that allows the examiner to ate the child's ability to perform skills based on the type of assistance the hild needs to accomplish the task.[83] The Performance Analysis Scale can be ised to show progress in a horizontal manner, indicating a greater degree of ndependence in task completion, even if the child is not performing new, higher evel, skills in a retest situation. Such information can be beneficial in dem- nstrating improvement in severely involved children who cannot be expected o show progress using standard measurements.

Contractures and Deformities

One of the primary effects of treatment on children with cerebral palsy night well be preventing contractures and deformities. This part of the as- essment includes a recording of existing contractures and deformities. Joint ange of motion should be recorded with a goniometer. The position for testing hould be included if tone or reflexes influence the child's passive or active ange of motion. Perry and colleagues[91,92] have shown that tone is influenced y position, and range of motion assessments will vary according to the position f the child during testing. Second, this section includes information on the otential influence of current posture and movement on future development f deformities and contractures. For example, if a child sits between his heels, e is at great risk for hip adductor contractures and medial femoral torsion.

Splinting and Surgery

If the child has splints, braces, casts, or has had surgery, this is included n the assessment. First, there is a description of surgical procedures and their nfluence on the child's current movement. Second, a description of splints, races and casts includes how long they are worn, for what purposes they are vorn, and a description of movement with appliances and how it differs from he movement without the devices.

Adaptive Equipment and Assistive Devices

Children who currently use adaptive equipment, assistive devices, or mo- ility aides to increase function and independence are included in the assess- nent. Depending on the setting, these data may be gathered by asking the arents about the child's function with equipment and without. The equipment r device is described with the goals for use of the equipment and the differences n function with and without the equipment.

Other Areas of Development

Analysis of the basic sensory functions and behavioral and physiologic haracteristics are also recorded but will not be discussed in this chapter.

Summary of Assessment

The assessment summary includes, first, a list of the child's strengths. This may include information regarding both internal and external resources, intelligence, interest, attention, cooperativeness, self-concept, sensorimotor skills, and activities of daily living as they apply to the specific child. The family's size, interest, level of understanding of the child's abilities and disabilities, time and energy available for interaction and therapy, and financial resources may be noted. Following a list of strengths, problems are noted. The procedure of enumerating strengths and problems allows the reader to focus on how the strengths can be used to facilitate development in the problem areas and facilitates integration of all aspects of the child's functional abilities.

Listing the problems leads directly to a list of goals for therapy and of treatment methods designed specifically to meet the goals listed. In the following section, Planning Treatment, a sample of how the evaluation and problems list are integrated with a treatment plan is illustrated.

PLANNING TREATMENT

Treatment for the child with cerebral palsy must be individualized based on his or her specific problems, age, degree of involvement, intelligence, associated problems, and family involvement; however, certain guidelines are important to follow if treatment is to remain effective over time.

1. *Treatment goals are designed to meet specific problems.* These will vary with age and extent of symptoms at onset of treatment.

2. *Treatment goals must be changed with changes in the presenting problem.* For example, an infant with hemiplegia may initially present with hypotonicity in the upper extremity and by 6 to 8 months present with hypertonicity once he begins to move against gravity.[82] The goal therefore changes from increasing tone in the involved upper extremity to decreasing tone in the involved upper extremity.

3. *Treatment methods and techniques change with the child's age, need for independence and function, as well as motor symptoms.* A young baby enjoys being held for play, therapy, dressing, and feeding. A natural environment is mother's lap and a great deal of baby treatment can effectively take place there. Because a 2-year-old needs to develop independence, dressing can be done on a bench or chair (with appropriate support) and treatment requires much more mobility, exploration, and self initiation. A 10-year-old needs to function independently. Treatment changes to provide the child with methods to monitor his or her own movements, maintain range of motion and perform movement independently. Teenagers are assisted in finding methods through recreation to integrate movement into their lifestyle.

4. *Families need to be given information regarding the child's problem and treatment as they are able to understand and assimilate the information.*

The role of the family in treatment is described in detail in the section on family involvement in this chapter.

5. *Suggestions to the family should be as practical as possible*, remembering that parents have responsibilities toward their other children and to each other as well as to their handicapped child.

6. *Therapy should be designed to provide active response from the child.* Passive movement is less effective in producing changes in tone or movement patterns. Active movement does not necessarily mean voluntary movement. For example, postural reactions performed automatically require a great amount of strength and endurance.

7. *Whenever possible movement should be initiated by the child.* Control of movement is maintained by the therapist, but the child should lead the treatment and initiate the activity.

8. *Repetition is an important component in motor learning.* Motor activities repeated throughout the session and repeated in functional ways at home have a better chance of becoming part of the child's habitual repertoire.

9. *The environment should be conducive to cooperative participation and support of the child's efforts.* Because therapy will be an active part of a cerebral palsy child's life, it should be pleasurable. If the child enjoys movement, he or she will be more inclined to make movement, through exercise and recreation, part of his or her lifestyle.

10. *Treatment must be geared to the functions the child needs as s/he grows and develops.* Functions used in activities of daily living, including dressing, feeding, and personal grooming, are important therapeutic techniques.

11. *Play should be integrated into therapy to provide motivation and purpose in order to reinforce and direct movement responses.* Play must be carefully monitored during treatment so that it does not overstimulate the child and interfere with the desired movement response or produce abnormal tone.

12. *Sensory stimulation must be integrated with motor output.* Loud or vigorous auditory and visual stimuli can be used to call attention and produce forceful movement. Multisensory stimuli, however, should not be used with highly distractible or emotionally volatile children. Tactile or vestibular hypersensitivity or hyposensitivity can have a profound effect on the movement outcome. Changing the type and level of sensory input can have a direct effect on improving the quality of motor response.

13. *Therapy should be designed to utilize the child's strengths to build on problem areas.* If a child has good imaginary play and language skills, story telling can focus the child's attention and imaginary play can provide a framework for moving.

14. *A single treatment progresses from positions in which the child has the most normal tone and movement to ones which are more challenging.* Within each treatment session a child should have the opportunity to work in various developmental positions appropriate to his or her age, but the progression from one position to another must be carefully controlled so that as the child is challenged by the force of gravity he or she continues to produce movement with normal postural tone. Treatment should end with positions and

activities which are functional for the child and which provide a cooldown period after a vigorous exercise session.

15. *Movement in one position prepares for movements in another.* Through experience with an individual child, the therapist will find positions and activities which change tone and provide greater variety in the child's movements. These activities are used early in a treatment session to give the child the feeling for control in positions where movement is easier prior to attempting movement in positions which are difficult or new for the child.

16. *As a child is able to perform movements independently, the therapist provides time in a treatment for the child to move freely.* It is important for the child to feel movement produced through his own efforts without the control of the therapist. Only in this way will the child incorporate these movements into his or her daily living.

17. *Individual treatment sessions should be designed to evaluate the effectiveness of treatment within the session.* This can be done informally by motivating the child to demonstrate an activity, movement or posture, at the beginning of treatment and again at the end to determine if changes have occurred or through more formalized methods (see Treatment Evaluation section). Knowing that change has occurred is motivating to the child and reinforcing for the therapist.

18. *Physical therapy treatment should be coordinated with all other medical and educational disciplines involved with the child.* Treatment should be integrated with the goals and methods of occupational and speech therapy, orthopedic management, and educational and home management. While the roles of these disciplines are very important in the total management of the child, they will not be discussed in this chapter. At different times in the child's life, the focus and importance of the various disciplines will change so that one discipline will have a higher priority than another. Interdisciplinary communication is essential to maintain a consistent approach to meeting the changing needs of the child and the family.

ILLUSTRATION OF TREATMENT

In order to illustrate how these principles of treatment are integrated into a specific program, a case study is presented, following the child from assessment through a treatment progression and treatment evaluation.

Summary of Assessment

Michael A. is a 3-year, 1-month-old boy, born 10 weeks prematurely with history of respiratory distress syndrome. He presents with the moderate-severe spastic diplegic type of cerebral palsy. The following summarizes his strengths and problem areas:

Strengths

1. Intelligent, cooperative, inquisitive child. No standardized testing done to date.
2. Uses speech to express wants and desires
3. Motivated to move
4. Not fearful of movement
5. Normal vision and hearing
6. Supportive, intelligent family, interested and able to provide appropriate care

Problem Areas

1. Abnormal tone: Increased extensor tone more on left than right, lower extremities more than trunk and upper extremities, distal parts more than proximal parts. Poor cocontraction in trunk muscles with intermittent extensor tone.
2. Abnormal sensory responses: Heighten response to tactile stimulus unanticipated touch produces generalized extensor response.
3. Abnormal patterns of movement: Michael's lower extremities are dominated by extension and adduction of the hips and plantar flexion at the ankles. Movement is initiated primarily from head and shoulders. More movement on the right side. More stability with abnormal tone on left side.
4. Persistent primitive reflexes: Limit variety of movements, asymmetric tonic neck reflex influences posture of upper extremities.
5. Delayed postural reactions: All components of the postural reactions are disturbed, preventing movement and maintenance of posture against the force of gravity. Inadequate postural reactions inhibit weight shift, ability to maintain or regain normal postural alignment, and produce isolated movements of body parts. Often the primitive reflex patterns override Michael's postural reactions, so that balance is inadequate in any position.
6. Oral motor dysfunction: Michael has slowly articulated single words and phrases. His voice is very low in volume. Open mouth posture is seen frequently in association with maintaining antigravity postures or stress in movement. Occasional drooling is observed.
7. Delay in motor development: Michael's independent gross motor development is at approximately a 6-month level, fine motor, 18 months to 2 years, and activities of daily living skills, 12 to 15 months. These delays are clearly related to motor dysfunction.
8. Limited range of motion: This child's active range is often limited by tone. Passive range is limited to 65 degrees in hamstrings, 60 degrees in hip adductors, and to neutral in gastrocnemius-soleus muscle group bilaterally.

Figures 11-1 to 11-8 illustrate Michael's problems.

Treatment Goals

Based on the problems described and illustrated in the assessment summary, the following immediate goals for therapy were established:

1. Change amount and distribution of abnormal tone

(*Text continues on page 378*).

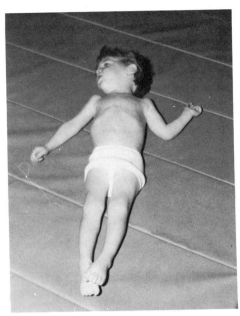

Fig. 11-1. Supine: extensor tone evident, more in lower extremities, more in distal parts. Asymmetric tonic neck reflex posturing assumed with head turning. Flaring of ribs indicates inactivity of abdominal muscles.

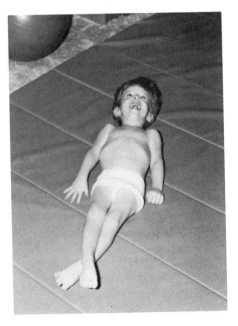

Fig. 11-2. Excitement increases extensor tone throughout. Scapular elevation, shoulder medial rotation, legs adducted, extended, feet plantar flexed. This pattern will be repeated with little variation with position changes.

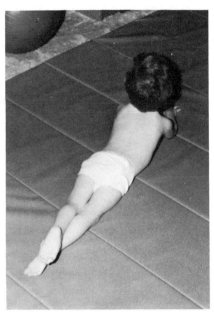

Fig. 11-3. Prone on elbows: Movement initiated from head and shoulders. Legs still dominated by extension, adduction, and plantar flexion. Limited equilibrium prevents good alignment. Can maintain position only if center of gravity is kept well within base of support.

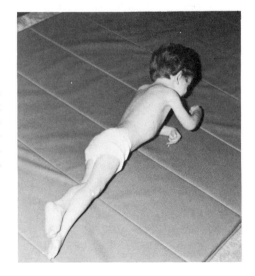

Fig. 11-4. Crawling: Asymmetries are noted, movement initiated with right side. Left side used to stabilize, right side for progression. Effort of progression increases scapular elevation, humeral medial rotation. Little variation in lower extremities.

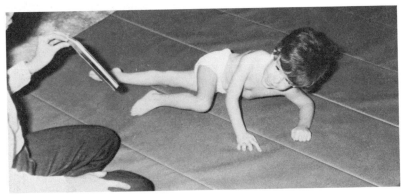

Fig. 11-5. Transition from prone to sit: Again initiation of movement from right side. Effort to stabilize and balance produces increased tone on left. Unable to rotate trunk over lower extremities or shift weight from left shoulder to left hip therefore cannot move the rest of the way to sitting.

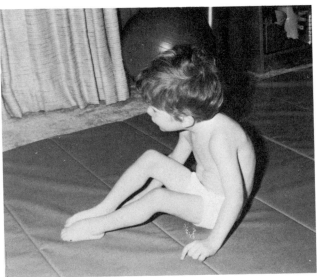

Fig. 11-6. Placed in sitting: Michael cannot assume sitting. Placed in sitting extensor tone evident in lower trunk and hips pulling him back onto sacrum. Hamstring spasticity contributes to hip extension and knee flexion. Plantar flexion persists. Lack of equilibrium evidenced by hands on floor to maintain position. Upper trunk and neck flexion in attempt to counteract excessive hip extension and bring center of gravity forward over base of support. Weight primarily on left side.

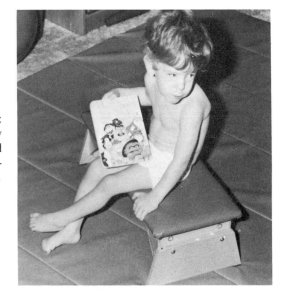

Fig. 11-7. Placed on a bench: Stress of position and insecurity increases extensor tone in hips and pelvis. Asymmetric tonic neck reflex again evident. Weight on left.

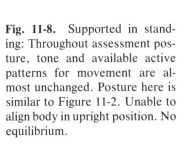

Fig. 11-8. Supported in standing: Throughout assessment posture, tone and available active patterns for movement are almost unchanged. Posture here is similar to Figure 11-2. Unable to align body in upright position. No equilibrium.

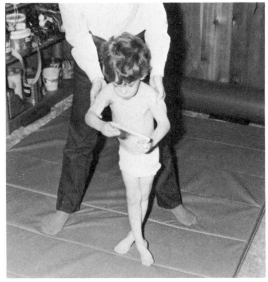

    a. Decrease excessive extensor tone in lower extremities

    b. Increase cocontraction patterns in trunk and shoulder girdle

    c. Decrease tone in distal muscles, plantar flexion of feet and flexion of hands

2. Develop symmetry in weight bearing through upper and lower extremities for normal posture alignment

3. Develop greater variety of movement patterns, particularly in the trunk and lower extremities

4. Develop rotation within the body axis to assist with transitions from one position to another

5. Develop weight shift through upper extremities for weight bearing while reaching out, and in the lower extremities in preparation for locomotion

6. Initiate movement with appropriate body parts for the task of the moment, for example, ability to use one part for movement while using another for weight bearing and stability

7. Develop better disassociation of movements of one body part from another for coordinated movements

8. Develop postural adaptations and alignment to improve equilibrium in all positions

9. Develop better freedom of movement to decrease influence of primitive reflexes seen with stress

10. Increase upper thoracic extension to prevent possible structural deformities

11. Provide opportunities for age-appropriate skills of self-help, play, and locomotion

Figures 11-9 to 11-20 show a progression of treatment activities designed to meet the goals described. Photographs were taken in a single treatment session. (See pages 380–386.)

Treatment Evaluation

Informal evaluations can be made during treatment if the therapist observes a particular skill, movement or position prior to treatment, later in treatment (compare standing alignment in Figure 11-8 with posture during therapy in Figure 11-20. Compare sitting posture in Figure 11-7 with Figure 11-19), and again at the end of treatment. By observing changes in tone, posture, and movement, it is possible to assess whether the goals for treatment are appropriate, whether the methods selected are meeting these goals, and what problems continue to exist. Figure 11-21 was taken prior to therapy demonstrating Michael's problem in independent sitting which contrasts with Figure 11-22 taken at the end of the treatment session.

FAMILY INVOLVEMENT

Involvement of the family in the intervention program for a child with cerebral palsy is an important aspect of treatment. In order to be effective in involving the family in an intervention program, physical therapists must recognize that a family consists of a system of relationships. The needs of the family and their resources to cope with these needs change over time, reflecting both continuity of family development as well as changes in structure and function of the family unit.[93]

When planning the home management aspect of the sensorimotor program, the therapist must recognize and accept that children grow up in different subcultures that have their own values, expectations, patterns of interpersonal relations, manners, and styles of intellectual operations and communications.[94] Programs for groups of culturally distinct or economically disadvantaged families have been notable failures when planned by white middle-class professionals, partly because of the lack of attention to individual needs and failure to understand attitudes of the group to be served.[95] The therapist must ask the parents what *they* would like to know about the child and what they would like to be able to do for him. Redman-Bentley,[96] in a study of 66 parents of children diagnosed with physical or mental disabilities or developmental delay, found that parents of young handicapped children do have specific needs and priorities as well as expectations for professionals with whom they were involved. She reported that parents wanted a more active role in the rehabilitation process of their handicapped children, a say in decisions concerning their child's program, as well as information regarding test results, and changes in the child's progress and program.

Recognizing and responding to the parents' needs may require the therapist to reorder priorities in order to initiate realistic plans for meeting the family's goals. According to Schaefer,[97] the most effective way to influence the development of children is to provide professional support for parental care of children. The family spends the greatest amount of time with the child; therefore, keeping the total child in mind, it makes sense to teach the parents to understand normal and abnormal development and make use of the available knowledge about care and management that is pertinent to their child. When beginning home management, it is important, when appropriate, to imitate the interactive style of the parents rather than requiring the parents to give up their accustomed methods of handling their child to follow a prescribed approach which may be incompatible with their own natural style. The parents can learn child care routines which will reinforce and maximize the child's skills while continuing to feel adequate as parents.[67] The parent who is taught basic concepts of development and who understands general principles of intervention is better equipped to generalize handling techniques to accommodate various situations which arise as the child grows and develops, as well as to assimilate these methods of management into their own parenting style.

Evidence is accumulating that the child's own parents are the best choice as caregivers to facilitate long-term gains. If, however, the internal and external

(*Text continues on page 387.*)

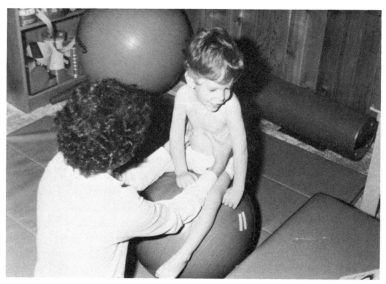

Fig. 11-9.   Therapy begins on a ball. Therapist's forearms inhibit adduction while hands facilitate trunk alignment, symmetrical weight bearing, and increased tone in trunk. Slow movement on the ball reduces extensor hypertonus while preparing for movement. This activity is designed to meet treatment goals 1, 2, 4, 5, 6, and 11.

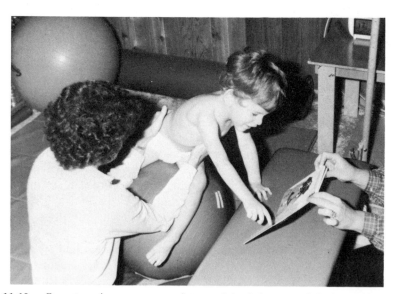

Fig. 11-10.   Once tone is more appropriate, activity is begun to left since Michael takes weight more easily on left and can produce movement while maintaining normal tone. This will prepare for rotation and weight bearing on right. Therapist facilitates trunk rotation while weight bearing through left hip, continuing to inhibit adduction. This activity is designed to meet treatment goals 1, 2, 3, 4, 5, 6, and 11.

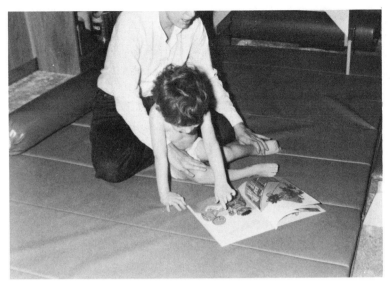

Fig. 11-11. Michael is placed in side sitting on right, an unfamiliar position. Stress of the position is shown in increased tone in right hand. Therapist inhibits trunk flexion on right while facilitating rotation of trunk to right. This activity is designed for treatment goals 1, 3, 4, 6, 7, 8, 9, 10, and 11.

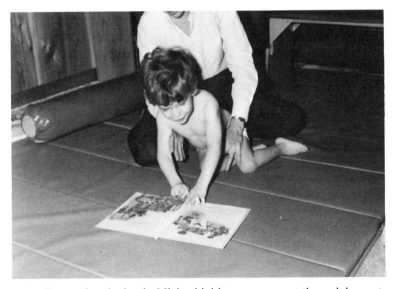

Fig. 11-12. By moving the book, Michael initiates movement through lower trunk and hip as he moves into a hands-knees position. Michael is not accustomed to moving over right side and could not perform this activity independently. Stress shows as increased tone in right upper extremity. Therapist facilitates transition while assisting appropriate weight bearing. This activity is designed for treatment goals 1, 3, 4, 6, 7, 8, 9, 10, and 11.

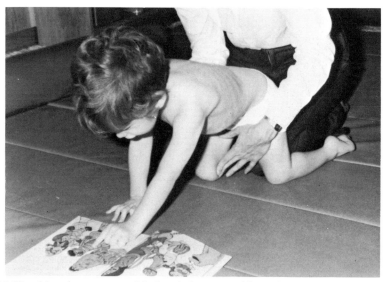

Fig. 11-13. Now in a more stable hands-knees position, right hand shows less stress; weight shift forward and back is facilitated by reaching out to identify characters in the book. Lateral weight shift is facilitated at pelvis by therapist's hand. This activity is designed for treatment goals 1, 3, 6, 7, 8, 9, 10, and 11.

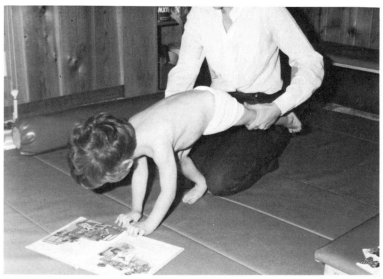

Fig. 11-14. From hands-knees, Michael is brought onto right foot with left leg extended, requiring flexion of right leg with weight bearing and extension of left leg. This is a very difficult position for Michael to assume or maintain because of his inability to adapt to positions requiring a high degree of disassociated movements while maintaining equilibrium over a very narrow base of support. This activity is designed for treatment goals 1, 3, 6, 7, 8, 9, 10, and 11.

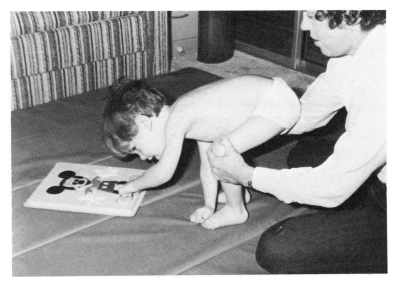

Fig. 11-15. The left leg is brought forward for weight bearing on hands and feet, again a position that increases tone distally in effort to maintain equilibrium. Active hip extension with knee flexion is required to maintain this position. Michael would collapse into squat if hip extensors were inactive. This activity is designed for treatment goals 1, 3, 6, 7, 8, 9, 10, and 11.

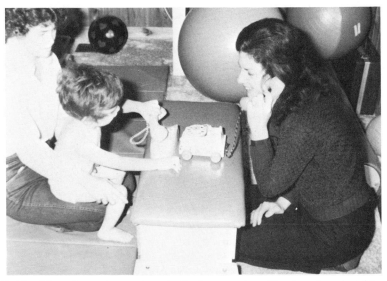

Fig. 11-16. Now that extensor tone in the lower extremities is reduced and trunk tone is increased, play activities are incorporated with moving to standing. Initially sitting in good alignment, Michael has a phone conversation with his mother. This activity is designed for treatment goals 1 to 9 and 11.

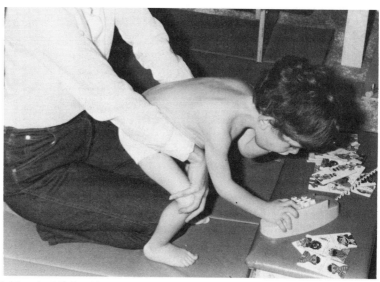

Fig. 11-17. As Michael begins to come to standing, the therapist assists in keeping his weight well forward over his feet while maintaining hip abduction to control extensor tone. This activity is designed for treatment goals 1 to 9 and 11.

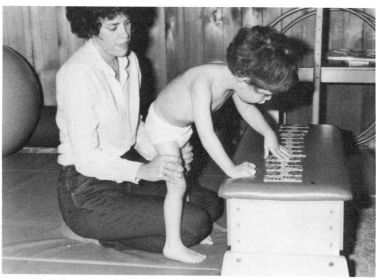

Fig. 11-18. By positioning toys on a low support surface, Michael ends with legs extended by trunk leaning forward. This keeps his weight forward over his feet while preventing excessive extension and adduction of his legs. This activity is designed for treatment goals 1 to 9 and 11.

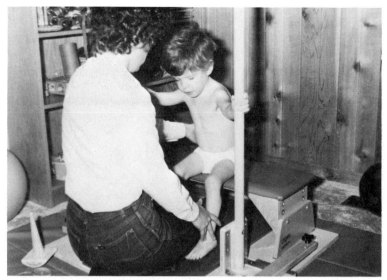

Fig. 11-19. In order to prevent increased flexor tone in the upper extremities which accompanies pulling with the arms, Michael uses parallel poles which maintain the shoulders at 90° flexion and abduction, elbows extended and forearms supinated. This will assist him in shifting his weight forward over his feet as he comes to stand. This activity is designed for treatment goals 1, 2, 3, 4, 5, 8, and 9.

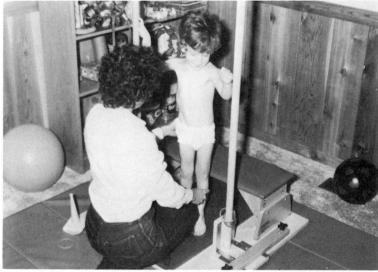

Fig. 11-20. In standing, trunk alignment is facilitated by the therapist's hand on the hip extensors. In this position Michael still has excessive extensor tone in the lower extremities, but body and head alignment is good and balance is sufficient that he can let go with one hand at a time to drop rings over the top of a stick (compare to Fig. 11-8). These activities represent a typical treatment session. This activity is designed for treatment goals 1, 2, 3, 4, 5, 8, and 9.

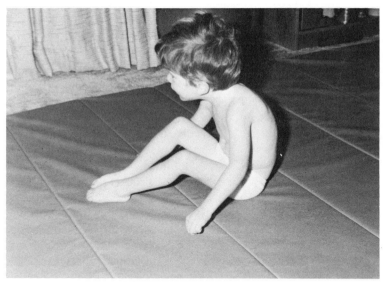

Fig. 11-21. This picture was taken prior to beginning the treatment session illustrated in the previous series of pictures. It illustrates well the problems described in the assessment summary: abnormal extensor tone with compensatory abnormal alignment, lack of equilibrium, and delayed development.

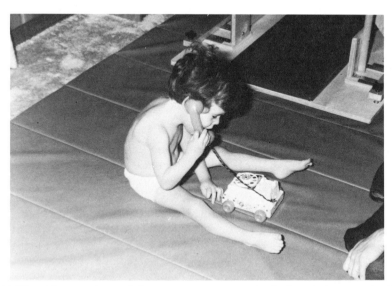

Fig. 11-22. After one hour of therapy, extensor tone in the legs is decreased, allowing a posture of hip flexion, abduction, and knee extension. With a wider base of support and his weight more evenly distributed, Michael can free one hand for play. Problems still persist. Extensor tone dominates pelvic posture and lack of cocontraction in the trunk prevents the pelvis being maintained in vertical position so that compensatory upper trunk flexion persists. These problems will continue to be addressed in therapy and home management.

resources of the family are inadequate to provide an optimal learning environment, a parent-surrogate can be substituted if the person can provide a stable, stimulating situation.[98] Extended family members and day care personnel are common sources of help.

Some of the success of the home management aspect of the intervention program depends on how effectively the parent is instructed. The author reported previously on a project that involved teaching 16 families of severely motor-handicapped children various activities to be done at home.[99] The initial interaction of the parents with the therapist, and his or her attitude and concern were as important to the overall performance of the parents as the actual method of written or oral instructions. Redman-Bentley[96] also found that the professional's personal traits were important. Parents preferred a professional who was honest, knowledgeable, and who listened to information provided by the parents. The physical therapist must realize, in deciding which daily care routines or therapeutic techniques should be included as part of the home program, that parents represent the entire range of social, emotional, and intellectual behaviors. Some parents have high intellect, good motor skills, and learn easily, but children sometimes have parents who are retarded, emotionally disturbed, alcoholic, or preoccupied with basic physiologic or financial needs.

Many therapists have a preconceived notion that managing a child with cerebral palsy places additional stress on the family, but the validity of this statement is unclear from the literature. Lonsdale[100] interviewed the parents of 60 developmentally delayed children about their reactions and the effect of the child on family relationships. More than half the parents interviewed reported marriage difficulties resulting from the birth of the handicapped child.[100] This is consistent with the findings reported by Gath.[101] High rates of physical and mental ill health among parents of handicapped children have been reported both by McMichael[102] and by Tizard and Grad.[103] Reports by Butler and colleagues[104] and Burden[105] have also stressed the likelihood of mental ill health in mothers.

On the other hand, the majority of studies reviewed by Dunlap and Hollingsworth[106] did not support the perception that the handicapped member, has a substantial effect on family life. Wishart and colleagues[107] compared the reports of regular family activities obtained from parents of developmentally delayed children and from parents of normal children acting as controls. These results showed little difference between the control and handicapped groups, and the presence of a delayed child in the family did not appear to change the family routine to any large extent. This study did not include families with children with significant motor handicaps. A comparison of families with children who have different degrees of physical and mental dysfunction may provide more information regarding the effects of motorically handicapped children on family routines and activities.

Simeonsson and McHale[108] reviewed the effects of a handicapped child on sibling relations. This review demonstrates that there is a great diversity of effects on the sibling relationship. Some studies showed that the presence of a handicapped child in a family results in problems of adjustment and development for siblings,[109] while other studies indicate that siblings of handicapped children may benefit from their experience and are often well adjusted.[100,110,111]

What are the implications for the therapist? First, the therapist should not assume that the presence of a handicapped child necessarily disturbs the structure, function, or development of the family unit. However the handicapped child is perceived by his or her own family, parents are able to accommodate the problems of raising a child with a handicapping condition to a considerable extent, assuming a successful parenting role with their child.

Second, the therapist must be able to achieve effective parent involvement as appropriate for the individual family. Therapists should not have preconceived ideas about what parents should do for their children, but should rather accept what a parent can do for their child and capitalize on these abilities. Scherzer and Tscharnuter state that, whenever possible, family involvement should go beyond intervention methods of home management to include treatment procedures, but that the therapist must help the parents put the home management program into the proper perspective so as not to disturb the parent-child relationship or the family unit and its functions.[67] Focusing attention exclusively on the infant's disabilities may hamper rather than foster overall development and place undue focus on the parent's inability to parent the handicapped child. All efforts must be made, rather, to stress the competencies of the child and the parents.

Third, handling techniques must be adapted to the skills of the parents and may consequently differ from the techniques and standards the therapist applies to the same activity. Some parents have the time, energy, and skills to carry out complicated therapeutic techniques on a regular basis, while other families will need constant instruction and support to modify feeding, dressing or daily care routines.

Fourth, while there is no prescribed method to assure successful teaching, methods of instruction include demonstration, written programs, verbal instructions, repetition and continual support. The intensity of instruction and need to adhere to a systematic teaching method will vary from family to family. The therapist must be able to evaluate the family's resources and vary his or her style of instruction, as well as goals for the home program, to meet the current level of skill, knowledge, and attitudes of the family.

Finally, the individual family's involvement in a home program varies. First, it may vary based on when they have their initial contact with the intervention program. Parents who have a young baby with suspected central nervous system dysfunction may not initially see the infant as different from other babies. All babies need to be dressed, bathed, diapered, and loved. The parents, therefore, may not see the need to change their method of caring for their infant, particularly if the child is comfortable in the present interaction and protests with imposition of new positions and movements. Parents who first begin therapy with an 18-month-old child diagnosed with cerebral palsy may be quite anxious to have activities to do at home to "help their child walk" or achieve some other obviously delayed motor milestone.

The family's involvement with a home program varies with the age of the child. Babies, toddlers, and preschool children generally spend a great deal of time with their own parents and are usually assisted with daily care routines. Parents have the opportunity to provide continued input for facilitating activities involving dressing, feeding, self-care, as well as functional motor skills. A school-age child has a greater need for independence and may refuse assistance from a parent once they have discovered some way to accomplish the task independently. The parents at this point may be more involved with transporting the child to after-school activities, assisting with homework, and, in their need to be parents, are realistically less involved with therapeutic intervention. Home programs for preteens and teenagers often involve instructing the child to carry out mobilizing techniques independent of adult assistance, or stressing recreational activities which encourage mobility and reinforce functional movement. The home management program does not decrease as the child grows older; however, the goals, activities, and persons responsible for the program must change if it is to remain an effective method of intervention. As an example, Figures 11-23 to 11-26 describe some of the activities included in Michael A.'s home program which includes activities to position for self-help skills (Fig. 11-23 illustrates dressing), play (Fig. 11-24), and use of adaptive equipment to promote social interaction with family (Fig. 11-25) and independent mobility (Fig. 11-26).

ADJUNCTS TO THERAPY

Tone-Reducing Casts

Short leg tone-inhibiting casts are designed to maintain normal alignment of the foot and ankle while inhibiting toe grasp as an habitual or compensatory stabilizing effort. They are currently used as an adjunct in therapy and during selected intervals of treatment and management at home and school. Sussman and Cusick[112] described the basic hypotheses in the use of tone-reducing casts. First, extending the toes inhibits the plantar grasp response. Second, firm fixation of the subtalar joint provides a stable base to reduce tone and facilitate mobility of the hips, knees, and trunk. Third, prevention of ankle dorsiflexion inhibits use of extensor thrust. As a result, tone-reducing casts allow development of desirable movement components of the trunk, hips, and knees with relatively full mobility during standing and walking.

Cusick and Sussman[113] described the use of tone-reducing casts with 145 children over a 46-month period. They developed specific criteria for patient selection, considerations for treatment, and follow-up. The casts were not used to correct foot deformity or to reduce contracture at the foot or ankle; they were implemented when passive foot and ankle range was complete and only during a closely supervised program of positioning and movement training when it was believed that gains in movement control could be made faster or sooner if the foot was stabilized in good alignment. The majority of cases were children

(*Text continues on page 392.*)

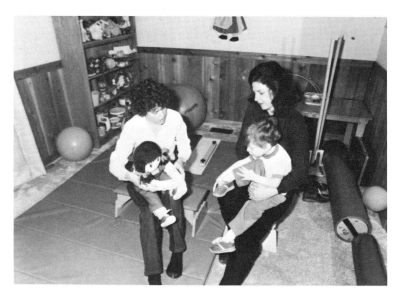

Fig. 11-23. In addition to Michael's active therapy program, his family has been instructed in positioning and assisting with daily care which reinforces his therapeutic goals. Here Michael's mother learns to facilitate trunk rotation and disassociated movements of one leg from the other while Michael assists with undressing.

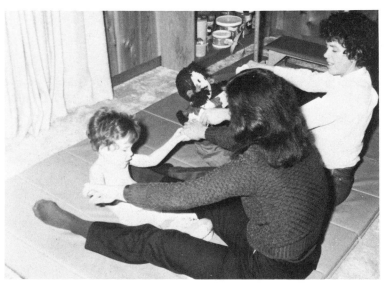

Fig. 11-24. Mother is shown a variation on a play activity that she and Michael do at home. By changing her way of holding his arms, a better pattern of head, neck, and trunk flexion can be encouraged.

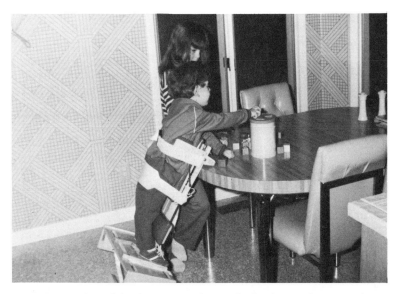

Fig. 11-25. Presently, Michael uses two pieces of adaptive equipment at home to provide him with a larger variety of movement patterns. This prone stander is attached to the kitchen table so that Michael can stand and play with his sister. Since he does not need to take weight on his hands to balance or support in standing, his hands are free for play.

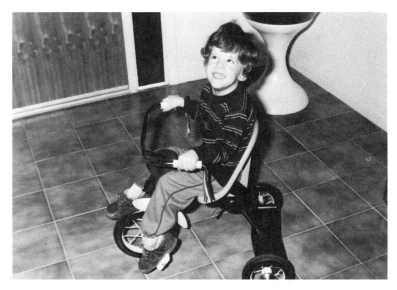

Fig. 11-26. Michael's father adapted his tricycle which provides him with a normal mobility activity. The seat from a "Hot Wheel" was attached to the standard seat, providing better pelvic and trunk control. An old pair of shoes, which were large enough to hold Michael's feet with his own shoes on, were attached to the foot pedals. This provides good support and alignment so Michael's feet stay on the foot pedals. Michael can ride his bike in the neighborhood, enjoying an experience of moving independently with other children.

with spastic cerebral palsy; however, use of casts with hypotonia and mixed athetoid-spastic cerebral palsy was also reported.

Embry[114] presented a preliminary report on a study designed to evaluate the effectiveness of inhibitory casts when used concurrently with a neurodevelopmental approach to children with cerebral palsy. Ten matched pairs of subjects between the ages of 6 months and 5 years were selected to receive 8 weeks of treatment. The experimental group wore casts during weight-bearing activities in treatment and at home. Data on step length, stride length, foot angle, walking base, and symmetry of gait were obtained from a weight-sensitive paper. While the data were not analyzed statistically at the time of reporting, early findings based on a small number of subjects appeared to support the effectiveness of inhibitory casting in achieving improved ambulation when used concurrently with a neurodevelopmental treatment approach. Figures 11-27 to 11-32 demonstrate the differences in postural alignment, tone, and independence in balance and movement achieved during therapy when tone reduction casts were used with Michael A.

Use of Adaptive Equipment

Adaptive equipment has become an integral part of therapeutic, educational, and home management programs for preschool children with motor dysfunction resulting from central nervous system deficit.[71,72,115–117] Recently, attempts have been made to document changes in posture or function in children using adaptive equipment.

Nwaobi and colleagues[118] reported on a study designed to determine whether tonic myoelectric activity of low-back extensors of children with spastic cerebral palsy changed in response to changes in seating. Electromyograms recorded less electrical activity when the seat surface elevation was 0 degree and backrest 90 degrees.

In a single-case study design, Cristarella[119] compared the sitting posture of a normal 3-year-old child with the sitting posture of a child with spastic cerebral palsy of the same age. While seated in small chairs, the children were filmed during play, and line drawings were made from a frame selected at random. In the normal child, the angles at the hips, knees, and ankles approximated 90 degrees, while the child with cerebral palsy showed significantly less than 90 degrees at the same joints. Spinal alignment was also compared. In the normal child, the pelvis was vertical and the spine showed normal curves. In the child with cerebral palsy, the upper spine was excessively rounded and the pelvis was not vertical. The child with cerebral palsy was then placed in a straddle position on a special chair which provided hip abduction. Film analysis showed the joint measurements of hip and knee flexion, and ankle dorsiflexion were much closer to 90 degrees, and the spinal curves approximated those of the normal subject. These studies suggest that tone and postural alignment can be influenced by adaptive equipment.

Hulme and colleagues[120] reported on the results of a survey constructed to assess the benefits of adaptive equipment used in homes of primarily non-

(*Text continues on page 396.*)

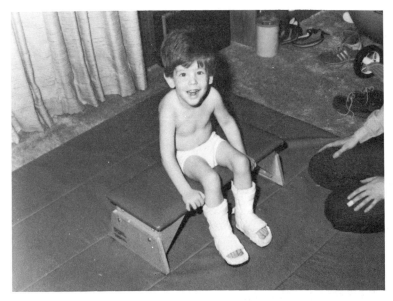

Fig. 11-27. With casts on, Michael sits with better alignment and hip abduction (compare with Fig. 11-7).

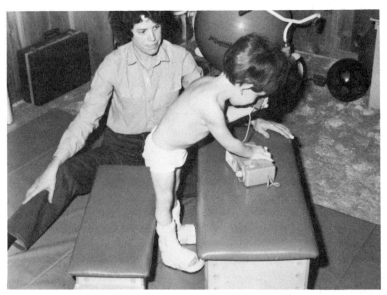

Fig. 11-28. Michael is able to demonstrate greater independent mobility with his casts on in therapy. The now stable base of support allows Michael to stand unassisted by the therapist.

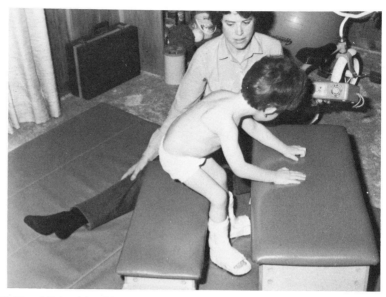

Fig. 11-29. Michael is able to move from standing to sitting independently, keeping his weight forward over his feet as he lowers himself to the bench. Still unable to balance in standing, it is necessary for Michael to use the bench for support.

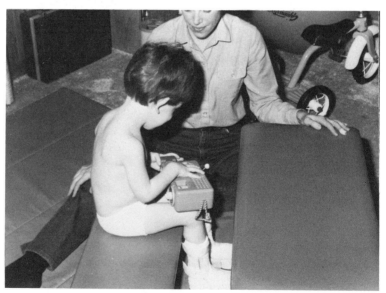

Fig. 11-30. Sitting balance is improved as tone is reduced at hips so that Michael sits more squarely on his bottom with trunk aligned over his pelvis. With improved postural alignment, Michael can use his hands for play rather than balance.

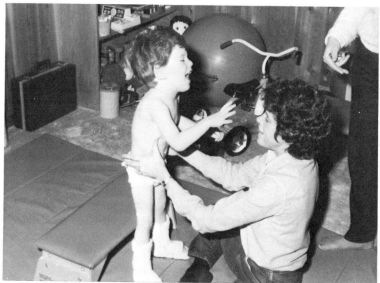

Fig. 11-31. Standing can be easily facilitated with better trunk and hip alignment. A wider base of support is possible and tone in the lower extremities is more appropriate for this task (compare to Fig. 11-20).

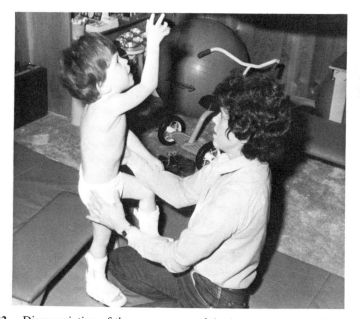

Fig. 11-32. Disassociation of the movements of the lower extremities is now possible. Michael can take weight on the right leg while maintaining hip and trunk alignment. Left leg is forward and flexed in preparation for stepping. The therapist facilitates weight shift and balance reactions.

ambulatory multiply handicapped clients ranging from 1 to 68 years old. Significant improvements were noted in social interactions and motor coordination. Adaptive chairs were the most consistently used types of equipment. A significant increase in independent eating and drinking was also found, along with a significant decrease in the time needed to eat a meal and time client spent in the bedroom. In the areas of social interaction, there was significant improvement in the number of times the client left the home and an increased variety of places visited by the client in the community.

In general, the current literature describes the selection, construction, and uses of various commercially available as well as custom-designed products to solve a particular problem of positioning, mobility, or activities of daily living function.[121-133]

Selection of Adaptive Equipment

Adaptive equipment should be carefully selected in consultation with a physical or occupational therapist to make certain that it meets the goals for which it is intended. Adaptive equipment is used to meet the following goals:

1. Adaptive equipment is used in homes to provide greater opportunities for independence in activities of daily living. By properly positioning a child so that he or she feels secure and motivated to practice newly acquired skills, many children are able to participate in feeding, toileting or other self-help skills.[115,134]

2. To prevent contractures and deformities by positioning a child to prevent the deforming influence while encouraging active movement.[121,135]

3. To provide greater variety of movement experiences and prevent habit patterns which limit the development of normal variations of posture and movement.[115]

4. To reinforce normal movement components, providing an opportunity for more normal alignment, weight shift, and postural adjustment during functional movement.[121,136]

5. To increase the child's opportunity to participate in social interaction and educational programs.

6. To provide mobility and encourage exploration. This is often the goal of providing adapted standard or electric wheelchairs for children who have no means of mobilization or whose movements are so slow that the effort is not worth the goal toward which the movement is directed.

Appropriate equipment provides enough support so that the child can direct his or her energies toward participation in the educational or social environment rather than exclusively toward maintaining posture. This reason alone may warrent the use of adaptive equipment for severely handicapped children.[117,137,138] Severely handicapped children are often unable to experience any degree of interaction or independence in school, recreation centers, or shopping areas without the assistance of adaptive chairs.[137]

Adaptive equipment, whether individually designed or commercially available, must meet the needs of the child as he or she grows, gains better control of posture and movement, and develops educational and daily living skills. Several books are available on planning, designing, and building adaptive equipment.[115,121,139–143] Appropriate selected adaptive equipment allows movement and encourages the child to make postural adaptations necessary in any given situation. It should not restrict the child's movements, but rather increase the child's possibilities to practice and use movements s/he is developing. Adaptive equipment limits the environment to the extent that movement is possible without stress or effort which produces abnormal tone and movement patterns. By assessing the needs of the child, the caregivers and the environment, and becoming familiar with possibilities for obtaining and building adaptive equipment, therapists should be better able to make decisions regarding use of adaptive equipment to help meet the needs of children with central nervous system dysfunction.

EVALUATION OF OUTCOME

Evaluating treatment presents a dilemma to those involved in treating children with cerebral palsy. The dilemma exists because therapists hold a strong belief, on the one hand, that early intervention is essential and effective and, on the other hand, documenting effectiveness is difficult because of the complex problems characterizing this population. The dilemma is heightened by the fact that the state of the art of evaluation of patients with cerebral palsy is not far advanced and results of clinical studies present confusing and sometimes contradictory results.[144] The confusion is partly caused by differences among studies in the subject selection, sample size, criteria for diagnosis, rigorousness of experimental design, and methods of evaluating and documenting change.

However, parents and consumer groups as well as granting agencies increasingly demand accountability. While it may not yet be possible to rigidly apply scales and measures to quantify program results, efforts must be made to document and compare various strategies of intervention. Numerous measures of effectiveness have been used to determine the long-term effect of treatment. These measures include assessment of general motor development,[145,146] standardized scales,[147] maturation of developmental reflexes,[148,149] increase in passive joint range of motion,[148,150] age of onset of walking and quality of gait,[73,150] improvements in home management,[151] and changes in functional abilities.[146,150] Many studies have used multiple evaluation measures because it is not clear in which realms changes can be expected.

Individual case histories and case review series have been used to evaluate the effectiveness of therapy. Paine[150] presents a case review follow-up study of 117 patients comparing treated with nontreated children from 1930 to 1950. The treated and untreated groups were comparable as to type, severity of involvement, and intelligence. Outcome assessments included gait, hand use, presence of contracture, and frequency of orthopedic surgery. The data presented suggest that intensive physical therapy of the type available from 1930 to 1950 had its chief effect on the patient with moderately severe spastic hemiparesis or quadriparesis, who developed a better gait if treated and had fewer contractures. Among the athetoids, no difference in gait or hand function in the treated group was found. Some data suggested that children with spastic cerebral palsy who began treatment prior to two years of age had better gait, fewer contractures and less orthopedic surgery. No evidence suggested that early treatment was beneficial in athetosis.

Köng[73] performed clinical case review of 69 patients receiving a specific therapeutic approach (Bobath) for at least 1 year. Degree of involvement at the end of the treatment period provided the only basis for comparison. Degree of involvement prior to treatment was not described. After one to four years of treatment, 53 (75 percent) had a normal gait and showed only minimal neurologic signs. No specific test instruments for outcome measures were described. No controls were used.

Several attempts have been made to use a more standard study design involving a control group. Hochleitner compared groups of children with and without Bobath therapy.[152] Direct matching of the two groups was not attempted; diagnoses varied as did severity and associated disabilities. Results demonstrated significant reduction in degree of disability among the treated group in comparison with the control group. Specific outcome measures were not described.

Wright and Nicholson[149] studied 47 spastic children under 6 years of age selected at random for immediate treatment, delayed treatment or no treatment groups. This study showed no evidence after one year that physical therapy affected the range of dorsiflexion of the ankle or abduction of the hip, nor that it had any effect on the retention or loss of primitive reflexes.

Scherzer and colleagues[151] used a double-blind design to study the effects of physical therapy on 22 children with cerebral palsy under 18 months of age. The treatment group received a combination of several modalities of neuro-developmental physical therapy and the control group received passive range of motion exercises. Assignment to group was by random selection. Group matching was not attempted with such a small sample size. The treatment group showed significant improvement in all areas evaluated, including motor development, social maturity, and ease of home management.

Sommerfeld and associates[148] compared the effect of two methods of providing physical therapy services in 19 severely mentally impaired students with cerebral palsy. In a school setting, the students were paired and assigned to either a direct therapy group or a supervised therapy management group. A group of 10 students from a school in which there was no physical therapy available served as a control comparison. The results of this study showed no significant differences in maturity of development reflexes, gross motor skills, or passive joint range of motion among students placed in direct, supervised or comparison groups.

Several studies have attempted to compare the effectiveness of one method of intervention with another. Sparrow and Zigler[147] utilized three groups, each with 15 profoundly retarded institutionalized children, to evaluate a modification of the sensorimotor patterning treatment (developed at the Institutes for the Achievement of Human Potential). The treatment group received a program developed after the IAHP method, a matched group participated in motivational activities for the same duration and intensity. A no treatment group received standard care of the institution. A wide variety of behavioral measures were employed. On the majority of measures, no differences in posttest performance among the three groups were found. All three groups showed some improvement in performance between the beginning and end of the study.

d'Avignon and colleagues[153] studied three groups of children who showed signs of central nervous system dysfunction prior to 6 months of age to compare the effectiveness of early physical therapy according to Bobath or Vojta versus a control group. Of the total 30 children, an evaluation at 33 months to 6 years showed 15 children with cerebral palsy and 15 who were considered normal. Vojta's criteria for "complicated" cerebral palsy (with sensory problems, seizures or mental retardation) and "uncomplicated" cerebral palsy were used for comparison among the three groups. The difference in distribution of these types was not significant. The intervention for the treated groups is not clearly described and the control group received "a less strictly performed and combined form of physiotherapy."

Abdel-Salam and colleagues[154] compared the effects of physical therapy on seven children with infantile spastic cerebral palsy with seven children with postencephalitic spastic paralysis. Both groups received the same therapeutic intervention. After four months, the group with infantile spastic cerebral palsy showed more significant improvement in function, as measured by decreased time to begin a movement and increased tempo of the movement, as well as improvement in activities of daily living and perceptual motor performance (as measured by tests devised by the authors) than did the group with postencephalitic spastic paralysis.

In addition to evaluating the long-term effects of treatment, it is valuable to document the immediate effects. Using a single-case study design, Watube and associates[155] used serial photographs to document changes in posture and gait in a spastic diplegic child during the course of a single treatment session. Palisano,[156] using a single-case design, utilized surface electrode EMG recordings to demonstrate changes in the phase of muscle activity during gait of a ten-year-old child with spastic diplegia following a 1-hour treatment session using neurodevelopmental techniques (Bobath). In both of these studies, changes in gait could be identified immediately after therapy. When combined with temporal information to coordinate the electrical activity with particular phases in the gait cycle, electromyography is able to provide information on dynamic patterns of muscular activity during walking.[157–159] It cannot, however, adequately record the force generated by muscle activity. Cinematography has been combined with electromyography to provide information on joint displacement, velocity, and acceleration.[160–161] Letts and colleagues[162] used videotape analysis and electromyography to obtain similar information.

Holt[163] advocated the use of electromyography in children with cerebral palsy, as early as 1966. He noted that the action of a muscle during a functional activity may be different from its action in response to conscious effort, and that a muscle's state of activity could not be reliably predicted from observation or clinical examination alone. Perry and her associates[92] confirmed these findings. In the evaluation of 23 ambulatory children with spastic diplegia, muscle activity patterns during gait could not be anticipated based on muscle activity in muscle test positions. While it is not possible for most clinics to use electromyography during clinical treatment, this method of evaluation has been shown to provide objective data for evaluating change in children with cerebral palsy, as well as for making decisions regarding orthopedic surgery.

The need to document changes and progress in children as a function of specified intervention still exists as a primary problem in evaluating effectiveness of treatment.

CONCLUSION

The treatment of the child with cerebral palsy presents an ongoing challenge and commitment by the physical therapist for several reasons. First, intensive care of newborn infants is changing this population and their presenting symptoms. Second, earlier identification and recognition of motor dysfunction brings the child to therapy at a much younger age; and third, better understanding of normal and abnormal development provides the therapist with greater possibilities for planning treatment. The physical therapist must be prepared to deal with all aspects of motor dysfunction and the associated problems of cerebral palsy as well as all aspects of normal child development in order to continue effective treatment as the child grows and develops. However, there remains a lack of systematic, longitudinal data on the development of handicapped children and on strategies to measure developmental changes related to programming. Therapists who believe that intervention is effective and essential must assume the professional responsibility to document treatment methodology and changes in motor outcomes. Only through objectively documenting these changes will the treatment of children with cerebral palsy advance. As caring professionals we have ahead of us the important task of documenting support for our strong commitment to the improvement of function in physically handicapped children.

REFERENCES

1. Bax MC: Terminology and classification of cerebral palsy. Dev Med Child Neurol 6:295, 1964.
2. Bobath K: A Neurological Basis for the Treatment of Cerebral Palsy. Clin Dev Med 75, 1980.
3. Ellenberg J, Nelson K: Early recognition of infants at high risk for cerebral palsy: Examination at age four months. Dev Med Child Neurol 23:705, 1981.

4. Dale A, Stanley FJ: An epidemiological study of cerebral palsy in Western Australia, 1956–1975. II: Spastic cerebral palsy and perinatal factors. Dev Med Child Neurol 22:13, 1980.

5. Hagberg B, Hagberg G, Ingemar O: Gains and hazards of intensive neonatal care: an analysis from Swedish cerebral palsy epidemiology. Dev Med Child Neurol 24:13, 1982.

6. Stanley FJ, Hobbs MST: Neonatal mortality and cerebral palsy: The impact of neonatal intensive care. Aust Paediatr J 16:35, 1980.

7. Kiely J, Paneth N, Zena S, et al: Cerebral palsy and newborn care I: Secular trends in cerebral palsy. Dev Med Child Neurol 23:533, 1981.

8. Lagergren J: Children with motor handicaps. Epidemiological medical and socio-paediatric aspects of motor handicapped children in a Swedish country. Acta Paediatr Scand Suppl 289, 1981.

9. Hagberg B: The epidemiological panorama of major neuropaediatric handicaps in Sweden. In Apley J (ed): Care of the Handicapped Child. Clinics in Developmental Medicine, No. 67. Lippincott, Philadelphia, 1978.

10. O'Reilly D, Walentynowicz J: Etiological factors in cerebral palsy: An historical review. Dev Med Child Neurol 23:633, 1981.

11. Koch B, Braillier D, Eng G, et al: Computerized tomography in cerebral palsied children. Dev Med Child Neurol 22:595, 1980.

12. Pape K, Wigglesworth J: Haemorrhage, ischaemia and the perinatal brain. Clin Dev Med 69/70, 1979.

13. Hill A, Volpe J: Seizures, hypoxic-ischemic brain injury and intraventricular hemorrhage in the newborn. Ann Neurol 10:109, 1981.

14. Churchill J, Masland RL, Naylor AA, et al: The etiology of cerebral palsy in preterm infants. Dev Med Child Neurol 16:143, 1974.

15. Minear WL: A classification of cerebral palsy. Pediatrics 18:841, 1956.

16. Quinton MB, Wilson JM: Competition of movement patterns applied to the development of infants. In Slaton DS, Wilson JM (eds): Caring for Special Babies. University of North Carolina, Chapel Hill, 1983.

17. Milani-Comparetti A, Gidoni EA: Pattern analysis of motor development and its disorder. Dev Med Child Neurol 9:625, 1967.

18. Milani-Comparetti A: Pattern analysis of normal and abnormal development: The fetus, the newborn, the child, In Slaton D (ed): Development of Movement in Infancy. University of North Carolina, Chapel Hill, 1980.

19. Crothers B, Paine RS: The Natural History of Cerebral Palsy. Harvard University Press, Cambridge, MA, 1959.

20. del Mundo-Vallarta J, Robb JP: A follow-up study of newborn infants with perinatal complications: Determination of etiology and predictive value of abnormal histories and neurological signs. Neurology 14:413, 1964.

21. Prechtl HFR: Prognostic value of neurological signs in the newborn infant. Proc R Soc Med 58:3–4, 1965.

22. Stanley FJ: Spastic cerebral palsy: Changes in birthweight and gestational age. Early Hum Dev 5(2):167, 1981.

23. Ziegler AL, Calame A, Marchand C, et al: Cerebral distress in full-term newborns and its prognostic value. A follow-up study of 90 infants. Helv Paediatr Acta 31:299, 1976.

24. Amiel-Tison C: Birth injury as a cause of brain dysfunction in full-term newborns. Adv Perinat Neurol 1, 1978.

25. Capute AJ: Identifying cerebral palsy in infancy through a study of primitive reflex profiles. Pediatr Ann 8:589, 1979.

26. Ingram TTS: The new approach to early diagnosis of handicaps in childhood. Dev Med Child Neurol 11:279, 1969.

27. Paine RS, Brazelton TB, Donovan DE, et al: Evolution of postural reflexes in normal infants and in the presence of chronic brain syndrome. Neurology 14:1036, 1964.

28. Nelson KB, Ellenberg JH: Neonatal signs as predictors of cerebral palsy. Pediatrics 64:225, 1979.

29. Campbell SK, Wilhelm IJ: Developmental sequence in infants at high risk in central nervous system dysfunction: The recovery process in the first year of life. In Stack J (ed): The Special Infant: An Interdisciplinary Approach to the Optimal Development of Infants. Human Sciences Press, New York, 1982.

30. Campbell S, Wilhelm I: Development of infants at risk for central nervous system dysfunction: Progress report. In Slaton DS, Wilson JM (eds): Caring for Special Babies. University of North Carolina, Chapel Hill, 1983.

31. Thompson T, Reynolds J: The results of intensive care therapy for neonates. I. Overall neonatal mortality rate II. Neonatal mortality rates and long-term prognosis for low birth weight neonates. J Perinat Med 5:59, 1977.

32. Fitzhardinge PM: Follow-up studies in the low birth weight infant. Clin Perinatol 3:503, 1976.

33. Stewart A, Turcan D, Rawlings G, et al: Outcome for infants at high risk major handicap. Ciba Found Symp 59:151, 1978.

34. Kamper J: Long-term prognosis of infants with severe idiopathic respiratory distress syndrome I. Neurological and mental outcome. Acta Paediatr Scand 67:61, 1978.

35. Rajani K, Goetzman BW, Kelso GF, et al: Prognosis of intracranial hemorrhage in neonates. Surg Neurol 13:433, 1980.

36. Williamson WD, Desmond MM, Wilson GS, et al: Early neurodevelopmental outcome of low birth weight infant surviving neonatal intraventricular hemorrhage. J Perinat Med 10:34, 1982.

37. Krishnamoorthy KS, Shannon DC, DeLong GR, et al: Neurologic sequelae in the survivors of neonatal intraventricular hemorrhage. Pediatrics 64:233, 1979.

38. Milla PT, Jackson ADM: A controlled trial of Baclofen in children with cerebral palsy. J Intern Med Res 5:398, 1977.

39. Hudgson P, Weightman D: Baclofen in the treatment of spasticity. Br Med J 4:15, 1971.

40. McKinlay I, Hyde E, Gordon N: Baclofin—A team approach to drug evaluation of spasticity in childhood. Scott Med J Suppl 1:526, 1980.

41. Young JA: Clinical Experience in the use of Baclofen in children with spastic cerebral palsy: A further report. Scott Med J Suppl 1:523, 1980.

42. Minford A, Brown JK, Minns RA, et al: The effect of baclofen on the gait of hemiplegic children assessed by means of polarized light goniometry. Scott Med J Suppl 1:529, 1980.

43. Joynt R, Leonard J: Dantrolene Sodium suspension in treatment of spastic cerebral palsy. Dev Med Child Neurol 22:755, 1980.

44. Carpenter E, Sietz D: Intramuscular alcohol as an aid in management of spastic cerebral palsy. Dev Med Child Neurol 22:497, 1980.

45. Samilson R (ed): Orthopaedic Aspects of Cerebral Palsy. Clin Dev Med 52/53, 1975.

46. Bleck EE: Orthopedic Management of Cerebral Palsy. Saunders Philadelphia, 1979.

47. House JH, Gwathmey FW, Fidler MO: A dynamic approach to thumb-in-palm deformity in cerebral palsy. Evaluation and results in 56 patients. J Bone Jt Surg 63A:216, 1981.
48. Goldner LJ: The Upper Extremity in Cerebral Palsy. In Samilson RL (ed): Orthopaedic Aspects of Cerebral Palsy. Clinics in Developmental Medicine, No. 52/53. Lippincott, Philadelphia, 1975.
49. Zancolli EA, Zancolli ER: Surgical management of the hemiplegic spastic hand in cerebral palsy. Surg Clin North Am 61:2 395, 1981.
50. Hoffer MM, Perry J, Melkonian GJ: Dynamic electromyography and decision making for surgery in the upper extremity of patients with cerebral palsy. J Hand Surg 4:424, 1979.
51. Bleck E: Deformities of the spine and pelvis in cerebral palsy. In Samilson R (ed): Orthopaedic Aspects of Cerebral Palsy. Lippincott, Philadelphia, 1975.
52. Bonnett C, Brown JC, Grow T: Thoracolumbar scoliosis in cerebral palsy. Results of surgical treatment. J Bone Jt Surg 58:328, 1976.
53. MacEwen GD: Operative treatment of scoliosis in cerebral palsy. Reconstr Surg Traumatol 13:58, 1972.
54. Allen BL, Ferguson RL: L-rod instrumentation for scoliosis in cerebral palsy. J Pediatr Orthop 2:87, 1982.
55. Truscelli D, Lespargot A, Tardieu G: Variation in the long-term results of elongation of the tendo achillis in children with cerebral palsy. J Bone Jt Surg 61B:466, 1979.
56. Castle ME, Reyman TA, Schneider M: Pathology of spastic muscle in cerebral palsy. Clin Orthop 142:223, 1979.
57. Root L, Spero CR: Hip adductor transfer compared with adductor tenotomy in cerebral palsy. J Bone Jt Surg 63A:767, 1981.
58. Cooper IS, Riklan M, Amin I, et al: Chronic cerebellar stimulation in cerebral palsy. Neurology 26:744, 1976.
59. Davis R, Barolat-Romana G, Engle H: Chronic cerebellar stimulation for cerebral palsy: Five year study. Acta Neurochir Suppl (Wien) 30:317, 1980.
60. Ivan LP: Chronic cerebellar stimulation in cerebral palsy. Appl Neurophysiol 45:51, 1982.
61. Penn RD, Etzel ML: Chronic cerebellar stimulation and developmental reflexes. J Neurosurg 46:506, 1977.
62. Wong PKH, Hoffman HJ, Froese AB, et al: Cerebellar stimulation in the management of cerebral palsy: Clinical and physiological studies. J Neurosurg 5:217, 1979.
63. Penn RD, Myklebust BM, Gottlieb GL, et al: Chronic cerebellar stimulation for cerebral palsy. Prospective and double-blind studies. J Neurosurg 53(2):160, 1980.
64. Gahm NH, Russman BS, Cerciello RL, et al: Chronic cerebellar stimulation for cerebral palsy: A double-blind study. Neurology 31:87, 1981.
65. Whittaker CK: Cerebellar stimulation for cerebral palsy. J Neurosurg 52:648, 1980.
66. Penn RD: Chronic cerebellar stimulation for cerebral palsy. A review. Neurosurg 10(1):116, 1982.
67. Scherzer A, Tscharnuter I: Early Diagnosis and Therapy in Cerebral Palsy. Pediatric Habilitation. Vol 3. Marcel Dekker, New York, 1982.
68. Sparling JW: The transdisciplinary approach with the developmentally delayed child. Phys Occup Ther Pediatr 1:3, 1980.
69. Levine MS, Trost-Miller T: Minimal diagnostic criteria for cerebral palsy: a single-blind study. Dev Med Child Neurol 23:114, 1981.

70. Bobath K: The normal posture reflex mechanism and its deviation in children with cerebral palsy. Physiotherapy 11:1, 1971.

71. Shepherd RB: Physiotherapy in Paediatrics. 2nd Ed. Heinemann, London, 1980.

72. Farber SD: Neurorehabilitation, A Multisensory Approach. Saunders, Philadelphia, 1982.

73. Kong E: Very early treatment of cerebral palsy. Dev Med Child Neurol 8:198, 1966.

74. Hoessly M: Normal and abnormal movement patterns in the newborn and young infant. Physiotherapy 65:372, 1979.

75. Saint-Anne Dargassies S: Neurological development in the full-term and premature neonate. Excerpta Medica, New York, 1977.

76. Amiel-Tison C: Neurological evaluation of the maturity of newborn infants. Arch Dis Child 43:89, 1968.

77. Brazelton TB: Neonatal Behavioral Assessment Scale. Clin Dev Med 50, 1973.

78. Dubowitz L, Dubowitz V: The Neurological Assessment of the Preterm and Full-term Newborn Infant. Clinics in Developmental Medicine. Vol 79. Lippincott, Philadelphia, 1981.

79. Prechtl H: The Neurological Examination of the Full-Term Newborn Infant. 2nd Ed. Clinics in Developmental Medicine. No 63. Lippincott, Philadelphia, 1977.

80. Bly L: The components of normal movement during the first year of life. In Slaton D (ed): Development of Movement in Infancy. University of North Carolina, Chapel Hill, 1980.

81. Provost B: Normal development from birth to four months: Extended use of the NBAS-K. Part I. Phys Occup Ther Pediatr 1:39, 1980.

82. Bobath B, Bobath K: Motor Development in the Different Types of Cerebral Palsy. Heinemann, New York, 1975.

83. Vulpe S: Vulpe Assessment Battery. NIMR, Toronto, 1977.

84. Molnar G: Motor deficit of retarded infants and young children. Arch Phys Med 55:393, 1974.

85. Fiorentino MR: Reflex Testing Methods for Evaluating Central Nervous System Development. 2nd Ed. Charles C Thomas, Springfield, IL, 1973.

86. Wilson J: Developmental Reflex Test. In Vulpe S (ed): Vulpe Assessment Battery, ed. NIMR, Toronto, 1977.

87. Capute AJ, Accardo PJ, Vining EP, et al: Primitive Reflex Profile. University Park Press, Baltimore, 1978.

88. Barnes M, Crutchfield C, Heriza C: The Neurophysiological Basis of Patient Treatment. Reflexes in Motor Development. Stokesville Publishing, Morgantown WV, 1978.

89. Morris SE: Assessment and treatment of children with oral motor dysfunction. In Wilson JM (ed): Oral-Motor Function and Dysfunction in Children. University of North Carolina, Chapel Hill, 1977.

90. Morris SE: The Normal Acquisition of Oral Feeding Skills: Implications for Assessment and Treatment. Therapeutic Media, Central Islip, NY, 1982.

91. Perry J: Rehabilitation of spasticity. In Feldman RG, Young RR, WP Koella (eds): Spasticity: Disordered Motor Control. Year Book Medical Publishing, Chicago, 1980.

92. Perry J, Hoffer MM, Antonelli MS, et al: Electromyography before and after surgery for hip deformity in children with cerebral palsy. J Bone Jt Surg 48A:201, 1976.

93. Simeonsson RJ, Simeonsson NE: Parenting handicapped children: Psychological perspectives. In Paul J (ed): Parents of Handicapped Children. Holt, Rinehart, & Winston, New York, 1981.
94. Lambie D, Bond J, Welkart DP: Home Teaching with Mothers and Infants. the Ypsilanti-Carnegie Infant Education Project. High/Scope Educational Research Foundation, Ypsilanti MI, 1974.
95. Campbell S, Wilson J: Planning infant learning programs. Phys Ther 56(12):1347, 1976.
96. Redman-Bentley D: Parent expectations for professionals providing services to their handicapped children. Phys Occup Ther Pediatr 2(1):13, 1982.
97. Schaefer E: Evaluating intervention effects on children, parents and professionals. In Wilson J (ed): Planning and Evaluating Developmental Progress. 2nd Ed. University of North Carolina, Chapel Hill, 1979.
98. Etaugh C: Effects of maternal employment on children: A review of recent research. Merrill-Palmer Q Behav Dev 20:71, 1974.
99. Wilson J: Help Your Child—A home management program for children with CNS dysfunction. In Wilson J (ed): Infants at Risk: Medical and Therapeutic Management. 2nd Ed. University of North Carolina, Chapel Hill, 1981.
100. Lonsdale G: Family life with a handicapped child: The parents speak. Child Care Health Dev 4:99, 1978.
101. Gath A: The impact of an abnormal child upon the parents. Br J Psychiatry 130:405, 1977.
102. McMichael J: Handicap. A Study of Physically Handicapped Children and Their Families. Staples Press, London, 1971.
103. Tizard J, Grad JC: The Mentally Handicapped and Their Families. Maudsley Monograph No. 7, London, 1961.
104. Butler N, Gill R, Pomeroy D, et al: Handicapped Children—Their homes and life styles. Department of Child Health, University of Bristol, 1978.
105. Burden RL: Measuring the effects of stress on the mothers of handicapped infants. Must depression always follow? Child Care Health Dev 6:111, 1980.
106. Dunlap WR, Hollingsworth JS: How does a handicapped child affect the family? Implications for practitioners. Fam Coord 26(3):286, 1977.
107. Wishart MC, Bidder RT, Gray OP: Parents' report of family life with a developmentally delayed child. Child Care Health Dev 7:267, 1981.
108. Simeonsson RJ, McHale SM: Review: Research on handicapped children: Sibling relationships. Child Care Health Dev 7:153, 1981.
109. Tew B, Laurence KM: Mothers, brothers and sisters of patients with spina bifida. Dev Med Child Neurol 15(6):69, 1973.
110. Caldwell BM, Guze SB: A study of the adjustment of parents and sibblings of institutionalized and non-institutionalized retarded children. Am J Ment Defic 64:845, 1960.
111. Grossman FK: Brothers and Sisters of Retarded Children: An Exploratory Study. Syracuse University Press, Syracuse, NY, 1972.
112. Sussman M, Cusick B: Preliminary Report: The role of short-leg, tone reducing casts as an adjunct to physical therapy of patients with cerebral palsy. Johns Hopkins Med J 145:112, 1979.
113. Cusick B, Sussman M: Short leg casts: Their role in the management of cerebral palsy. Phys Occup Ther Pediatr 2:93, 1982.
114. Embry O: Preliminary Report: Inhibitive tone casts used in conjunction with neurodevelopmental treatment. NDT Newsletter, August 1982.

115. Finnie N: Handling the Young Cerebral Palsied Child at Home. 2nd Ed. Dutton, New York, 1975.
116. Conner FP, Williamson GG, Siepp JM: The First Three Years: A Curriculum Guide for Infants and Toddlers with Sensorimotor and Other Developmental Disabilities. Appendix A. Columbia University Press, New York, 1978.
117. Fraser B, Galka G, Hensinger RN: Gross Motor Management of Severely Multiply Impaired Students. Vol 1: Evaluation Guide. University Park Press, Baltimore, 1980.
118. Nwaobi OM, Burbaker CE, Cusick B, et al: Electromyographic investigation of extensor activity in cerebral palsied children in different seating positions. Dev Med Child Neurol 25:2, 175, 1983.
119. Cristarella M: Comparison of straddling and sitting apparatus for the spastic cerebral-palsied child. Am J Occup Ther 29(5):273, 1975.
120. Hulme JB, Poor R, Schillein M, et al: Perceived behavioral changes observed with adaptive seating devices and training programs for multihandicapped, developmentally disabled individuals. Phys Ther 63:2204, 1983.
121. Bergen A, Colangelo C: Positioning the Client with CNS Deficits: The Wheelchair and Other Adaptive Equipment. Valhalla Rehabilitation Publishers, Valhalla, NY, 1982.
122. Breed A, Ibler I: The Motorized Wheelchair: New freedom, new responsibility, and new problems. Dev Med Child Neurol 24:366, 1982.
123. Carlson J, Winter R: The 'Gillette' sitting support orthosis for nonambulatory children with severe cerebral palsy or advanced muscular dystrophy. Minn Med 61(8):469, 1978.
124. Carmick J: High chair adaption. Totline 7(4):15, 1981.
125. Carrington E: A seating position for a cerebral palsied child. Am J Occup Ther 32(3):179, 1978.
126. Coletti T, Weaver J, Jacquard S: Adaptive kneeler for handicapped children. Phys Ther 59:886, 1979.
127. Dunkel R, Trefler E: Seating for cerebral palsied children—The Sleek Seat. Phys Ther 57:524, 1977.
128. Gajdosik C, Gajdosik R: Spool roll for positioning the child prone. Phys Ther 61:1288, 1981.
129. Ivey A, Roblyer DD: Rollermobile for children with cerebral palsy. Phys Ther 60:1162, 1980.
130. Ottenbacher K, Malter R, Weckwerth L: Toilet seat arrangement for children with neuromotor dysfunction. Am J Occup Ther 33(3):193, 1979.
131. Susko G, Rice H, Williams J: Orthopedic cart for severely handicapped persons. Phys ther 56:1132, 1976.
132. Trefler E, Hanks S, Huggins P, et al: A modular seating system for cerebral palsied children. Dev Med Child Neurol 20:199, 1978.
133. Wilbur S: Foam rubber sidelying support for children with cerebral palsy. Phys Ther 55(12):1345, 1975.
134. Wilson J: Selection and use of adaptive equipment for preschool children. In McLaurin S (ed): The Preschool Special Child. University of North Carolina, Chapel Hill, in press.
135. Rang M, Douglas G, Bennet G, et al: Seating for children with cerebral palsy. J Pediatr Orthop 1:279, 1981.
136. DiCarlo C, Forbis A: A chair for the child with hypertonic CNS dysfunction. Phys Ther 56(10):1151, 1977.

137. Hulme JB, Gallacher MA, Hulme RD: The Montana Adaptive Equipment Project: A cost efficient model for the delivery of adaptive equipment services in rural settings. Phy Occup Ther Pediatr 1:59, 1981.

138. Sontag ED (ed): Educational Programming for the Severely and Profoundly Handicapped. CEC, Div on MR, Boothwyn, 1977.

139. Except Child, suppl 9(1):4, 1979.

140. Hofmann R: How to Build Special Furniture and Equipment for Handicapped Children. Charles C Thomas, Springfield IL, 1970.

141. Lowman E, Klinger J: Aids to Independent Living. McGraw-Hill, New York, 1969.

142. Macey P: Mobilizing Multiply Handicapped Children: A Manual for the Design and Construction of Modified Wheelchairs. University of Kansas, Lawrence, 1974.

143. Robinault I (ed): Functional Aids for the Multiply Handicapped. Harper & Row, Hagerstown, MD, 1973.

144. Simeonsson RJ, Cooper DH, Scheiner AP: A review and analysis of the effectiveness of early intervention programs. Pediatrics 69:635, 1982.

145. Ingram AJ, Withers E, Speltz E: Role of intensive physical and occupational therapy in the treatment of cerebral palsy: Testing and results. Arch Phys Med Rehabil 40:429, 1959.

146. Footh WK, Kogan KL: Measuring the effectiveness of physical therapy in the treatment of cerebral palsy. J Am Phys Ther Assoc 867, 1963.

147. Sparrow S, Zigler E: Evaluation of a patterning treatment for retarded children. Pediatrics 62(2):137, 1978.

148. Sommerfeld D, Fraser B, Hensinger RN, et al: Evaluation of physical therapy service for severely mentally impaired students with cerebral palsy. Phys Ther 61(3):338, 1981.

149. Wright T, Nicholson J: Physiotherapy for the spastic child: An evaluation. Dev Med Child Neurol 15:146, 1973.

150. Paine R: On the treatment of cerebral palsy—The outcome of 177 patients, 74 totally untreated. Pediatrics 29:605, 1962.

151. Scherzer A, Mike V, Ilson J: Physical therapy as a determinant of change in the cerebral palsied infant. Pediatrics 58:47, 1976.

152. Hochleitner M: Vergleichende Untersuchung von Kinder mit zerebraler Bewegungsstörng, mit und ohme neurophysiologischer Frühtherapie. Oesterr Aerzt 32:1108, 1977.

153. d'Avignon M, Noren L, Arman T: Early physiotherapy ad modum vojta or Bobath in infants with suspected neuromotor disturbance. Neuropaediatrics, 12:232, 1981.

154. Abdel-Salam E, Maraghi S, Tawfik M: Evaluation of physical therapy techniques in the management of cerebral palsy. J Egypt Med Assoc 61:531, 1978.

155. Watube S, Otabe T, Kii K, et al: Improving the walking patterns of a spastic diplegic child. Totline 7(1):14, 1981.

156. Palisano RJ: Investigation of Electromyographic Gait Analysis as a Method of Evaluating the Effects of Neurodevelopmental Treatment in a Child with Cerebral Palsy. Master's Thesis, Division of Physical Therapy, School of Medicine, University of North Carolina at Chapel Hill, 1981.

157. Chong KC, Vojnic CD, Quanbury AO, et al: The assessment of the internal rotation gait in cerebral palsy. Clin Orthop 132:145, 1978.

158. Perry J, Hopper M, Giovan P, et al: Gait Analysis of the triceps surae in cerebral palsy. J Bone Jt Surg 56A:511, 1974.

159. Woltering H, Guth V, Abbink F: Electromyographic investigations of gait in cerebral palsied children. Electromyogr Clin Neurophysiol 19:519, 1979.

160. Sutherland DH, Schottstaedt ER, Larsen LJ, et al: Clinical and electromyographic study of seven spastic children with internal rotation gait. J Bone Jt Surg 51A:1070, 1969.
161. Sutherland DH, Cooper L: Crouch gait in spastic diplegia. Orthop Trans 1:76, 1977.
162. Letts RM, Winter DA, Quanbury M: Locomotion studies as an aid in clinical assessment of child gait. Can Med Assoc J 112:1091, 1975.
163. Holt KS: Facts and fallacies about neuromuscular function in cerebral palsy as revealed by electromyography. Dev Med Child Neurol 8:255, 1966.

APPENDIX

Classification of Cerebral Palsy by Topographical Distribution of Tone and Abnormal Movement

Spasticity is characterized by increased muscle tone, stereotyped and limited patterns of movement, decrease in active and passive range of motion, tendency to develop contractures and deformities, persistence of primitive and tonic reflexes, and poor development of the postural reflex mechanism.

Spastic hemiplegia is the most common type of spastic cerebral palsy.[1] Characteristics:

1. One side of the body shows abnormal muscle tone and movement.
2. The entire side of the body is involved, including the face, neck, and trunk, as well as the extremities. The upper extremity is significantly more involved than the lower extremity. There is no preference for side.[2]
3. Often strabismus, oral motor dysfunction, somatosensory dysfunction (akinesia, astereognosis), and perceptual and learning disorders are associated problems.
4. Sensory deficit may be as detrimental to ultimate function as spasticity and motor deficit.
5. The child often ignores the involved side and uses the sound side for activities and weight bearing (Fig. A-1).[3]
6. Seizures often develop as the child grows older.[4]

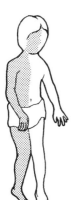

Fig. A-1. Right spastic hemiplegia.

Spastic diplegia is most frequently related to problems of prematurity, with increasing prevalence.[5,6] Characteristics:

1. The total body is affected, with greater involvement in trunk and lower extremities than upper extremities and face (Fig. A-2).

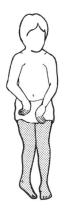

Fig. A-2.   Spastic diplegia.

2.   Often the child has associated bilateral esotropia, along with oral motor and speech problems.

3.   Often one side is more involved than the other (double hemiplegia), particularly in the lower extremities.

Spastic quadriplegia is often related to birth asphyxia in term infants[5] or grade 3 and 4 intraventricular bleeds in very immature infants.[7,8] Characteristics:

1.   The total child is involved—head, neck, trunk, and arms equally or more involved than legs.

2.   The infant often presents first with hypotonia.

3.   If the disorder is severe, tone dominates the child's posture and movement, either totally extended (Fig. A-3a) or totally flexed (Fig. A-3b). The ability to move against gravity is very slight.

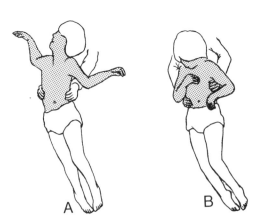

Fig. A-3.   Spastic quadriplegia.

4. Associated problems include vision, hearing defects, seizures, mental retardation, and oral motor problems.

5. Often the involvement is asymmetrical, leading to contractures and deformities, particularly scoliosis and dislocation of the hip on the more involved side.[9]

Athetosis (dyskinetic syndromes) is related to erythroblastosis and birth asphyxia.[1]

Types of dyskinetic syndromes:

1. *Nontension athetoid*: involuntary movements without increased muscle tone

2. *Dystonic athetoid*: abnormal positioning of limbs, head, and trunk with unpredictable increased tone

3. *Choreoathetoid*: involuntary, unpredictable small movements of the distal parts of the extremities

4. *Tension athetoid*: increased muscle tone, which actually blocks involuntary movements

Characteristics:

1. Muscle tone is variable.
2. Purposeful movement is poorly executed and coordinated.
3. The child lacks the ability to sustain postural alignment (Fig. A-4).
4. Involvement is often asymmetrical.
5. Tonic reflexes dominate posture.[10]
6. Hypotonia precedes onset of athetosis.
7. Involuntary, unpredictable movements are exaggerated by voluntary movement, postural adjustments, changes in emotions and anxiety or speech.[11]
8. The child usually has severely impaired speech, poor respiratory control, and other oral motor problems. High-frequency hearing loss is common.

Ataxia is associated with developmental deficits of the cerebellum.

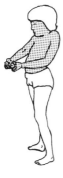

Fig. A-4. Athetosis.

Characteristics:

1. Low postural tone, markedly defective postural function resulting in disturbed equilibrium, and cocontraction make sustained control against gravity difficult.[10,12]
2. Diplegic distribution affects trunk and legs more than arms and hands.
3. Balance is poor when standing and walking; stance and gait are wide-based (Fig. A-5).
4. Intention to use the hands produces tremor.
5. Movement is uncoordinated for both gross and fine motor tasks.
6. Stress or attempts to speed up movement increases incoordination.
7. Spastic diplegia or athetosis is often concomitant.
8. Ataxia often follows the initial stage of hypotonia.
9. Associated problems include nystagmus, poor eye tracking, and delayed and poorly articulated speech.

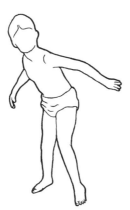

Fig. A-5.   Ataxic cerebral palsy.

Flaccid, hypotonia is often a transient stage in the evolution of athetosis or spasticity.[13]
Characteristics:

1. The child has decreased muscle tone, real or apparent weakness, and increased range of motion, but has little power to move against gravity.
2. Excessive joint flexibility is indicative of severe hypotonia.
3. The child lies in "frog-leg" position when placed on back (Fig. A-6a).
4. If the child develops enough tone to sit up, he often stabilizes the body with the hands and sits between the legs to provide a wider base of support and accommodate for postural instability in the trunk (Fig. A-6b).

Mixed types is the term used most commonly to indicate spastic diplegia mixed with athetosis, but it may be used to describe any child who does not fit characterizations described above.

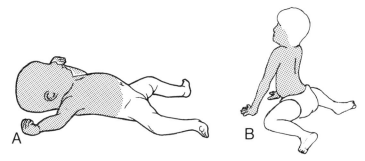

Fig. A-6.   Atonic cerebral palsy. a: Supine. b: Sitting.

Appendix References

1. O'Reilly D, Walenlynowicz J: Etiological factors in cerebral palsy: A historical review. Dev Med Child Neurol 23:633, 1981.
2. Michaelis R, Rooschuz B, Dopfer R: Prenatal origins of congenital spastic hemiparesis. Early Hum Dev 4(3):243, 1980.
3. Knutsson E: Muscle activation patterns of gait in spastic hemiparesis, paraparesis and cerebral palsy. Scand J Rehab Med (Suppl) 7:47, 1980.
4. Cohen ME, Duffner PK: Prognostic indicators in hemiparetic cerebral palsy. Ann Neurol 9:353, 1981.
5. Bennett FC, Chandler LS, Robinson NM, et al: Spastic diplegia in premature infants, etiologic and diagnostic consideration. Am J Dis Child 135:732, 1981.
6. Russell EM: Correlation between birth weight and the clinical findings on diplegia. Arch Dis Child 35:548, 1960.
7. Pape K, Wigglesworth J: Haemorrhage, ischaemia and the perinatal brain. Clin Dev Med 69/70, 1979.
8. Scott H: Outcome of very severe birth asphyxia. Arch Dis Child 51:712, 1976.
9. Bleck EE: The hip in cerebral palsy. Orthop Clin North Am 11:79, 1980.
10. Carr JH, Shepherd RB: Physiotherapy in Disorders of the Brain. Heinemann, London, 1982.
11. Kabat H, McLeod M: Athetosis: Neuromuscular dysfunction and treatment. Arch Phys Med 40:285, 1959.
12. Hagbert B, Sanner G, Steen M: The dysequilibrium syndrome in cerebral palsy. Acta Paediatr Scand Suppl 61:226, 1972.
13. Lesny IA: Follow-up study of hypotonic forms of cerebral palsy. Brain Dev 1(2):87, 1979.

Index

Page numbers followed by f indicate figures; page numbers followed by t indicate tables.